0
20,00

S0-BIV-994

290 129 570 3

155.2   2901295703
ZUC Zuckerman, Marvin
Psychobiology of
Personality

Psychobiology of Personality

SECOND EDITION, REVISED AND UPD

Praise for the first edition

"An up-to-date review of thinking and research dealing with personality, primarily from a psychobiological point of view ... provides the reader with a broad grasp of the field as well as an understanding of some of the important conceptual and methodological problems inherent in much of the research described."

American Journal of Psychiatry

"Presents a wealth of data supporting the idea of consistency of traits over the lifetime of an individual. This is an important book for the student of human behavior.... Its strength lies in its thoroughness."

Human Ethology Bulletin

"Effectively brings the integration of psychology and biology closer to a reality ... a valuable addition to undergraduate libraries."

Choice

"By far the best introduction to the field, and will undoubtedly be the textbook chosen by the adventurous souls who decide to lecture on the psychobiology of personality."

Personality & Individual Differences

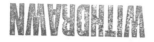

Psychobiology of Personality

SECOND EDITION, REVISED AND UPDATED

MARVIN ZUCKERMAN
University of Delaware

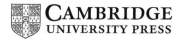
CAMBRIDGE
UNIVERSITY PRESS

CAMBRIDGE UNIVERSITY PRESS
Cambridge, New York, Melbourne, Madrid, Cape Town, Singapore, São Paulo

Cambridge University Press
40 West 20th Street, New York, NY 10011-4211, USA

www.cambridge.org
Information on this title: www.cambridge.org/9780521815697

© Marvin Zuckerman 1991, 2005

This book is in copyright. Subject to statutory exception
and to the provisions of relevant collective licensing agreements,
no reproduction of any part may take place without
the written permission of Cambridge University Press.

First edition first published 1991
Second edition first published 2005

Printed in the United States of America

A catalog record for this publication is available from the British Library.

Library of Congress Cataloging in Publication Data
Zuckerman, Marvin.
    Psychobiology of personality / Marvin Zuckerman. – 2nd ed., rev. and updated
        p.   cm.
    Includes bibliographical references and indexes.
    ISBN 0-521-81569-X (hardcover) – ISBN 0-521-01632-0 (pbk.)
    1. Personality.   2. Psychobiology.   I. Title.
    BF698.Z825   2005
    155.2 – dc22   2004020557

ISBN-13   978-0-521-81569-7 hardback
ISBN-10   0-521-81569-X hardback

ISBN-13   978-0-521-01632-2 paperback
ISBN-10   0-521-01632-0 paperback

Cambridge University Press has no responsibility for
the persistence or accuracy of URLs for external or
third-party Internet Web sites referred to in this book
and does not guarantee that any content on such
Web sites is, or will remain, accurate or appropriate.

To Rae

Contents

Preface

The first edition of *Psychobiology of Personality,* published in 1991, provided a comprehensive treatment of a subject about which most psychologists have only a fragmentary knowledge, if any. Most behavior geneticists
know a lot about the genetics of personality but little about its psychophysiology or psychopharmacology. Conversely, most psychopharma-
cologists know a lot about the psychopharmacology of personality and psychopathology but little about behavioral genetics. Most social and many
personality psychologists know a lot about traits and their assessment but
little about the psychobiology of traits. The first edition was based on a
levels approach to personality (see Figure 7-1) that attempts to explore all
levels of personality, from the genetic to the trait with stops at the neurological, biochemical, physiological, conditioning, and behavioral levels of
explanation. The goal was not reductionism but a connectivism that respects the mode of explanation at each level and attempts to understand,
as much as possible, the connections between phenomena at all levels. Although causation is usually assumed to work up from the more basic levels
to the behavioral ones, it can work in the opposite direction. Only experimentation can decide the issues of causation; correlation cannot do this,
as we patiently explain to students in introductory psychology (although
clinicians sometimes forget this).

The psychobiology of personality has been explored by "top-down" and
"bottom-up" approaches. The top-down approach is to identify basic personality traits in humans and then see what correlates of these traits can be
found in physiology, biochemistry, neurology, and genetics. Anthropomorphic extensions may be made to behavior in other species because much
of the basic knowledge about the biological bases of behavior come from
experimentation that is only possible using nonhuman species. Bottom-
up approaches start with biobehavioral knowledge and definitions from

work with other species and attempt to extend these to humans. Animal models for human personality traits and behavior are used. Eysenck (1967) was an exemplar of the top-down approach and Gray (1982) is one for the bottom-up approach. This book and its predecessor are based on a top-down approach. The previous edition, however, devoted many pages to exploring the viability of work and concepts developed from research with other species, whereas this volume will put more emphasis on the human psychobiology with only a few animal models included. The ones included are those in which a shared biological marker goes beyond mere analogy when identifying behavioral traits shared by humans and rats or monkeys.

The last edition included a chapter on the "consistency of personality," which discussed the research on the reliability of behavioral or personality traits over time and across situations, as well as the trait–state distinction and the question of the relative importance of person, situation, and their interactions in behavior. Although not entirely resolved, there is less preoccupation with these issues than in previous decades. The trait concept seems "alive and well," despite attacks on it during the 1970s. The trait-versus-state distinction is widely accepted, as is the idea that traits represent states aggregated across time and situations. The idea that the personality–situation interaction is basic to most kinds of behavior also is acknowledged by most of us. Although I spent many years engaged in these metapsychological controversies, I have become bored by them and I think most personality psychologists also have gone on to other things. Readers still interested in these issues should see my chapter in the first edition.

Chapter 1 discusses this general approach and then starts with definitions of the system of traits at the top level. When the first edition was written, the so-called Big-Five approach was largely confined to lexical studies of adjectives and Costa and McCrae's definition by questionnaire was limited to a three-factor model. With the publication of the revised NEO (Costa & McCrae, 1992a) with five-factor scales, including subtrait facet scores, research on the five-factor model has grown at an exponential rate. Investigators in some areas, such as behavioral genetics, have rushed to redefine their trait dimensions within the context of the Big-Five. However, psychobiological research based on three-factor models such as those of Eysenck (1967), Tellegen (1985), and Cloninger (1987), and an "Alternative-Five" model of Zuckerman and Kuhlman as well as a newer eight-factor model by Cloninger and his colleagues has continued, despite the appeal of Costa and McCrae (1992b) that all other systems should be translated into the "longitude and latitude" system of the Big-Five. Since then, many empirical comparisons have been made of these various systems, and there is indeed some moderate to substantial correlation between the primary three components of most systems. Although there are some crucial differences in details, the subsequent chapters are grouped by these commonalities. The first chapter describes the major trait systems and research comparing them. The chapter also describes systems of temperament developed on children and possible connections between these and adult personality traits.

Chapter 2 describes the methodologies and concepts in the psychobiological areas of the book: psychophysiology, psychopharmacology, neurology of the brain, and genetics. The first edition of this book was organized by level of psychobiology. For instance, there was a chapter on psychophysiology introduced by a discussion of the methods used in this field, followed by a presentation of the theory and research in all areas of personality using psychophysiological methods. In this revised volume, all of the psychobiology methods are presented in Chapter 2, and the remaining chapters are organized by four basic personality traits. Readers who are already familiar with all or any of the psychobiological methodologies and concepts described in subsequent chapters can, of course, skip those sections. Readers may have to turn back to this chapter, at times, when reading later chapters, but I feel that this new organization will provide more continuity to the psychobiological story.

Chapters 3 to 6 each represents a basic dimension of personality. The groupings of the traits are based on the empirical findings on the relationships among factors described by different systems. Four of five basic factors are comparable, if not identical, in most of the systems: Extraversion/Sociability (Chapter 3); Neuroticism/Anxiety/Harm Avoidance (Chapter 4); Psychoticism/Unsocialized Impulsive Sensation Seeking/Novelty Seeking/Conscientiousness/Constraint (Chapter 5); Aggression-Hostility/Agreeableness/Cooperativeness (Chapter 6). The fifth factor in the Big-Five is Openness to Experience and in the Alternative-Five it is Activity. These two have no relationship to each other and are not represented in other personality systems, although activity is a trait in most temperament systems. For these reasons, and because the fifth factors are not prominent in psychobiological research with human adults, they are not included in this book; the discussion is limited to the four basic dimensions described earlier.

Psychopathology, as defined by psychiatric criteria, is discussed within each of the trait chapters in which it is most relevant, rather than in separate chapters as in the previous edition. Research and theory on anxiety disorders are treated in the chapter on neuroticism/anxiety, and research on disinhibitory and antisocial disorders is discussed in the chapters on impulsive sensation seeking and aggression-hostility. Much of the psychobiological research using human subjects has come from the field of psychiatry. Psychologists are increasingly coming around to the idea that most forms of psychopathology, particularly the personality and anxiety and mood disorders, can be conceptualized in terms of specific patterns of personality dimensions (Widiger, 1991; Zuckerman, 1999). If this is true, then personality and psychopathology probably share certain kinds of psychobiological characteristics. Neuroticism, for instance, seems to be a predisposing trait for anxiety and depressive mood disorders, and impulsive sensation seeking and aggression are found as traits from which antisocial personality develops.

Chapter 7 will attempt to examine the entire pattern of levels from the genes to personality traits. To what extent is reductionism possible? In this chapter, I consider a field that has flourished since the first edition, evolutionary psychology. This is a field that attempts to describe broad selected patterns of behavior among the species and is only secondarily interested in individual differences within the species. However, it deals with such differences in terms of different evolved strategies for adapting to the basic challenges of survival and mating. Although evidence of such patterns may be inferred from studies of extant humans, I believe that the real evolutionary hypotheses are better tested by observations of our cousins on our branch of the evolutionary tree who differentiated from early hominids millions of years ago. Personality differences based on behavior among primates and other mammalian species are reviewed in this chapter.

The neurosciences move ahead at a much faster rate than the social sciences. Progress in the latter often consists of substituting new areas of research interest for older ones, rather than an increased depth of understanding of the earlier ones. These are not new paradigms but new fads. Scientists merely become bored with the old areas of research. In the neurosciences the models change, impelled by advances in methodology, but the area of research, such as brain function, remains constant.

Advances in research, particularly that on psychobiology of humans, have accelerated during the last decade because of new methodologies such as brain imaging. Previously, the main method for studying brain function was the EEG. Using the EEG to study the brain is like studying the ocean only from the surface depths. The PET scan and, more recently, the functional MRI, opened the entire brain to view. Unfortunately (from our perspective), the expense of this research has resulted in a funding priority to studies of psychopathology rather than personality. Methodological advances in other areas also have occurred. In the area of psychopharmacology, assessment of receptors for neurotransmitters has become increasingly central to an understanding of the functions of specific neurotransmitter systems. Behavior genetics, based on biometric studies of twins and adoptees and family studies, has moved into the area of molecular genetics with the identification of specific genes associated with personality traits.

All of these developments in the psychobiology of personality justify this revision of the older book. Fifty-five percent of the 655 references in this edition were published since the first edition went to press (1991–2004). My intention is not to discard all of the previous theory and research described in the last volume but to build on it. This is the way of science – and of evolution itself.

CHAPTER 1

Temperament and Personality: Trait Structure and Persistency

As in the 1991 first edition of this book, I begin with a discussion of temperament and personality and their basic dimensions. This is a necessary first step in a top-down approach because one cannot begin a levels analysis of psychobiology without a classification of traits at the top level. It would be like a science of astronomy without distinctions between planetary bodies such as asteroids, planets, stars, and galaxies; geology as a science of "rocks" sorted by size; or biology that makes distinctions only between two-legged and four-legged creatures – putting humans and chickens in the same category. Classification of phenomena is basic to any science. Without it, all is chaos.

There is a difference, however, between the classification of behavioral traits and other types of scientific classification. We are not defining "types" in the sense of clear-cut assortment of individuals. The concept of continuous, normally distributed trait dimensions is not widely understood outside of psychology. I purposely use the labels "high" and "low" sensation seekers, rather than type terms, such as "Big-T" and "Little-t," to define persons falling near the extreme ends of the continuum on this trait. Types, however, may be defined from a combination of independent dimensions as particular combinations of high or low scores on these dimensions in the same way that syndromes of psychopathology are defined by particular combinations of symptoms.

In the earlier volume, I discussed certain issues about traits that preoccupied personality researchers in the 1970s. Among these issues were whether to use narrow or broad trait concepts, states versus traits, and whether there was any consistency of traits or states across situations (Mischel, 1968). These issues no longer fascinate personality psychologists, and I do not deal with them at all in this book. In the last volume, an entire chapter was devoted to the question of consistency. In this book, I discuss consistency within systems of traits in every chapter rather than in a separate chapter. Readers who wish to revisit these issues can refer to the 1991 volume.

The current preoccupation of personality psychologists concerns arguments over which traits are the basic ones and which system best describes them (Costa & McCrae, 1992; Eysenck, 1992; Zuckerman, 1992). Costa and McCrae and other advocates of the Big-Five model claim that their five traits are the final answer and that all other systems should be reinterpreted within their dimensions. This preemptive assertion was questioned by several investigators, including Eysenck (1994), Zuckerman (1994), and Block (1995, 2001). As will be seen, there are some similarities across systems, particularly on four of the major factors, but there also are differences in which factors are considered major and which are merely subfactors in the hierarchy dominated by the major factors.

TEMPERAMENT

The distinctions between temperament and personality are not always clear. Strelau (1983, 1998) has made what are, perhaps, the clearest distinctions. Temperament is

a) distinguished by basic, relatively stable personality traits
b) expressed in the energetic and temporal (rather than the motivational or goal-directed) aspects of behavior
c) present from early childhood
d) known to have behavioral counterparts in other species of animals
e) primarily determined by inborn (genetic) biological mechanisms
f) but subject to changes caused by maturation and the interaction of the genotype with specific life experiences.

These distinctions do not completely distinguish temperament and personality and contain certain contradictions.

With distinction regard to (a): How stable must temperament traits be and over what time periods? There is little consistency of behavioral traits in the first year of life and prediction of behavior from 1 to 5 years is very low for most temperament traits (Thomas & Chess, 1986). Consistency does not appear until about age 3 and is still low until age 6 (Kagan & Moss, 1962). Consistency estimates for adult personality traits are higher than those for measures of temperament (Roberts & DelVecchio, 2000). Criterion (f) would explain the greater consistency of adult personality. If temperament is changeable by maturation, most of these changes will occur in childhood. By late adolescence – after personality is shaped by genetic and maturational differences – life experiences may have less impact than those occuring when the personality is still malleable.

With regard to (b): This distinction in the type of measures used is the clearest of Strelau's distinctions. General activity and emotionality are expressive aspects of temperament. But, many temperament theorists include sociability or aggression as factors of temperament and these are goal-directed and motivated. In fact, expressive and goal-directed are not mutually exclusive. Extraversion has the goal of making and keeping friends and is expressed in positive emotions such as joy and elation. Neuroticism has the goal of being secure in relationships and avoiding rejection and is expressed in negative affects like anxiety and depression.

With regard to (c): It is true that some traits are more easily observed and defined in infancy than in adulthood. However, this may be more a function of maturation than a way of defining temperament. Sociability, for instance, becomes more observable when the child enters school, simply because it offers the first opportunities to interact with peers for any length of time. Sexual interest and desire may depend on inborn characteristics, but it cannot be reliably determined until early pubescence. Many genes are not expressed at birth, but they are activated by a maturational timetable and even by environmental stimulation.

With regard to (d): I agree that temperament traits in humans should show analogues in other species (Zuckerman, 1984). Ideally, this should be in species that are closer to us genetically, like the other primates. However, over 90% of the experimental research is done with rodents, and we must rely mostly on nonexperimental observational research on primates living in natural colonies for analogues of personality. Even so, sociability, aggression, fearfulness, and sensation seeking (approach, exploration, play) can be observed in many species. Their equivalence to human analogues, however, cannot be assumed. The discovery of common biological markers for behavior in animals and humans provides some confidence in the animal models.

With regard to (e): With few exceptions, no temperament or personality traits are completely determined by heredity. Few are "primarily determined" unless one defines "primarily" as any trait with a heritability above .50. Heritability is not a static statistic, but it may show changes with age. Intelligence, for example, shows higher heritabilities in adolescents and adults than in young children. Heritabilities for temperament may be high in early childhood, but they decrease in adult life as environmental influences become more potent. Angleitner et al. (1995) and Strelau (1998) found little difference in heritabilities of classical types of temperment scales and personality scales in adults, and they even found low heritabilities for some of the temperament scales. It is clear that temperament cannot be distinguished from personality in terms of higher genetic influences in the former.

In the final analysis, the main way we can distinguish temperament from personality is that temperament is defined by the type of variables, such as behavioral observations or parental ratings, used to study individual differences in infants and young children, whereas personality is assessed by methods typically used with older children and adults suggest as questionnaires. Some of these traits are similar at all ages, whereas others are unique to a specific stage of development.

SYSTEMS OF TEMPERAMENT

Thomas and Chess

The first longitudinal study of temperament in infancy was conducted by Thomas and Chess (1977; Chess & Thomas, 1984). Like Strelau, Thomas and Chess distinguished temperament from personality, abilities, and motivation in terms of style or expression of response ("how") as opposed to its content ("what") or goals ("why"). The study, which was initiated in 1956, began with infants between 2 and 3 months of age who were reassessed at various intervals into adulthood. Parental ratings were used at the earlier stages and other methods were used at later ages.

Nine categories of behavior initially were established based on a rational classification of parent interview protocols. The categories are listed below in order of the rater reliabilities (in parentheses). The lower reliabilities indicate variables that were difficult for raters to define.

1. *Approach-Withdrawal*: Reactions to novel stimuli such as new foods, toys, and strangers (.84).
2. *Activity Level*: Activity in various situations, such as bathing, eating, playing, crawling, and walking (.71).
3. *Rhythmicity (regularity)*: Regularity in functions such as feeding, elimination, and sleep (.62).
4. *Distractibility*: The ease of changing the direction of attention from one activity to another (.61).
5. *Adaptability*: Long-term responses to new or altered situations; modifiability of behavior (.58).

6. *Attention Span and Persistence*: The length of time a particular activity is pursued and the continuation in an activity in spite of attempts at interference (.43).
7. *Quality of Mood*: The amount of pleasant, joyful, and friendly behavior contrasted with the amount of unpleasant, crying, and unfriendly behavior (.37).
8. *Threshold of Responsiveness*: The intensity of stimulation in any sensory modality that is necessary to evoke a response (.15).
9. *Intensity of Reaction*: The energy level of responses regardless of their quality or direction (.00).

It is apparent that raters had a difficult time translating parental interview data into variables 8 and 9. Activity level and approach-withdrawal had good reliabilities, and the other variables were low to moderate in reliability.

Rational and factor analyses led Thomas, Chess, and Birch (1968) to define three types:

1. "Easy Temperament" is defined by high scores on regularity, approach, adaptability, mild or moderate intensity of reaction, and predominance of positive mood.
2. "Difficult Temperament" is the polar opposite of "Easy Temperament," with irregularity, withdrawal, nonadaptability, intense reactions, and negative mood. This type is on the opposite end of a continuum with "easy temperament."
3. "Slow-to-Warm-Up Temperament" consists of mild negative reactions and slow adaptation to new stimuli or persons but only mild intensity of emotional reactions and no irregularity.

Consistency of the nine temperament categories from 6 to 8 months (Huttunen & Nyman, 1982) and 1 to 4 years (Thomas & Chess, 1986) to the ratings at 5 years of age did not show very high prediction. Although some of the correlations were significant, very few exceeded .30. The most reliable were activity and Adaptability. Prediction of adult ratings on the nine variables from ratings at 1 to 5 years of age was even worse. None of the correlations exceeded .30. Adaptibility, and approach-withdrawal at 3 and 4 years of age did correlate low but significantly with their manifestations in adults. Intensity and mood at 4 years also correlated significantly. The adjustment factor at ages 4 and 5 predicted a clinical diagnosis at adulthood, and at 3 and 4 predicted an easy versus difficult rating derived from interviews and a questionnaire given to adults. The nine child temperament variables accounted for about 7 to 9% of the variance in ratings derived from the interview

but 15 to 18% of the adult temperament data derived from the questionnaire. Mood and adaptability were the most successful in predicting adult
adjustment.

Rothbart and Derryberry

Thomas and Chess did not speculate on the biological or genetic origins of
their basic traits of temperament. Rothbart and Derryberry constructed a
developmental theory of temperament using more sophisticated statistical,
observational, and laboratory methods and current psychobiological models. They defined temperament as constitutional differences in reactivity
and self-regulation, influenced over time by heredity, maturation, and experience (Rothbart & Derryberry, 1981). Reactivity, which refers to arousability
of physiological and behavioral systems by stimulus intensity, novelty, and
other signal qualities, may be positive or negative in terms of affective response. Self-regulation refers to the processes that modulate reactivity such
as approach-avoidance/withdrawal, attack, inhibition, orienting toward or
away, self-soothing versus self-stimulation, and seeking excitement versus
seeking comfort from others.

Figure 1-1 shows their developmental model (Rothbart, Derryberry, &
Posner, 1994). Traits are arranged from top to bottom in order of emergence
in developmental age and the biological loci in the brain. *Negative emotionality* or discomfort is observable from the newborn period. *Frustration/
anger* in response to goal-blocking, and *Approach* to cues of reward or novelty with positive affect, can be seen from 2 months on. *Fear* in response to
cues for punishment or novelty, and expressed in distress, avoidance, and
behavioral inhibition, develops from 6 months on. The last developing traits
are *affiliation* and *effortful control*. Effortful control represents a more conscious cognitive control system operating through attention and cognitive
processing of information. It is important in the inhibition of aggression
and the modulation of fear.

Buss and Plomin

Buss and Plomin (1975, 1984) define temperament as earlier occuring traits
(observable by 2 years of age) that are strongly genetic in origin. No one
would argue with the first criterion, but the second is more problematic.
Certainly, temperament traits should show some degree of heritability, but
how much? Heritabilities can vary with age. A trait that appears to be highly
heritable during infancy may have attenuated heritability with age, or vice
versa.

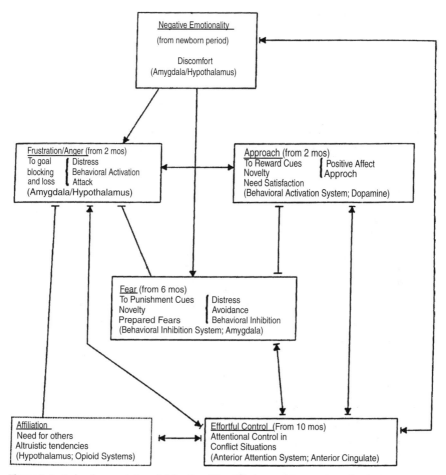

Figure 1-1. A developmental model for the differentiation and integration of temperament systems. From "A psychobiological approach to the development of temperament," by M. K. Rothbart et al., 1994. In J. E. Bates and H. D. Wachs (Eds.), *Temperament: Individual differences at the interface of biology and behavior* (p. 107). Washington, DC: American Psychological Association. Copyright 1994 by the American Psychological Association. Reprinted by permission.

Buss and Plomin developed rating scales of temperament for parents to describe their children and a self-report test for adults. In the 1975 versions, there were four basic traits of temperament, described as follows:

Parent Rating Scales

1. *Emotionality:* gets upset and cries easily, is easily frightened and/or has a quick temper, and is not easygoing.

2. *Activity:* always on the go from the time of waking, cannot sit still for long, fidgets at meals and similar occasions, prefers active games to quiet ones.
3. *Sociability:* likes to be with others, makes friends easily, prefers to play with others rather than alone, is not shy.
4. *Impulsivity:* difficulty in learning self-control and resistance to temptation, gets bored easily, goes from toy to toy quickly.

Factor analyses of items showed good factorial validity; most of the items loaded on the scales to which they had been rationally assigned.

Self-Report Questionnaire (for older children and adults)

1. *Emotionality:* general, fear, anger
2. *Activity:* tempo (fast), vigor (energy, forcefulness)
3. *Sociability:* makes friends easily vs. shy, likes to play with others vs. alone
4. *Impulsivity:* inhibitory control (lack of), decision time (quick), sensation seeking, persistence (lack of)

Factor analyses confirmed the assignment of items to each of the four scales, but questions about the factorial unity and heritability of the impulsivity scale led the researchers to drop it from their system. In our opinion, this was a mistake. Our own factor analyses consistently have shown that impulsivity and sensation seeking are joined in a common factor in both three and five factor levels: Impulsive Sensation Seeking. Socialization also is included (Zuckerman, Kuhlman, Thornquist, & Kiers, 1991). This factor is similar to those found in other adult personality systems (Zuckerman, Kuhlman, Joireman, Teta, & Kraft, 1993). By excluding I from EASI, the investigators removed a vital part of personality structure and possibly the one most rooted in genetics and biology.

Strelau

Strelau was the most powerful influence in reviving the interest in temperament in the West. The conferences he organized in Poland beginning in the 1970s brought together temperament researchers from the United States and Western and Eastern European countries. Strelau was influenced by Neo-Pavlovian theorists such as Teplov and Nebylitsyn. Before Strelau's approach, the concepts of nervous system traits such as excitation, inhibition, and mobility of nervous processes had been operationally defined by laboratory methods such as conditioning, psychophysical, and psychophysiological methods. Dogs and humans were diagnosed into personality types based on these methods. Strelau was the first to try to translate these into behavioral terms using ratings and questionnaires. The Strelau Temperament

Inventory (STI, Strelau, 1983) was his first attempt to operationalize Pavlovian constructs in behavioral terms. The basic three scales were:

Strength of excitation, or the ability to work under intense, distracting, or disturbing conditions. This also was called "strength of the nervous system" and persons with such strong nervous system were called "low reactives."

Strength of inhibition, or the ability to exercise behavioral restraint and to remain calm under provocation. In Western slang, such persons might be called "cool."

Mobility of nervous processes, or the ability to shift from states of excitation to inhibition or back to excitation. It could be expressed in quickness of starting work and ease of relaxing and falling asleep.

An additional variable, *Activity*, was added to the theoretical structure. Strelau's theory is one of stimulus regulation by behavior. Activity was defined as driven by the need for stimulation and the regulation of arousal level. It sounds very much like Zuckerman's (1979, 1994) construct of sensation seeking and the earlier model of an "optimal level of arousal."

The items for the test were rationally derived without item or factor analysis. A consequence was high correlations between the three subscales and a lack of correspondence with the real factorial structure among the items. Some of these admitted deficiencies were psychometrically remedied in a revised STI (Strelau, Angleitner, Bantelmann, & Ruch, 1990). However, a more detailed analysis of the theory of temperament led away from Pavlovian constructs to a new temperament system that looks more like Western dimensions (Strelau & Zawadzki, 1993). These new scales are described here:

Formal Characteristics of Behavior Temperament Inventory (FCB-TI)

1. *Briskness*, or the tendency to react quickly, to keep a high tempo in activities, and to shift easily in behavior according to situational demands.
2. *Perseveration*, or the tendency to continue behavior when the situations eliciting the behavior are no longer present.
3. *Sensory Sensitivity*, or the ability to sense or react to low-intensity sensory stimulation.
4. *Emotional Reactivity*, or intense emotional reactivity to provocative stimuli; emotional sensitivity and low emotional endurance.
5. *Endurance*, or the capacity to react adequately in situations of intense and long-lasting stimulation.
6. *Activity*, or the seeking of high stimulation through behavior or stimulating surroundings.

The new scales are factor analytically derived and have good reliabilities, although they are as yet not extensively studied. Strelau describes his system as one of adult temperament, but it could easily be applied to children and seems to draw on earlier concepts of "reactivity" or "strength of the nervous system."

Goldsmith and Campos

Goldsmith and Campos (1986) used a variety of methods for infant temperament including inventories, laboratory methods, and caretaker interviews. The theory suggests that temperaments are initially related to emotional responses and represent emotional or affective traits. Their Toddler Behavior Assessment Questionnaire includes five scales, all of which include an emotional dimension. (Activity is regarded as always related to emotional arousal, a dubious assumption):

1. Activity Level
2. Pleasure
3. Social Fearfulness
4. Anger Proneness
5. Interest Persistence (Interest is regarded as an emotion in Izard's (1993) system of classification of emotions.)

Kagan

Kagan's earlier work involved a long-term longitudinal study of 44 boys and 45 girls from "birth to maturity" (Kagan & Moss, 1962). The cohort was studied at ages 0–3, 3–6, 6–10, 10–14, and as adults, 19–29 years of age. The variables were dynamic interpersonal ones reflecting the psychoanalytic zeitgeist during the 1950s, that is, aggression, dependency, sexuality, anxiety, and repression. This study is more thoroughly reviewed in the 1991 edition of this book. One notable result was that practically no child variables from birth to age 3, and few from ages 3 to 6, were predictive of the adult ratings. Whether this was because of the inappropriateness of some of the variables used for children or to a real lack of connection between temperament at early ages and adult personality is hard to say. At the time, Kagan regarded these traits as an outcome of parent-child environment, but later, like others of us from that generation of personality psychologists, he became convinced that temperament had primarily biological roots.

In the 1980s, Kagan began primarily to use laboratory methods to define what he described as the *inhibited* temperament. Behavioral methods consisted of infant and child reactions to novel stimuli, situations, or strangers as defined by approach, withdrawal, inhibition, and physiological arousal, such as heart rate. Maternal separation combined with the appearance of a stranger was one of the methods. The methods were adjusted to age and sometimes supplemented by parent reports and maternal interviews (Kagan, 1989).

The child with the inhibited temperament was consistently timid, fearful, and cautious in an unfamiliar situation, particularly in the presence of strangers. The uninhibited child was consistently sociable, fearless, and spontaneous with positive emotions in the same situations. Kagan did not regard these as extremes on a dimension but treated the uninhibited children as normal or a different type (Kagan, Reznick, & Snidman, 1988). He did not study this other type as an extreme like undercontrolled or overactive. In view of the adult dimensions of personality, to be discussed later, the two types seem to be a combination of introversion and neuroticism (inhibited type) and stable extraversion (uninhibited type).

Reactions to novel situations, such as the open field test, in studies of rodents, seem to confound fearfulness or anxiety and explorativeness or sensation seeking (Zuckerman, 1984). In humans, however, one type of inhibition is associated with the trait of anxiety, whereas the disinhibition or lack of behavioral control is associated with either extraversion or surgency or sensation seeking.

Most of the children in the study who were inhibited at 2 to 3 years of age were still socially inhibited at 7.5 years of age (Kagan et al., 1988). However, these early samples were selected from extremes of the distribution. There was little prediction in a third group of children who were unselected on the dimension. Many of the inhibited children later developed anxiety disorders (Hirshfeld et al., 1992), which tends to indicate that the primary dimension assessed by these early behavioral and physiological measures was neuroticism or anxiety trait.

Caspi and Moffitt

Caspi (2000, Caspi, Moffitt, Newman, & Silva, 1996) followed a complete cohort of children born in a city in New Zealand from ages 3 to 21. They cluster analyzed scales of temperment ratings at age 3 into three types: *inhibited, undercontrolled,* and *well-adjusted.* The inhibited type resembles the type studied by Kagan. When children of this type reached age 21, they were described as shy, fearful, cautious, and not affectionate, outgoing, or confident. When the undercontrolled children reached young adulthood, they were seen as reckless, careless, aggressive, alienated, impulsive, thrill seeking, untrustworthy, and unreliable. Uncontrolled children were more likely to develop an antisocial personality and inhibited children were more likely to develop depression. Both of these types were more likely to become alcoholic than well-adjusted children.

Caspi and Moffit's concepts of temperament have excellent predictive value for later personality and psychopathology. The undercontrolled type is lacking in most of the other childhood temperament classifications, but it is prominent in most adult personality classifications to be described next.

Mischel

Like Kagan, Mischel used behavioral methods to define a temperamental category based on the ability to delay gratification. Mischel, Skoda, and Peak (1988) observed 4-year-old children in an experiment in which the subjects were offered a choice between a small reward that they could take immediately and a larger, more desirable reward given if they could resist taking the smaller reward. The subjects were evaluated later when they were 16 years of age using trait ratings. The simple behavioral measure, seconds of delay in a single situation at 4 years of age, correlated positively with trait descriptions of the adolescents such as attentive, planful, and competent, and negatively with trait descriptions such as immature behavior under stress. The preschool response also predicted parents' ratings of social competence in their adolescent children. Correlations as high as .49 were obtained.

It is ironic that Mischel (1968), who earlier maintained that there was little consistency of trait-relevant behaviors from one situation to another over much shorter periods of time, found a consistency from a laboratory reaction in early childhood to behavioral traits in adolescence of a magnitude higher than most studies of childhood temperament and adult personality. Judging from the descriptions of the outcome of the childhood temperament, the capacity to delay gratification in childhood might be a precursor of adult traits like conscientiousness or impulsivity.

COMPARISONS OF TEMPERAMENT TRAIT SYSTEMS

Table 1-1 compares the major childhood temperament classifications that have been discussed with the exception of those only involving one or two types, such as Kagan's, Caspi and Moffitt's, and Mischel's. I have taken the liberty of using Buss and Plomin's 1975 EASI system instead of their 1984 EAS, because the excluded trait of Impulsivity in the old one included many facets that have much in common with the other trait systems.

Four of the trait systems include an Approach factor that includes readiness to approach novel stimuli or strange persons. Buss and Plomin call this

Table 1-1. Comparisons of Temperament Systems

	Thomas & Chess (1977)	Rothberg et al. (1994)	Buss & Plomin (1975)	Strelau & Zawadzki (1993)	Goldsmith & Campo (1986)
*Approach	Approach-Withdrawal	Approach	Sensation Seeking*	*Activity	–
*Activity	Activity	Activity	Activity	Briskness	Activity
*Negative Mood	Negative Emotionality	Fear	Emotionality	Emotional Reactivity	Social Fearfulness
*Persistence	Persistence	–	*Persistence	Perseveration	Interest Persistence
*Sociability	–	Affiliation	Sociability	–	Pleasure
*Anger	–	Frustration-Anger	Anger*	–	Anger Proneness
Sensitivity	Threshold Response	–	–	Sensory Sensitivity	–
Strength of Reaction	Intensity of Reaction	–	Vigor*	–	–
Distractibility	Distractibility	–	–	–	–
Rhythmicity	Rhythmicity	–	–	–	–
Adaptability	Adaptability	–	–	–	–
Control	–	Effortful Control	–	–	–
Endurance	–	–	–	Endurance	–

*These are subtraits within the earlier Buss and Plomin (1975) EASI system.

13

factor sensation seeking, and Strelau and Zawadzski call it activity. Block (1995) described the tendency of different theorists to give different names to the same trait as the "jingle-jangle" factor. It is even more confusing when that name is used by others for a different factor. Of course, there sometimes are differences between concepts. For instance, Strelau's Activity factor refers to "the tendency to undertake activities of high stimulative value," and this definition does not directly include the idea of novelty.

Activity level is a factor in all systems, except Strelau calls it "Briskness." Negative mood is a factor in all systems although some explicitly include fear, sadness, or anger, whereas others simply refer to general emotionality. Goldsmith and Campos call it "Social Fearfulness" and use "Pleasure" and "Anger Proneness" to describe other factors. Similarly, Rothberry and Derryberry call the factor "fear" and describe another factor as "anger." The factor of Persistence, or the capacity to maintain attention and continue an activity in spite of distractions, is common to all systems except that of Rothberg and Derryberry.

Sociability is common to three of the theories if one includes Goldsmith and Campos's Pleasure factor in this category. There may be less agreement on the inclusion of this factor, because it is not observable in young infants. Anger emerges from general distress at a fairly early age (2 months), but it is still not distinguished from general emotionality in the Thomas and Chess and Strelau and Zawadzki systems. Thomas and Chess's Threshold of Response and Intensity of Reaction are included in only one other system for each. These two are not at all reliable in Thomas and Chess's study, and sensory sensitivity is the least reliable of Strelau's traits. The remaining traits of Thomas and Chess have no clear match in the other systems, although Distractibility seems like the other pole of persistence. Rhythmicity only may be appropriate for feeding and sleeping in early infancy. Adaptability has some resemblance to a previous Pavlovian concept of Strelau – Mobility of Nervous Processes.

These comparisons of theories have been made on a rational rather than an empirical basis. Ultimately, a comparison of systems must be made by empirical correlational analyses. But a more important problem is the relationship between measures of temperament in infancy and childhood with measures of personality in adults. Longitudinal studies must be used to answer the question of the continuity between early temperament and later personality. Few such studies have been done. Let us first examine the different systems currently in use for the description of adolescent and adult personality.

ADOLESCENT AND ADULT PERSONALITY

In a symposium in which the participants were Eysenck, Costa, and myself, the title of my presentation was: "What is a basic factor and which factors are basic?" (Zuckerman, 1992). The answer to the second question, of course, depends on the answer to the first. A basic personality factor, in my opinion, is almost the same as the definition of temperament defined earlier, except that it may or may not be directly observable in the same form in infants or very young children. My criteria are: (1) reliable identification of the dimension factor across methods, genders, and ages; (2) at least moderate heritability; (3) identification of similar kinds of behavioral traits in nonhuman species; (4) association of the trait with biological trait markers; and (5) consistency of the trait in some form from childhood through a significant portion of the life span. Some systems never get far beyond the first criterion, and others believe the job is finished when they demonstrate the second one.

For many years, books on personality only presented Sheldon's (1942) system of temperament types based on body builds, Cattell's (1957) 16-personality factor system, and Eysenck's two or three factors. Today, most texts focus on Costa and McCrae's version of the Big-Five model. However, a great deal of the psychobiological literature reports studies based on other systems. The question of which are the basic factors must depend on the psychobiological validity of systems. I believe that there is sufficient overlap between at least four factors among systems, regardless of differences in the precise constitutents of these factors, to perceive a system of basic personality trait organization.

Unlike the temperament traits discussed previously, there is a great deal of research comparing the personality traits from different systems.

TWO- OR THREE-DIMENSIONAL SYSTEMS

Eysenck

In the years just after World War II, Eysenck (1947) defined a three dimensional system for personality: *introversion-extraversion* (E), *neuroticism* (N) or emotional instability versus stability, and *psychoticism* (P), or tough-minded antisocial and psychotic tendencies versus socialized humaneness (called "tendermindedness" by Eysenck, a somewhat pejorative term). Although P was conceptually part of the system from the beginning, it was not included in the standard questionnaire methods used to assess the basic traits until much later (Eysenck & Eysenck, 1976).

Unlike other theories of the time, Eysenck devised a theoretical model for the traits, although he used psychometric methods to build the personality scales. The model was based on psychobiology and learning theories. The psychobiology of the early 1950s was primitive compared to modern understanding of brain and behavior. The learning theories influencing his work originally were Pavlovian and later Hullian. The concept of differences in response to cortical arousal and basic arousability later became central to his concept of extraversion and autonomic arousal to introversion. The biological basis of psychoticism was only vaguely postulated and never developed fully (Eysenck & Eysenck, 1976). Behavior genetic approaches to personality dominated his thinking during his last years.

The wide range of theory and research on his theories can be found in many publications with the best summaries in his two major books (Eysenck, 1967; Eysenck & Eysenck, 1985). Although a full definition of his traits encompasses all levels of personality from the genetic to the trait, the primary definitions are from the trait level. Eysenck's model of personality was a hierarchic one going from behavior, to habits, to first-order traits, and finally to the supertraits, or types (but in a quantitative sense), E, N, and P. In his more recent comprehensive volume he defined the supertraits in terms of their narrower trait constituents (Eysenck & Eysenck, 1985). Eysenck, Barrett, Wilson, and Jackson (1992) later incorporated these facets of the supertraits into a questionnaire that permitted their measurement within the three-factor model. The theoretical definitions from the 1985 work are:

E: sociable, lively, active, assertive, sensation seeking, carefree, dominant, surgent, venturesome.

N: anxious, depressed, guilt feelings, low self-esteem, tense, irrational, shy, moody, emotional.

P: aggressive, cold, egocentric, impersonal, impulsive, antisocial, unempathic, creative, tough-minded.

The nature of the E factor, in terms of its component subtraits, has been a matter of dispute since the early 1960s. The earlier form of his questionnaire included two main types of items, sociability and impulsivity ones. Carrigan (1960) and Guilford (1975) both claimed that these were two independent dimensions and did not belong together in a broad E factor, but Eysenck and Eysenck (1963) initially defended the combination. With the introduction of the P scale into their questionnaire, new factor analyses of items showed that impulsivity items tended to move from the E into the P dimension. Eysenck and Eysenck (1985) seem to have conceded this change in the nature of E when they assigned impulsivity to the P factor in the classification described earlier. However, they point out that some types of impulsivity correlate more highly with E, whereas others are closer to P.

The problem with E, even now, is that it subsumes two related but distinguishable types of factors. Depue and Collins (1999) call one "interpersonal engagement" or affiliation and warmth, and the other "agentic," which includes dominance, exhibitionism, and achievement. The agentic type also has been called "surgency." Hogan (1982) has a six-factor model in which surgency and sociability constitute two separate major factors. The distinction could be important for the psychobiology of E because Depue and Collins claim that the neurotransmitter dopamine is more strongly related to the agentic kind of E than to the affiliative type.

The core of neuroticism is negative emotions, anxiety, depression, guilt, and hostility, together with character traits such as low self-esteem. Longitudinal studies show that it is the personality precursor of anxiety and unipolar mood disorders (Zuckerman, 1999). Measures of this trait from many kinds of tests, including pure anxiety trait tests, are highly correlated. N and anxiety and depressive traits are virtually indistinguishable. However, hostility has a higher relationship with an aggression factor when one includes such a factor (Zuckerman, Joireman, Kraft, & Kuhlman, 1999).

The nature of the P dimension has been more widely disputed than E or N (Block, 1977; Zuckerman, 1989). Block and Zuckerman suggested that if a clinical term must be used, it should be "psychopathy" rather than "psychoticism." The idea that the scale measures a kind of latent psychoticism, in addition to antisocial, egocentric, and aggressive tendencies, came from the conceptual origin of P in studies of psychiatric patients in which neurotic disorders were distinguished from psychotic ones (Eysenck, 1955).

An earlier version of the P scale contained a number of items suggestive of psychotic delusional thinking in addition to the other types of items. But most of these items were dropped in a revised P scale (Eysenck, Eysenck, & Barrett, 1985), because they were so infrequently endorsed in normal populations that they skewed the scale toward zero producing a non-normal distribution. There are now only a few mild paranoid types of items. The rest of the items are a mixture of impulsivity, sadism, lack of empathy, aggressiveness, sensation seeking, lack of conscientiousness about work, finances, and punctuality, and unconventional social attitudes (e.g., marriage should be abolished). All of these suggest the traits of the psychopath. In line with this hypothesis among the highest scoring groups on P are criminals and successful artists (creativity is supposedly associated with P and successful modern artists are perhaps more likely to be egocentric and aggressive).

Eysenck (1992), however, noted that certain psychophysiological and bio-chemical markers associated with schizophrenia also correlated with P.

Longitudinal studies of Eysenck's Big Three over long periods of time are rare, but data from the Berkeley Guidance and Oakland Growth studies conducted in the San Francisco bay area are relevant to the question of consistency. The data consisted of a variety of Q-sort type ratings of children (Bronson, 1966) and follow-up ratings of these children at adolescent and adult ages (Block, 1971). In my 1991 volume I grouped these results into three categories reflecting the Eysenck three: extraversion/sociability, neuroticism/emotionality, and psychoticism/impulsivity/unsocialized sensation seeking.

Predictions from 5 to 7 years to adolescence (14–16) were quite low for N and P but moderate for E. Predictions from junior high to senior high school were moderate (around .40) for all three traits but lower for the longer term prediction from senior high school to adult ages (rs = .18–.36). However, these correlations were much higher when corrections for attenuation were used; around .60 for short-term and .3 to .5 for long-term prediction to adulthood.

Haan/Bronson/Block

My grouping of the variables in the studies by Bronson and Block were rationally guided in view of the subtraits known to be included in E, N, and P factors. Haan (1981) actually factor analyzed these ratings in order to find factors that were the same at all age periods. Some of these resembled factors in Costa and McCrae's Big Five and some resembled factors in other systems.

1. *Cognitively Invested:* Interest in ideas resembling one facet of Costa and McCrae's Openness to Experience factor.
2. *Open/Closed to Self:* Resembling the broader factor.
3. *Emotionally under/overcontrolled:* Aggressive, rebellious, and unpredictable at one extreme and emotionally guarded at the other. This resembles Eysenck's P factor.
4. *Under/overcontrolled Heterosexual:* Reflects control in the sexual sphere.
5. *Nuturant versus Hostile:* Resembles the Agreeableness factor in the Big Five.

There are two control dimensions. Block conceives of self-control as a major dimension of personality and views it as a bipolar factor with under-control and overcontrol both maladaptive extremes of adjustment. Block and Block (1980) devised a questionnaire measure of ego control and gave it to students in high school. Twenty-five years later as adults, he gave them the ego-control scale from another instrument. The two measures correlated .52–.53 for men and women, a very good degree of prediction over such a long time span. Prediction for Haan's (1981) factors between adolescence and 30–37 years of age also were high but only for women. For men, they were high in the short-term prediction (junior to senior high) but, with the exception of the Cognitively Involved factor, were insignificant over the long term.

Block (2001) seems to have what amounts to a two-factor theory of personality that includes *ego-undercontrol/overcontrol* and *ego-resilience*. The former could be characterized as impulsivity, and the latter as stable extraversion (high E, low N). These conclusions are based on correlations with other major systems (Zuckerman et al., 1993).

Gray

Jeffrey Gray has been the most influential modern theorist in the field of psychobiological personality. Unlike Eysenck, a top-down theorist whose neuropsychology was fixed in the arousal theory of the 1950s, Gray has been an active researcher in comparative neuropsychology. He has attempted to work up from neurobehavioral studies on rats to human personality traits, exploring the biochemical, neuropsychological, and behavioral mechanisms lying between genes and traits. These mechanisms will be discussed in subsequent chapters.

Gray's concepts of the basic dimensions of personality use Eysenck's as coordinates but suggest that the more basic behavioral dimensions lie between these coordinates. The *anxiety* dimension, for instance, went from stable extraversion to neurotic introversion, and the *impulsivity* dimension ran from stable introversion to neurotic extraversion as shown in Figure 1-2 (Gray, 1971). Gray drew these diagonals at 45-degree angles to Eysenck's E and N, but he now suggests that they are closer to a 30-degree angle, with anxiety closer to the N dimension than to E, and impulsivity closer to E than to N. Gray also had a third dimension that he called fight-flight, which he thought might be related to Eysenck's Psychoticism (P) dimension.

P, however, created a problem for Gray, because he now had to define anxiety and impulsivity in three rather than two of Eysenck's dimensions. His solution is illustrated in Figure 1-3 (Gray, 1987). Impulsivity is now defined as a dimension going from stable introversion and low P to high N, E, and P. Anxiety is now conceived of as a bipolar dimension with anxiety disorders at one pole and psychopathic types, characterized by an abnormal absence of anxiety, at the other. Anxiety is high N, low E (introversion),

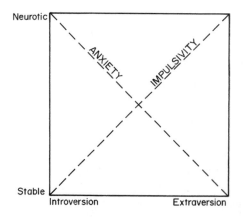

Figure 1-2. Rotation of Eysenck's dimensions of neuroticism and introversion-extraversion to dimensions of anxiety and impulsivity proposed by Gray. From J. A. Gray, 1987, *The psychology of fear and stress* (p. 351). Cambridge: Cambridge University Press. Copyright 1987 by Cambridge University Press. Reprinted by permission.

and low P, whereas psychopathy is a stable (low N) extravert with high P. Not shown here is fight-flight or aggression still identified with the P dimension only.

These categories were developed on a rational basis. Gray had not constructed special scales to define his dimensions, but when he or others extrapolated to the human level, they used combinations of Eysenck's dimensions. More recently, others have developed scales based on Gray's constructs regarding the underlying emotional-motivational bases of the

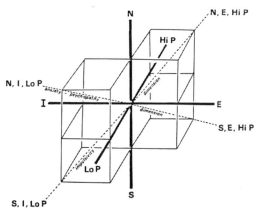

Figure 1-3. Gray's three-dimensional conceptualization of *anxiety-psychopathy* and *impulsivity dimensions* (dashed lines within coordinates of Eysenck's three dimensions (thick solid lines) of *extraversion-introversion* (E-I), *neuroticism-stability* (N-S), and *psychoticism* (P). From "The neuropsychology of emotion and personality," by J. A. Gray, 1987, In S. M. Stahl, S. D. Iverson, and E. C. Goodman (Eds.), *Cognitive neurochemistry* (p. 186). Oxford: Oxford University Press. Copyright Oxford University Press, 1991. Reprinted by permission.

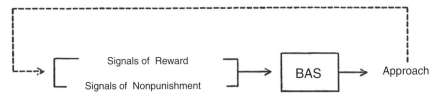

Figure 1-4. The Behavioral Approach System (BAS) as defined by its inputs and outputs. From "The neuropsychology of temperament," by J. A. Gray, 1991. In J. Strelau and A. Angleitner (Eds.), *Explorations in temperament* (p. 115). New York: Plenum Press. Copyright Plenum Press, 1991. Reprinted by permission.

dimensions (Ball & Zuckerman, 1990; Carver & White, 1994; Torrubia, Avila, Moltó, & Caseras, 2001; Wilson, Barrett, & Gray, 1989).

Underlying the impulsivity dimension is a *Behavioral Approach System* (BAS), which is activated by conditioned reward stimuli and cues signaling the termination of punishment. The BAS may be identified with the Approach temperament described earlier, except that Gray does not include novel stimuli as elicitors of approach but only stimuli that have been associated with previous reward or relief from punishment. BAS is reflected in *sensitivity to signals of reward* and relative insensitivity to signals of punishment (Figure 1-4).

Anxiety is based on a *Behavioral Inhibition Mechanism* (BIS), which is activated by conditioned signals of punishment or threat, novel stimuli, or cues associated with the termination of reward or frustrative nonreward (Figure 1-5). High anxiety is reflected in a sensitivity to signals of punishment, or nonreward and an aversive reaction to very novel stimuli

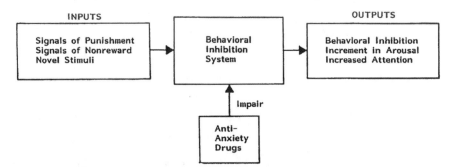

Figure 1-5. The Behavioral Inhibition System (BIS) as defined by its inputs and outputs. From "The neuropsychology of temperament," by J. A. Gray, 1991. In J. Strelau and A. Angleitner (Eds.), *Explorations in temperament* (p. 110). New York: Plenum Press. Copyright Plenum Press, 1991. Reprinted by permission.

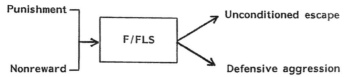

Figure 1-6. The Fight/Flight System (F/FLS) as defined by its inputs and outputs. From "The neuropsychology of temperament," by J. A. Gray, 1991. In J. Strelau and A. Angleitner (Eds.), *Explorations in temperament* (p. 114). New York: Plenum Press. Copyright Plenum Press, 1991. Reprinted by permission.

(or persons), and a relative insensitivity to signals of reward. The typical reaction to such stimuli is heightened alertness, physiological arousal, and inhibition of all ongoing behavior.

The fight-flight dimension (Figure 1-6) is actually more characterized by the fight option or aggressiveness. It is based on unconditioned responses to pain or punishment including the withdrawal of reward. Those who are high on this dimension have a strong unconditioned response to punishment or withdrawal of reward itself, but the response is likely to be aggressive or active avoidance, rather than inhibition as with the BIS.

Tellegen

Tellegen's (1985) model was a three-factor one with some similarity to Eysenck's model (E, N, P) but with the higher-order factors defined by addition of their facet scales as in the Costa and McCrae (1992) five-factor method. The model has assumed some importance in the psychobiological literature because of its use in the Minnesota Separated Twin Study (Bouchard, Lykken, McGue, Segal, & Tellegen, 1990), the psychopharmacology studies of Depue and Collins (1999), and the New Zealand longitudinal study (Caspi, 2000).

The three primary factors and their component subfactors are:

1. *Positive Emotionality* (PE): Well-being, social potency, social closeness, and achievement.
2. *Negative Emotionality* (NE): Stress reaction, alienation, and aggression.
3. *Constraint*: Control, harmavoidance, and traditionalism.

There is one additional scale called Absorption, or the capacity to become absorbed in altered states of consciousness or fantasy experience.

More recently, Tellegen and Waller (in press) proposed a four-factor approach, dividing the PE factor into PE agentic type (PEM-A) and PE communal type (PEM-C). Both types are characterized by well-being and social potency, but PEM-A is defined by achievement and absorption (but not by social closeness), whereas PEM-C is defined by social closeness (but not by achievement or absorption).

Church and Burke (1994) tested the models for the Tellegen scales using confirmatory factor analysis. The three-factor model was supported except for the social closeness scale loading (negatively) on the NEM instead of the PEM factor, and well-being loading on both factors. A respecified four-factor model fit Tellegen's revised model somewhat better, except that some scales loaded on more than one factor, for instance, alienation correlating positively with NEM and negatively with PEM-C.

Caspi (2000), using cluster analyses on temperament scales at age 3, defined three types: undercontrolled, inhibited, and well-adjusted. The undercontrolled children as young adults described themselves as reckless, careless (uncontrolled), and sensation seeking (low harm avoidance), and high in aggression and alienation (NEM). The inhibited children grew up to be cautious (overcontrolled), nonimpulsive and nonaggressive, and not affectionate, outgoing, or confident (low PE).

Cloninger

Cloninger's trait model, like Eysenck's, is based on a psychobiological theory of personality but differs from Eysenck's in that the scales were not developed from factor analyses of items. Cloninger's goal was to establish a personality system tied to basic dimensions of psychopathology. Cloninger is a biological psychiatrist who conceives of the monoamine neurotransmitter systems as the basis of personality traits. He started with three basic personality traits: novelty seeking, harm avoidance, and reward dependence (Cloninger, 1987). Two of these resemble dimensions in Gray's model, as can be seen in Table 1-2. Harm avoidance represents a trait of behavioral inhibition and sensitivity to signals of punishment or frustrative nonreward (Gray's anxiety dimension). Reward dependence is theoretically related to sensitivity to signals of reward or reduction of punishment, like Gray's impulsivity. However, the third dimension of novelty seeking is the one actually related to appetitive approach behavior, whereas reward dependence is related only to *social reward* sensitivity and is behaviorally descriptive of a dependent personality.

Novelty seeking behavior descriptions closely resemble those of sensation seeking trait (Zuckerman, 1979, 1994), particularly the last version of this trait: impulsive sensation seeking. In Gray's (1982) theory, novel stimuli are classified, along with stimuli associated with punishment, as sources of anxiety, and therefore a person who readily approaches such stimuli

Table 1-2. Cloninger's Three-Factor Model in Comparison with Gray's Model

Cloninger Personality Dimension	Gray Personality Dimension	Relevant Stimuli	Behavioral Response (Cloninger)
Reward Dependence	Impulsivity	Conditioned signals for reward or relief of punishment	Resistance to Extinction
Harm Avoidance	Anxiety	Conditioned signals for punishment, novelty or frustrative non-reward	Passive avoidance Extinction. Behavioral inhibition
Novelty Seeking	(Obverse of Anxiety?)	Novelty, potential reward, potential relief of monotony or punishment	Exploratory pursuit, appetitive approach, active avoidance

Adapted from "A systematic method for clinical description and classification of personality variants," by C. Robert Cloninger, 1987, *Archives of General Psychiatry, 44*, Table 1, p. 575. Copyright 1987 by American Medical Association. Reprinted by permission.

would be someone low on the dimension of anxiety or harm avoidance in Cloninger's system.

Cloninger later expanded his three-dimensional system to a seven-factor model, including one more personality factor, persistence, and three dimensions of character, self-directiveness, cooperativeness, and self-transcendence (Cloninger, Svrakic, & Przybeck, 1993). The distinction between temperament and character traits has a 19th-century flavor. Temperament is described as heritable dispositions affecting processing of information by the "perceptual memory system," whereas character traits are based on differences in the self-concept involving acceptance of self, others, and "nature in general." They develop from interactions of temperament with the environment and life experiences, and are presumably less heritable than temperaments.

Cloninger has developed subtrait or facet scales for each of the seven major traits as described here:

Novelty Seeking (NS): 1. exploratory excitability versus rigidity; 2. impulsiveness versus reflection; 3. extravagance versus reserve; 4. disorderliness versus regimentation.

Harm Avoidance (HA): 1. anticipatory worry versus optimism; 2. fear of uncertainty versus confidence; 3. shyness versus gregariousness; 4. fatigability versus vigor. It should be noted that subscales 1 and 2 resemble N scales in other tests, whereas 3 and 4 are usually measures of E in other models. Thus, HA might be expected to correlate with E as well as N in other tests.

Reward Dependence (RD): 1. sentimentality versus insensitivity; 2. persistence versus irresoluteness; 3. attachment versus detachment; 4. dependence versus independence: Note that *persistence*, regarded as a fourth trait of temperament is listed as a subtrait of RD, but later analyses showed it to be independent of the RD dimension.

Self-directiveness (SD): 1. responsibility versus blaming; 2 purposeful versus goal undirected; 3. resourcefulness versus apathy; 4. self-acceptance versus self-striving; 5. congruent second nature.

Cooperativeness (C): 1. social acceptance versus intolerance; 2. empathy versus social disinterest; 3. helpfulness versus unhelpfulness; 4. compassion versus revengefulness; 5. pure-hearted versus self-serving.

Self-transcendance (ST): 1. self-forgetful versus self-conscious; 2. transpersonal identification; 3. spiritual acceptance versus materialism.

Correlations among the seven factors showed that NS was fairly independent or uncorrelated with the other six. However, HA was substantially correlated ($-.47$) with SD, and RD and SD were highly correlated ($.54$ and $.57$) with C.

A factor analysis of the 25 subscales showed that novelty seeking and harm avoidance factors were reconstituted from their assigned subscales, as were the cooperativeness, self-directedness, and self-transcendance factors. However, only two of the four reward dependence scales loaded on a common factor, and persistence was only defined by that single scale on a weak seventh factor.

There is nothing wrong with developing a model for personality assessment using rational or theoretical criteria for initial item selection and scale construction. However, it is necessary to follow up with empirical psychometric techniques to see if the structure postulated does correspond to the reality of the actual relationships among items and scales.

The claim that the seven scales in Cloninger's system represent basic personality factors is questionable. All other analyses of personality have revealed extraversion and neuroticism as basic factors of personality. Extraversion or sociability is not a distinctive factor in this system but is only a part of the harm-avoidance factor in which it is confounded with neuroticism type subscales. Reward dependence is a misnomer for a social dependency factor. Cloninger may have included this, because it is an important factor in some of the personality disorders, but it is not a basic factor in other systems, and indeed is not a coherent factor identified by

Cloninger's own analyses. Cloninger's model is the only other one besides mine (to be discussed) that identifies novelty seeking and impulsivity as a basic personality factor. Perhaps he was influenced by the wide range of biological phenomena already related to sensation seeking.

FIVE DIMENSIONAL SYSTEMS

The Big-Five

The origins of the so-called Big-Five go back to early studies by Fiske (1949), Tupes and Christal (1961), and Norman (1963). These early investigators used personality relevant adjectives collected by Cattell (1957) to investigate the structure of personality. The data from peer ratings of subjects were subjected to factor analyses. The analyses revealed five strong and recurrent factors rather than the 16 postulated by Cattell. Goldberg (1990, 1994) extended these analyses using an even broader sample of trait-relevant adjectives and many analyses. The five factors, each illustrated by the highest loading terms from Goldberg (1994) are:

   I. *Extraversion or surgency:* talkative, extraverted, verbal, bold, and assertive, versus shy, quiet, introverted, untalkative, and bashful.
  II. *Agreeableness:* sympathetic, kind, warm, helpful, and considerate versus cold, unsympathetic, unkind, harsh, and rude.
 III. *Conscientiousness:* organized, neat, systematic, thorough, and efficient versus disorganized, careless, unsystematic, inefficient, and sloppy.
 IV. *Emotional Stability:* unenvious, relaxed, unemotional, unexcitable, and undemanding versus moody, temperamental, jealous, touchy, and envious.
  V. *Intellect or Openness to Experience:* creative, imaginative, intellectual, philosophical, and artistic, versus uncreative, unimaginative, unintellectual, unintelligent, and simple.

These factors are derived from the language, or lexical analyses of the terms people used in describing themselves or others. Translations of the scale into many languages have resulted in the same five factors. The method is based on the assumption that the language reflects the basic trait structures of personality. This assumption may not be entirely correct. Words have been devised to describe the more socially obvious traits that are important to people. Agreeableness is important and has many descriptive terms in language, whereas emotional stability or instability (neuroticism) has fewer terms, probably because negative emotions are often concealed and internal and expressed mainly in diagreeable behavior.

A trait like sensation seeking that is quite fundamental, in terms of genetic determination and biological roots, has few adjectives that can be used to describe it (e.g., adventurous, daring, playful). The strength of factors depends on the number of potential item markers going into the factor analyses. This is why sensation seeking emerges only as a subtrait of extraversion in this kind of analysis. The basic elements of science do not necessarily correspond to those that are most phenomenologically salient. If they did, we would use the ancient Greek classification, air, water, earth, and fire, instead of the periodic table of elements.

The popularity of the Big-Five model increased when Costa and McCrae (1985) added Conscientiousness and Agreeableness to their orginal three-factor questionnaire: Neuroticism, Extraversion, Openness to Experience (NEO) (Costa, McCrae, & Arenburg, 1980). Next, they defined each of the five factors in terms of six subtraits, or "facets," in a hierarchal model of traits (Costa & McCrae, 1992). Each facet contributes equally to the major trait to which it is assigned. Thus, the facets define the five supertraits as described here:

Neuroticism (N): 1. anxiety, 2. angry hostility, 3. depression, 4. self-consciousness, 5. impulsiveness, 6. vulnerability

Extraversion (E): 1. warmth, 2. gregariousness, 3. assertiveness, 4. activity, 5. excitement seeking, 6. positive emotions

Openness (O): 1. fantasy, 2. aesthetics, 3. feelings, 4. actions, 5. ideas, 6. values

Agreeableness (A): 1. trust, 2. straightforwardness, 3. altruism, 4. compliance, 5. modesty, 6. tender-mindedness

Conscientiousness (C): 1. competence, 2. order, 3. dutifulness, 4. achievement striving, 5. self-discipline, 6. deliberation

The initial extension of the three-factor model to the five-factor one was done on a rational basis rather than starting from a new scale and item analyses. The assignment of six facet scores to each major factor and the selection of these scores also was based on rational criteria. A factor analysis by the test authors showed some divergence of facets from the assignment of facet scales to the five major factors (Costa & McCrae, 1992a). Some facets loaded more highly or equally on other factors than the ones to which they had been rationally assigned. A number of studies had failed to replicate the general model of the revised NEO using confirmatory factor analyses. However, McCrae and his colleagues, using a different statistical method, were able to replicate the structure (McCrae, Zonderman, Costa, Bond, & Paunonen, 1996).

Costa and McCrae (1992) did a 7-year longitudinal study of peer ratings based on the NEO-PI. Stability coefficients for the five-factor scores ranged from .63 to .84. Stability was essentially the same for a middle-aged group, 31 to 51 years at the start of the study, and an older group, 58 to 81 at the start. Costa and McCrae assert that, by the age of 30, personality is "essentially fixed." Changes in level were assessed in another study using self and spouse ratings (Costa & McCrae, 1988). Only 3 of 26 facet scales showed a change in level over a 6-year period. Declines with age in activity, positive emotions, and openness to actions were found, although age accounted for only a minor proportion of variance for the last two of these.

The Alternative Five

The research on the Alternative Five began in the 1980s as an attempt to develop a system of personality description that could be used as a framework for the 1991 version of this book. The initial selection of scales for factor analyses were based on traits that were involved at that time in genetic and psychobiological studies of temperament and personality. Eysenck's Big Three were an obvious starting point, because they were based on a biological model of personality. Buss and Plomin's (1975) four factors of temperament and the subfactors comprising them and Strelau's Temperament Inventory with its Pavlovian type constructs were easily adapted to an adult population. The Sensation Seeking Scale (SSS) had demonstrated high heritabilities and many biological correlates (Zuckerman, 1979, 1994; Zuckerman, Buchsbaum, & Murphy, 1980) so its subscales also were included. Similarly, impulsivity has been assessed in a number of different scales so several of these were included. In total, we hypothesized eight factors that might comprise basic dimensions of personality including: sociability, general emotionality (neuroticism), anxiety, aggression/hostility, socialization, sensation seeking, impulsivity, and activity. Scales for social desirability were included on the chance that they would define a methodological ninth factor (they did not). At least three scale markers were included for each of the anticipated factors.

At the time we started these studies, the Big Five had not been been translated into a questionnaire by Costa and McCrae. However, even if it had, we would probably have not included their scales, because they were developed from a lexical basis and we were looking for scales that could be placed in an evolutionary, psychobiological framework. The Big-Five scales such as conscientiousness, agreeableness, and openness to experience (or culture) were framed entirely in human terms.

Factor analyses of the 46 scales included in the first study (Zuckerman, Kuhlman, & Camac, 1988) and 33 scales in the second study (Zuckerman,

Kuhlman, Thornquist, & Kiers, 1991) showed an optimal solution of five factors that were stable across samples and genders. The tracking of factors across three- to seven-factor solutions also showed that both three- and five-factor solutions were equally robust. The three-factor solution looked very much like Eysenck's conception of the three basic factors, and his E, N, and P scales were the strongest markers for these factors. However, we decided to adopt the robust five-factor solution for our scales, because it offered more specificity with no expense of lowered factor reliability. Finally, item analyses and factor analyses of items were used to develop a questionnaire, the Zuckerman-Kuhlman Personality Questionnaire (ZKPQ) with scales for each of the five factors (Zuckerman, Kuhlman, Joireman, Teta, & Kraft, 1993). Subsequent factor analyses of the items within each scale yielded subfactors within three of them.

The factor scales are described as follows:

1. *Impulsive Sensation Seeking (ImpSS)*. This scale includes two subfactors: impulsivity and sensation seeking. The impulsivity component is described by a lack of planning and a tendency to act impulsively without thinking. The sensation seeking items describe a general need for thrills and excitement, a preference for situations in which the outcome is unpredictable; exciting, unpredictable friends, and a general need for change and novelty. The same combination of impulsivity and sensation seeking was found in Buss and Plomin's (1975) classification of basic temperament, and research has demonstrated the basic utility of this "marriage of traits made in biology" (Zuckerman, 1993).

2. *Neuroticism-Anxiety (N-Anx)*. This factor is characterized by a tendency toward emotional upset, tension, worry, fearfulnes, obsessive indecision, lack of self-confidence, and sensitivity to criticism.

3. *Aggression-Hostility (Agg-Host)*. Included in this factor are verbal aggressiveness, rude, thoughtless or antisocial behavior, vengefulness and spitefulness, a quick temper, and impatience with others.

4. *Sociability*. This is a narrow extraversion factor with two subfactors: one indicating a liking for big parties and a lot of social interaction with many friends; the other part is an intolerance for social isolation in extraverts but an enjoyment of solitary activities in introverts.

5. *Activity*. One subfactor describes the need for general activity and impatience and restlessness when there is nothing to do. The other subfactor indicates a liking of hard and challenging work and plenty of energy for work and life's other activities. There has been little study of the consistency of this temperament trait from childhood to adult age, possibly because the trait has not been well defined in adult personality

tests. However, follow-up studies of children and adolescents with Attention Deficit Hyperactivity Disorder (ADHD) show that the core features of attention deficit and poor impulse control continue into adulthood (Gadow, 2001).

Many of what are regarded as basic factors in the Alternative Five are included as subfactors or facets of the Big Five in Costa and McCrae's hierarchal systems. "Gregariousness," activity, and "excitement seeking" are facets of E in their system, and anxiety, hostility, and impulsivity are facets of N. The disagreement is in which traits are regarded as basic and which are major, and, in some cases, in the placement of traits within the major ones.

The fifth trait in each system is totally different. We decided not to include an intellective factor like culture or openness to experience and instead included the activity factor that is basic to every system of child temperament. But despite these differences in the conceptions of the trait hierarchies there is still substantial similarity between four of the Big-Five and Alternative-Five systems, as will be discussed next.

COMPARISONS OF PERSONALITY TRAIT SYSTEMS

Personality traits in different systems with different names may sometimes be measuring the same trait and personality traits with the same name may be measuring different traits. We can tell more by examining the content of the different trait scales, but the ultimate test must be in the actual correlations and shared factors of the different scales within the same population. Many of the items used in personality scales have been handed down and borrowed with only some slight modifications from the original parent stock in the studies by Cattell (1957) and Guilford and Zimmerman (1956). It is therefore not surprising that there is a great deal of resemblance in scales derived from factor analyses or other methods of item analysis.

One study compared three of the structural models already described: Eysenck's Big-Three, Costa and McCrae's Big Five, and Zuckerman and Kuhlman's Alternative Five (Zuckerman et al., 1993). The major factor scales from the EPQ-R, the NEO-PI-R, and the ZKPQ were intercorrelated and factor analyzed. Three factors accounted for 63% and four factors for 74% of the variance among the 13 scales. Beyond the first four factors eigen values dropped below one, indicating little to be gained by analyses of factors beyond three and four. Therefore, three factors were rotated in one analysis and four in another. The results of these are shown in Tables 1-3 and 1-4.

Table 1-3. Three-Factor Analysis of NEO, ZKPQ, and EPQ
Personality Scales

Scale	Factor Loadings		
	Factor 1	Factor 2	Factor 3
NEO Extraversion	.89	−.17	−.07
EPQ Extraversion	.76	−.35	.23
ZKPQ Sociability	.75	−.19	.17
ZKPQ Activity	.60	.00	−.11
NEO Openness	.35	.11	−.21
ZKPQ N-Anxiety	−.10	.93	−.03
NEO Neuroticism	−.13	.90	.17
EPQ Neuroticism	−.12	.92	.03
EPQ Psychoticism	−.12	−.11	.80
NEO Agreeableness	.06	−.06	−.72
NEO Conscientiousness	.14	−.03	−.68
ZKPQ ImpSS	.46	.02	.65
ZKPQ Agg-Host	.27	.32	.63

From "A comparison of three structural models for personality: The Big
Three, the Big Five, and the Alternative Five," by M. Zuckerman, D. M.
Kuhlman, J. Joireman, P. Teta, and M. Kraft, 1993, *Journal of Personal-
ity and Social Psychology, 65,* Table 4, p. 762. Copyright 1993 by the
American Psychological Association. Reprinted with permission.

In the three-factor analysis (Table 1-3), the measures of extraversion or
sociability from the three systems were highly loaded on the same factor and
activity from the ZKPQ also loaded highly on this factor. The three measures
of neuroticism all loaded above .90 on the same factor with negligible loadings, on the other two factors. EPQ psychoticism had the highest loading
on factor 3 and ZKPQ impulsive sensation seeking (Impss) and aggression-
hostility (Agg-host) and NEO agreeableness and conscientiousness also had
substantial loadings, supporting Eysenck's (1992) assertion that the latter
two are part of psychoticism.

The dimensions of extraversion and neuroticism, especially neuroticism,
are quite similar if not identical in all three systems despite differences in
breadth of scale content and scale construction. Apparently, there is a core
similarity, perhaps sociability for extraversion and anxiety for neuroticism,
that overrides differences in other facets of the super traits.

The three factors fit within the framework of Eysenck's PEN model. But
two of the models are five-factor ones, so the four factor analysis may reveal
some greater similarities (Table 1-4). As can be seen, the E and N factors
remain unchanged but the P factor is now divided into one containing
conscientiousness, psychoticism, and impulsive sensation seeking, and the

Table 1-4. Four-Factor Analysis of NEO, ZKPQ, and EPQ Personality Scales

Scale	Factor Loadings			
	Factor 1	Factor 2	Factor 3	Factor 4
NEO Extraversion	**.88**	−.14	−.05	.17
EPQ Extraversion	**.79**	−.32	.17	−.08
ZKPQ Sociability	**.76**	−.16	.10	−.07
ZKPQ Activity	**.60**	.01	−.18	.02
ZKPQ N-Anxiety	−.13	**.92**	−.01	.08
NEO Neuroticism	−.15	**.90**	.10	−.11
EPQ Neuroticism	−.16	**.91**	−.04	−.08
NEO Conscientious	.15	−.07	**−.86**	−.02
EPQ Psychoticism	−.09	−.08	**.80**	−.28
ZKPQ ImpSS	.48	.08	**.74**	−.02
NEO Agreeableness	−.04	−.07	−.31	**.81**
ZKPQ Agg-Host	.35	.34	.24	**−.72**
NEO Openness	.27	.14	.18	**.67**

From "A comparison of three structural models for personality: The Big Three, the Big Five, and the Alternative Five," by M. Zuckerman, D. M. Kuhlman, J. Joireman, P. Teta, and M. Kraft, 1993, *Journal of Personality and Social Psychology, 65*, p. 762. Copyright 1993 by the American Psychological Association. Reprinted with permission.

fourth factor is NEO agreeableness and openness versus ZKPQ aggression-hostility. Thus, four of the five factors from the ZKPQ and the NEO show substantial factor identity. The fifth factors in the two systems (activity and openness) could not be confirmed because only the one marker for each was included in the analysis.

The primary factor scales from the three instruments were correlated, but not factor analyzed, with some other scales including the Buss and Plomin (1975) EASI and Block and Block's (1980) scales for ego-undercontrol and ego-resiliency. The EASI emotionality scale correlated very highly with all three N scales; the EASI sociability correlated very highly with all three E scales; and the EASI impulsivity scale correlated very highly with ZKPQ ImpSS and EPQ P, and moderately with NEO agreeableness and ZKPQ aggression-hostility. Thus, the EASI, conceived of as a scale of basic temperament, fits closely to the primary three factors in the personality scales. EASI activity correlated highly with ZKPQ activity but NEO openness did not correlate with any of the EASI scales.

The highest correlation of the Block and Block ego-undercontrol scale was with the ZKPQ impulsive sensation seeking scale ($r = .63$) and the highest correlation of their ego resilience scale was with the NEO extraversion scale ($r = .51$). However, ego resilience was also correlated negatively with all three N scales and positively with NEO scales for agreeableness, and openness. Ego-undercontrol also correlated negatively with NEO conscientiousness, agreeableness, and openness, and positively with EPQ P and ZKPQ aggression.

Stallings, Hewitt, Cloninger, Heath, and Eaves (1996) correlated the scales of Cloninger's TPQ with Eysenck's EPQ scales. The TPQ contains only the four temperament scales and not the three character scales. Harm avoidance correlated positively with N and negatively with E; novelty seeking correlated positively with E and P; and reward dependence correlated positively with E and negatively to P.

Zuckerman and Cloninger (1996) compared the scales of the ZKPQ and EPQ with those from Cloninger's TCI, which contains all seven of his personality traits. Three of the scales from the ZKPQ and the TCI measures were highly correlated: ZKPQ impulsive sensation seeking with TCI novelty seeking ($r = .68$), ZKPQ neuroticism-anxiety with TCI harm avoidance ($r = .66$), and ZKPQ aggression-hostility with TCI cooperativeness ($r = -.60$). ZKPQ activity correlated moderately with TCI persistence ($r = .46$). The results comparing the temperament scales with Eysenck's EPQ were like those obtained in the Stallings et al. (1996): harm avoidance was negatively related to E and positively correlated with N; novelty seeking was positively related to P and E; and reward dependence was negatively related to P and positively to E. Persistence showed a weak but significant negative correlation with P. Among the character traits, cooperativeness correlated negatively with P, self-directiveness was negatively related to P and N and slightly positively to E, and self-transcendence was not correlated with either E, N, or P.

Cloninger's temperament scales and cooperativeness (the obverse of aggression) are more directly related to four of Zuckerman and Kuhlman's personality scales than to Eysenck's Big Three. They seem to meaure dimensions lying between Eysenck's: novelty seeking between P and E, harm avoidance between E and N dimensions, and reward dependence between P and E but, unlike novelty seeking, low rather than high on P. On a theoretical basis, they could correspond more closely to Gray's model, which suggests that the dimensions of personality that correspond with underlying behavioral and psychobiological dimensions (anxiety and impulsivity) do lie between Eysenck's major axes. Gray, however, has more recently conceded that they are closer to one or another of Eysenck's major dimensions (anxiety to N and impulsivity to E) rather than lying at a 45-degree angle between E and N (see Figure 1-2).

Gray's Behavioral Activation and Behavioral Inhibition systems (BAS and BIS) have been operationalized in scales developed by Carver and White

(1994) and Torrubia et al. (2001). Carver et al. developed one scale for Behavioral Inhibition, but on the basis of item and factor analyses developed three scales to measure the BAS: (1) reward responsiveness, or positive reactions to the occurence or anticipation of reward; (2) drive, or the persistent pursuit of reward; and (3) fun seeking, similar to impulsive sensation seeking. They compared these scales with Eysenck's E scale, a measure of manifest anxiety (MAS) that correlates highly with N, and Cloninger's TPQ scales of harm avoidance, novelty seeking, and reward dependence. They also used scales of negative and positive affectivity as traits. Negative affectivity was expected to be related to the BIS scale and positive affectivity to the BAS scale. Tellegen and others have suggested that E and N dimensions of personality are measures of positive affect and negative affect respectively and even named his first and second factors accordingly.

As expected, E was related to all three BAS scales but not to the BIS, and MAS correlated with the BIS scale but with none of the BAS scales. Also as predicted, negative affectivity was related only to BIS and positive affectivity to all BAS scales but not to BIS. The results were less clear with Cloninger's TPQ scales, ostensibly based on Gray's theory. Harm avoidance was positively correlated with BIS as expected, but it also correlated negatively with drive and fun seeking BAS scales. Novelty seeking correlated only with one of the BAS subscales, fun seeking. Reward dependence correlated with both BIS and the reward subscale of the BAS.

Zuckerman, Joireman, Kraft, and Kuhlman (1999) did a study using Torrubia and others' measures of BAS and BIS called Sensitivity to Reward (SR) for the BAS and Sensitivity to Punishment (SP) for the BIS scale. The scales are based on Gray's theory that the BAS sensitizes one to cues associated with reward and BIS sensitizes to cues associated with punishment. They also included an affect test, the Multiple Affect Adjective Check List-Revised (MAACL-R; Zuckerman & Lubin, 1985; Lubin & Zuckerman, 1999). The MAACL is a more differentiated affect measure than the one used in the Carver et al. study, providing three measures of negative affect (anxiety, depression, and hostility) and two scales of positive affect (positive affect and sensation seeking, a kind of surgency, affect). The personality scales used were the EPQ and the ZKPQ. Table 1-5 shows the correlations obtained between the SR and SP scales and the personality and affect scales.

E and Sociability correlated positively with SR and negatively with SP. N and N-Anx correlated high and negatively with SP and did not correlate at all with SR. The P scale did not correlate with either motivational measure, but the Impulsive Sensation Seeking Scale showed the same pattern as

Table 1-5. Correlations between Personality and Affect Traits and Sensitivities to Reward (SR) and Punishment (SP) Scales

	SR	SP
EPQ Extraversion	.34***	−.43***
EPQ Neuroticism	.05	.60***
EPQ Psychoticism	.08	−.06
EPQ Lie	−.19*	−.01
ZKPQ Sociability	.30***	−.29***
ZKPQ Neuroticism-Anxiety	.02	.63***
ZKPQ Impulsive Sensation Seeking	.24**	−.28***
ZKPQ Aggression-Hostility	.23*	.12
ZKPQ Activity	−.02	−.13
MAACL Anxiety (A)	.02	.54***
MAACL Depression (D)	−.04	.42***
MAACL Hostility (H)	.07	.23*
MAACL Positive Affect (PA)	.11	−.36***
MAACL Surgent (SS) Affect	.33***	−.38***
MAACL Dysphoria (A + D + H)	.02	.44***
MAACL Positive Affect Total (PA + SS)	.22*	−.41***

*$p < .01$, **$p < .001$,***$p < .0001$
EPQ = Eysenck Personality Questionnaire, ZKPQ = Zuckerman-Kuhlman Personality Questionnaire, MAACL = Multiple Affect Adjective Check List

E, correlating positively with SR and negatively with SP. Aggression correlated positively with SR. The same pattern of correlation between E and N and SR and SP was obtained by Torrubia et al. (2001).

All three negative affect measures and the total Dysphoria score correlated significantly with SP but not at all with SR, similar to the specific correlation of N measures with SP. However, the correlation of SP with anxiety was much stronger than the one with hostility. Surprisingly, simple positive affect (e.g., happy, peaceful) was negatively related to SP but not at all to SR. However, the surgent type of affect (e.g., enthusiastic, daring, wild) was related positively to SR and negatively to SP, the same pattern as shown by E and Sy. The total positive affect score (PA + SS) showed the same pattern.

The replicated factor analyses of the data yielded three factors with Eysenck's E, N, and P as the best markers for them. Positive affect of both types loaded on the E factor and the surgent type loaded as highly as E itself on the factor. Negative affects loaded on the N and P factors but anxiety had the highest loading on N and hostility was the defining affect for P.

SP was as strong a marker as was N itself for the N factor and SR had a strong loading on the E factor with a secondary loading on P.

To the extent that Torrubia's scales are valid assessments of Gray's BAS and BIS systems, it can be concluded that BIS and susceptibility to cues for punishment are nearly identical with the personality factor of neuroticism and associated with negative affect traits, particularly anxiety and depression. The BAS and susceptibility to cues for reward are primarily associated with E and positive, surgent affect, and, second, to P, where it is associated with negative affect, particularly hostility.

The associations between the components of six systems of personality are given in Table 1-6. The parallel rows in the table are based on the highest correlations found in actual studies, rather than the theoretical descriptions of the system authors. For instance, although some have maintained that anxiety or negative affect is a combination of E and N (introverted neuroticism), almost all the empirical work shows that they are almost entirely N related and not related to E. Some traits correlate primarily with one trait in another system but also correlate to a lesser degree with other traits. The placement of the traits in rows parallel to traits in other systems is based on the highest correlations with traits in the systems represented in immediately adjacent columns. Novelty seeking, for instance, correlates very highly with impulsive sensation seeking in the ZKPQ and much lower with sociability. However, in the EPQ, it correlates nearly equally with E and P. ImpSS itself shows a primary loading on a P factor but a secondary loading on E in three of four factor analyses (Zuckerman et al., 1993).

Although there are differences between factors as defined by the six systems, four factors are found in some form in all systems of five or more factors and combined with others in the three factor models. These four are: Extraversion/Sociability, Neuroticism/Anxiety (or negative affect), Constraint versus Impulsive Sensation Seeking, and Aggression/Hostility versus Agreeableness. These same traits also are found in most temperament scales (Table 1-1): sociability, negative mood, anger, and approach. The latter involves both impulsivity and sensation seeking (reactions to novel stimuli or persons). The continuity from childhood temperament to adult personality only has been examined in a few studies. Some of these show continuity across long age intervals, particularly appproach versus fearful inhibition, and undercontrol versus overcontrol. Aggression and antisocial behavior show consistency in many individuals from conduct and oppositional disorders in childhood to antisocial personality disorder in adults.

Activity is a temperamental trait in almost every system for children that has been omitted in most adult systems or relegated to a secondary trait

Table 1-6. Correspondences between Primary Traits in Six Systems

Eysenck	Tellegen	Gray	Costa & McCrae	Zuckerman & Kuhlman	Cloninger
Extraversion	Positive Affectivity	Behavioral Approach	Extraversion	Sociability	- Harm Avoidance
Neuroticism	Negative Affectivity	Behavioral Inhibition	Neuroticism	Neuroticism-Anxiety	Harm Avoidance
					- Self-Directive
Psychoticism	- Constraint	Fight/Flight	- Conscientiousness	Impulsive Sensation Seeking	Novelty Seeking
					- Reward Depend.
		Fight/Flight	Agreeableness	- Aggression-Hostility	Cooperativeness
				Activity	Persistence
			Openness		Self-Transcendence

A minus sign indicates that the trait is negatively related to the trait in the first left hand column. Block's two-factor system is not shown here. Ego resilience is negatively related to N and positively related to E; ego undercontrol is primarily related to ImpSS, but also to E, P, and Conscientiousness.

under extraversion. Persistence is another temperament trait neglected in adult personality systems. Some temperament traits such as sensitivity and adaptability may find expression in adult neuroticism, and others such as rhythmicity may simply have no direct relationship with adult personality.

SUMMARY

This chapter attempts to find some common factors that have been used to describe temperament or personality across the various systems for doing this. In the area of temperament, usually used to describe basic behavioral traits in infants and children, the factors appearing in all or most of the systems include: Approach, Activity, Negative Mood or Fearfulness, Anger, Sociability, and Persistence. All except the last of these resemble factors derived from some systems of adolescent or adult personality. Six systems of personality structure are presented. Correlations between traits in different systems reveal four major factors across systems: Extraversion/Sociability, Neuroticism/Anxiety (or Negative Affect), Constraint versus Impulsive Sensation Seeking, and Aggression/Hostility versus Agreeableness. Although Activity is always a major factor in temperament systems, in children it is either ignored or regarded as a subtrait of Extraversion in most adult systems, with the exception of the Zuckerman-Kuhlman model. Openness to Experience is unique to the Costa and McCrae Big-Five model. Self-Directiveness and Self-Transcendence are unique to the system developed by Cloninger.

The present volume will be organized around the basic four factors that are found in most systems of adult personality with a chapter devoted to each. But before proceeding to a psychobiological analysis of these four major factors of personality, I devote the next chapter to the methods used to study psychobiology in humans for the benefit of readers who may not be familiar with some or all of these.

CHAPTER 2

Psychobiological Methods

ADVANCES IN METHODOLOGIES

Ethical constraints restrict the scope of psychobiological methods used with living human beings. In other species, one can surgically or chemically destroy selected parts of the brain and observe the effects on behavior. Autopsy can be used to verify the brain alterations. One also can stimulate selected areas of the brain electrically or chemically through canulas to the brain areas. Brain stimulation in humans is usually done through external stimulation of the senses with stimulation varying in intensity, quality, or content. Chemical manipulation is done through infusion or ingestion of drugs, which can produce transient effects in these systems. Most psychopharmacological work with humans is done on abnormal populations with limited generalizability to normal personality variants.

Measurement of responses of specific brain areas to stimulation may be done directly, using implanted electrodes. Until recently, brain study in humans was limited to amplified electrical potentials from the scalp (EEG and cortical evoked potentials) indicating areas of cortical reactivity imprecisely located in areas under the surface electrodes. Newer brain imaging methods such as *positron emission tomography* (PET) and *functional magnetic resonance imaging* (fMRI) allow us to view activity at all levels of the brain at specific cortical and subcortical loci.

The peripheral autonomic system has been studied using physiological methods for measuring cardiovascular (heart rate, blood pressure, blood flow), respiratory, and electrodermal (skin conductance) methods. These methods have been widely used in studies of emotion, perception, and cognition, and some have used them to study personality traits such as neuroticism, and emotional traits such as anxiety and hostility. But emotions originate in the brain. There has been much recent interest in activity of parts of the limbic brain involved in emotions, such as the amygdala.

39

Newer imaging methods including PET and fMRI have been used in studies of emotional states in psychopathology and eventually will be used to study personality traits as well.

Neuropsychology in humans primarily has been done by autopsy findings correlated with behavioral evidence obtained before death. In living humans, simple neurological tests and more quantifiable psychological tests have been used in attempts to confirm and localize suspected brain damage. The results using tests sometimes were validated by exploratory surgery.

The new brain imaging methodologies can identify structural brain differences. These methods have progressed from the fuzzier images derived from *computed tomographic* (CT) scans to the sharper images obtained from *magnetic resonance imaging* (MRI). The 19th-century pseudoscience of phrenology suggested direct correlations between sizes of specific cortical brain areas, erroneously judged from the contours of the skull, and personality or character traits. The demise of phrenology led to a loss of interest in the possibilities of real relationships between personality and brain structure. Structural differences have been considered relevant only in neurological disorders or severe kinds of psychopathology. There are, however, findings in brain imaging research with abnormal populations that suggest that relative sizes of some brain areas could have some relationships to personality dimensions. Research in this area, however, is almost nonexistent.

Estimates of levels of changes in activity in brain neurotransmitter systems were obtained from metabolites of the neurotransmitters or their enzymes obtained from blood and urine. Fewer studies have been done on metabolites obtained from cerebrospinal fluid (CSF). Even though CSF is more directly in contact with the brain, and therefore a potentially better measure of brain neurochemical activity, the requirement of a lumbar puncture to obtain it limits its usefulness. The lumbar puncture usually is done only once on patients or well-paid volunteers and therefore cannot be used in experimental studies requiring a before-and-after assessment of the effects of a short-term experimental treatment. Blood and urine indirect measurements of neurotransmitter activity may reflect, in some part, peripheral system activity rather than brain activity. Newer methods use specific neurotransmitter stimulants (agonists) or blockers (antagonists) and measure the response of hormones obtained from blood but known to vary more directly with changes in brain neurotransmitter functions.

Studies of personality have been slow to utilize many of these newer methods for various reasons. The brain imaging methods, for instance, have been located in medical facilities and therefore require collaboration between personality psychologists and psychiatrists or other medical persons. Many of the methods are expensive, and grants supporting research have been given primarily to do research on clinical groups characterized by some form of psychopathology. Normals only have been studied in control groups matched to the patient group. Correlational methods used in personality research require large numbers of subjects to provide reliable findings, but most studies of patients and controls have been done using relatively small numbers of subjects so that correlations within groups between personality and biological traits have a large margin of error with consequent difficulties of replication.

Biometric behavior genetic studies on humans have utilized samples of twins and adoptees to separate the effects of genetic and environmental variation. Other studies used biologically related siblings or parents and children to estimate total familial effects combining genetic and environmental sources of variance. Some more recent studies have combined the twin and adoption methods using pairs of twins separated at or near birth and adopted into different families. Biometric studies of personality traits enable investigators to partial the total trait variance into that produced by: (1) genetics; (2) shared family and social environment; and (3) nonshared environment. To some extent, the methods also allow a differentiation between additive polygenetic mechanisms and other types such as Mendelian dominant-recessive and epistatic (specific combinations of genes) mechanisms. These biometric methods can answer the question of the relative effects of heredity and environment in a given population of a given age at a given time, but they cannot identify the actual genes associated with personality traits or forms of psychopathology. Identification of such genes is essential in understanding the biological variants produced by the genes, and it is these biological variants that directly affect the behaviors defining the trait.

Advances in molecular genetics in the last decades since the discovery of the DNA molecule at mid-century now permit identification of major genes associated with medical or psychopathological disorders. Even more recent studies, dating from the late 1990s, have applied these methods to personality traits.

The rest of this chapter will discuss the methods currently available for study of the psychobiology of personality. Readers already familiar with any or all of these methods can skip this chapter or the parts of it with which they are already familiar. Others may benefit from a reading of this material before going on to the subsequent chapters that deal with specific areas of personality. The reader occasionally may have to refer back to this chapter for the description of a particular method.

GENETICS

Until 1953, a half century ago, the gene was only a hypothetical unit of heredity. In 1953, James Watson and Francis Crick proposed that deoxyribonucleic acid (DNA) was the molecular basis of the gene. Since that landmark discovery, the molecular mechanisms of heredity have been extensively studied, the human genome has been deciphered, the genetic bases of many neurological disorders have been defined, and work in progress is searching for major genes associated with different forms of psychopathology and, most recently, personality traits. Long before these advances in molecular genetics, psychology was preoccupied with the "nature versus nurture" dichotomy. How much of our personality is a function of genetic determination and how much is due to environmental influences, particularly family and societal ones? Natural variations in genetic relatedness of individuals were used in an attempt to answer the nature-nurture question and statistical methods were devised to separate the two kinds of influence.

Biometric Methods

Quantitative genetics is based on the assumption that if genetic factors affect a quantitative trait, resemblance of relatives should increase with increasing degrees of genetic relatedness. Genetic relatedness varies with the degree of relationship:

Identical Twins: 100% of genes in common

First-degree Relations: fraternal twins, ordinary siblings, parents, children: 50%

Second-degree Relations: grandparents, grandchildren, half-siblings, uncles and aunts, nephews and nieces: 25%

Third-degree Relations: great-grandparents, great-grandchildren, first cousins: 12.5%

Adoptive Relations: parents, children, siblings, and so on: 0%

To the extent that a phenomenal trait is based on additive polygenetic mechanisms, inheriting half of their genetic material from each parent, the degree of similarity of any two relationships should show the same ratio, for example, identical twins to fraternal twins (2 to 1).

Twin Studies. Twins are frequently used to estimate the *heritability* of a trait. Heritability is the proportion of phenotypic variance that is a function of genetic sources. A frequent method is to compare either similarity (corre-lation) or variance between pairs of identical twins compared to similarity or variance between pairs of fraternal twins. On a genetic basis, the trait measure in identical twins would be expected to correlate twice as high as that for fraternal twins. If a trait were totally determined by genetic factors alone, identical twins would correlate 1.00 and fraternal twins .50. Corre-lations approaching these figures, indicating near total genetic determina-tion, are found only for certain physical characteristics such as height or some reliable physiological traits such as EEG alpha rhythms.

Fraternal twins are compared with identical twins in order to control the factor of *shared environment*. Like identical twins, fraternal twins are born at the same time into the same family and therefore share some broad features of their environments such as parents, other siblings and relatives, social class, neighborhoods, schools, and sometimes friends. Critics of the method point out that although both types of twins may share the same parents, the parents may respond differently to each twin, and there may be more of a tendency to treat identical twins the same than to do so with fraternal twins. Of course, this tendency may be because identical twins behave more similarly than fraternal twins, eliciting more consistent reac-tions from their parents. Another violation of the assumptions behind the comparison is that the interactions between the twins may either reinforce similar behavioral tendencies in one another or establish nonreciprocal types of patterns such as dominance and submission. The former is a shared environmental factor that might occur more frequently in identical twins and therefore show up as a genetic factor in the calculation of heritability. A third possible confound is that because identical twins are more likely to share a common placenta and chorionic sac, whereas fraternal twins never do so, the prenatal environment may have a differential effect in the two types of twins. This may be a factor in certain types of psychopathol-ogy in which there is more concordance among identical than fraternal twins.

In the calculation of *heritability* from comparisons of identical and fra-ternal twins the differences between the correlations of the two kinds of twins on the trait is used to estimate heritabilities. If the correlation is the same in both types of twins, heritability is zero and, to the extent that both correlations are high, the resemblance of both types of twin is assumed to be because of shared environment. A rough estimate of heritability may be obtained by doubling the difference between the correlations of identical and fraternal twins. The difference represents half of the genetic effect and is doubled to estimate the entire genetic effect.

The heritability calculated from identical twins is referred to as *broad heritability* because it includes additive, dominance, *and* epistasis types of genetic mechanisms. But fraternal twins and ordinary siblings in relation to each other and their parents only show the effects of additive genetic mechanisms. This type of heritability is called *narrow*. This difference between broad and narrow heritabilities may account for the marked differences between the higher heritabilities calculated from twin studies and those derived from parental-offspring and sibling studies. A nonadditive type of mechanism may reduce the correlations between siblings. Epistatic mechanisms, requiring special combinations of genes, are found in identical twins who share the same set of genes. Correlations of near zero in fraternal twins, or correlations much lower than half of the correlation between identical twins, may indicate the operation of nonadditive genetic mechanisms.

In the calculation of heritability, the genetic part of the variance in the trait is removed, then the proportion of variance due to *shared environment* is subtracted and the remainder is assumed to be because of *nonshared environment* and error of measurement. The nonshared environment is everything that influences one member of a family but not the others in the family. Different friends, mentors, life experiences, illnesses, or other factors constitute the nonshared environment.

Different treatment of siblings by the parents, or perception of such differences, is also part of the nonshared environment, although it may well be because of a reaction to real differences between siblings in their interactions with parents. One sibling may be conforming and well-behaved and elicit nothing but praise and reward from parents and teachers, whereas another may be rebellious and unsocialized and therefore draw more punishment and rejection from parents and others. The behavioral differences may have genetic sources but they affect the environment in different ways. These are problems in *genotype-environment correlation*. Plomin, DeFries, McLearn and Rutter (1997) call this type of genotype environment correlation *evocative*. They also describe two other types. If children inherit genotypes compatible or correlated with those of parents and siblings, they are likely to be reinforced for the traits emerging from that genotype. This is called *passive* genotype-environment correlation. If a child of academic parents is bright and shares their intellectual interests, he or she is likely to be esteemed and favored. But if another sibling did not inherit the ability and temperament traits favoring academic achievement, he or she may encounter disfavor or even rejection. The third type is *active* genotype environment correlation. Individuals cannot choose their parents but they can choose from alternative possibilities offered by the environment according to their genetically influenced propensities. They choose their friends, peer groups, activities and, eventually, spouses, from among those available. Two siblings may shape different kinds of environment because of differences in their genetically influenced temperaments. The friends they choose because of their compatibility in turn reinforce the traits they share with them. Adoption studies provide a method for better separation of effects due to genetics and environment and their interactions.

Adoption Studies. Adoption studies of humans are like the cross-fostering studies done with animals, although the studies of humans rely on natural selection and are therefore less controlled. In animal studies, an offspring born to a mother of one strain is taken at birth and transferred to a mother of another strain. The two strains differ in the trait for genetic reasons and the question is whether the similarities of offspring and parent are due to genes or rearing environment or their interaction. In the studies of humans, children who are adopted into other families at or close to birth are compared with their biological parents or siblings and their adopted parents or siblings.

The biological parents and siblings share genes but not environment with the adoptee, whereas the adoptive parents and siblings share an environmental influence but not a genetic one with the adoptee. The caveat is whether or not there has been some selective placement of the adoptee with other relatives or based on a match on the relevant trait. Usually only physical traits – coloring and health – influence adoption choices, as the adopting parents usually do not know the personal characteristics of the biological parents.

The correlation of the adoptee with the biological parents' traits can only be due to additive genetic causes if adoption occurred very early in life. There is, of course, some possibility of influence by the prenatal environment or the early mother-child interaction if the adoption did not occur right after birth. The correlation of the adoptee with the adoptive family relatives can only be due to the shared social environment of the family, assuming there has been no selective placement. Interaction effects are possible. The expression of the genetic influence of the biological parents may depend in some part on the characteristics of the adoptive parents or the kind of environment they provide. A child may inherit high intelligence from her biological parents, but if she is adopted into a family with little interest in academic achievement she may not show the achievement that she would have if she had been adopted into a family with stronger intellectual values.

To the extent that adoption agencies screen potential adopting parents for marital stability, motives for adoption, economic viability, and personal characteristics, the samples of adopting parents will have a restricted range of potential negative environmental influences. A restricted range could mean that shared environmental variance would also be restricted compared to genetic variance. If the families with negative characteristics are not considered for adoption then the full range of the potential influence of environment on the children will not be present. This is particularly important in the study of psychopathological traits.

It should be noted that the environmental influence represented by the adoptive family is not the total environmental effect but only the shared one. It does not include the nonshared environmental influences occurring outside of the family. The genetic influence represented by the biological parents and siblings is only that due to narrow genetic (additive) mechanisms and does not include that due to other mechanisms, dominance, and epistasis. To assess broad heritability, one can turn to another type of adoption study, separated twin adoptions.

Twin Adoptions. Studies of twins separated at or close to birth and raised in different families without any contact with each other during their formative years are particularly valuable in estimating the influence of broad heritability. Any similarity between identical twins separated in this manner could only be due to their shared total genetic makeup. The correlation of a trait between sets of separated identical twins is a direct estimate of heritability. The correlation for separated fraternal twins would have to be doubled because they share only half of their genes in common. A comparison of the correlation of separated identical twins can be contrasted with the correlation for twins raised together in the same family to give an estimate of the shared environmental influence. If the correlations are the same, there is no effect of shared environment. To the extent that the correlation of twins raised together is higher than the one for twins raised apart the shared environment does play a role. There are two major ongoing studies of twins reared apart (Bouchard, Lykken, McGue, Segal, & Tellegen, 1990; Pederson, Plomin, McClearn, & Frieberg, 1988). A surprising result of these studies is that the correlations of twins separated and those raised together are very close for most personality traits indicating little or minimal effect of shared environment.

As stated previously, the correlation of separated identical twins is a direct estimate of heritability. Figure 2-1 shows the correlations of separated identical twins on different kinds of traits in the Minnesota twin study (Bouchard et al., 1990). For physical characteristics such as height,

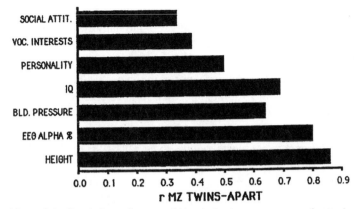

Figure 2-1. Correlations of separated identical twins on measures of attitudes, interests, personality, intelligence, blood pressure, EEG (alpha), and height (data from Bouchard et al., 1990).

the correlation approaches unity suggesting nearly total heritability. Some physiological characteristics, such as the predominance of the EEG alpha rhythm, also approach maximal heritability. Heritability of intelligence is about .70 whereas personality traits are about 50% genetic according to this criterion. Measures of vocational interests and social attitudes (along a liberal-conservative dimension) are lower in heritability but still show some influence of genetics.

An estimate of the heritability of personality traits using a broader range of studies of all types of twins on self-report personality tests suggests that 30 to 50% (average 40%) of the variance in personality is due to genetic factors and the rest is due to nonshared environment (Plomin et al., 1997). Peer ratings yield about the same results. Nontwin studies of familial relations do not yield heritabilities as high as these, perhaps because of the influence of nonadditive genetic mechanisms.

Cautions on Heritability

Heritability is often treated as a fixed, universal statement of causation. The following cautions should be emphasized in interpreting this statistic:

1. Heritability depends on the reliability of the phenotype measure. Obviously, if the measure is unreliable, the calculations based on it are unreliable.
2. Heritability can vary from one time to another. Changes in mores, such as in sexual permissiveness, from one generation to the next, can change heritabilities (Dunne et al., 1997).

3. Heritability can vary from one population to another. A trait such as disinhibition can show little heritability in a population characterized by a strict religious upbringing and high heritability in a nonreligious one (Boomsma, de Geus, van Baal, & Koopmans, 1999).
4. Heritabilities apply to populations, not to individuals. One cannot say that an individual's trait is some percentage due to heredity and some percentage due to environment.
5. One cannot generalize from heritabilities within populations to the source of differences between populations. This rule is violated by those who postulate that ethnic or racial differences must have genetic/evolutionary sources.
6. Heritability is an imprecise statistic and requires large *n*s for stable results.

The finding that most personality traits have a substantial heritability is only surprising to dogmatic environmental theorists who believe that personality is entirely shaped by family and culture. Such a view is no longer tenable in view of the overwhelming evidence from biometric behavioral genetic studies. However, all that these studies show us is that genetics is a factor in most personality traits, and the range of this influence among different traits is not broad. The next step is to find which genes are actually involved in a particular trait and which biological traits are affected by those genes. This brings us to the most recently developed area: molecular genetics.

Molecular Genetics

When I started graduate school in 1949, the gene was a hypothetical construct. By the time I graduated (1954), Watson and Crick (1953) had identified the molecular structure of the DNA molecule. Since that time, methods of identifying genes and their loci on chromosones have been developed allowing for an examination of the role of specific genes in forms of pschopathology and personality traits. The identification of genes with personality traits only began in the last half of the 1990s. Plomin et al. (1997) discussed the potential of molecular genetics for psychology as follows:

Psychology is at the dawn of a new era in which molecular genetic techniques will revolutionize genetic research in psychology by identifying specific genes that contribute to genetic variance for complex dimensions and disorders. (p. 277)

The DNA double helix consists of two strands that are held apart by pairs of four bases: adenine, thymine, guanine, and cytosine. The DNA replicates itself and synthesizes proteins according to the information coded in the particular sequence of bases. The DNA is converted to messenger RNA which forms amino acid sequences. The bases code for sequences of 20 amino acids. In various combinations the amino acids make up the specific enzymes and proteins which form the nervous system and other body structures.

Genes are segments of the DNA containing anywhere from thousands to millions of base pairs in length. Until recently, there were an estimated 100,000 genes in the human genome, but this has now been reduced to about 30,000. Some simpler organisms with less complex nervous systems have this many genes so that nervous system complexity cannot be a simple function of the number of genes but must be involved in their interactions. The brain is the most likely site of individual differences in behavior and it is probably significant that an estimated one third of our genes are expressed only in the brain. The vast majority of nucleotide base sequences are the same across most members of our species. Only about one thousandth (three million of three billion) nucleotide bases differ among people. We are very much more the same than different in our genetic makeup. However, those varying forms of genes, or polymorphisms, are a major source of individual differences. One way in which they differ is in the number of repetitions of the nucleotide base pairs. The number of repeats has been used to distinguish persons with different levels of personality traits. Although the number of repeats at a particular locus is inherited in a Mendelian fashion, many such genes are usually involved, and if the genetic mechanism is an additive one they may combine to produce a trait that is normally distributed.

Alleles are different forms of the same gene. A gene may have two or more alleles. Mendel's second law, independent assortment, states that the inheritance of one gene is not affected by the inheritance of another, or that there is no association between genes or alleles. The method of genetic analysis of animal or human traits called *linkage* is based on a violation of Mendel's second law. Although independent assortment works for genes on different chromosones or even widely spaced on the same chromosone, genes very close on the same chromosone do not assort independently. This nonindependent assortment enables investigators to search the entire genome in order to find linkages between DNA markers and genes involved in disease or behavioral traits and to eventually locate these genes by their proximity to the marker. Linkage for single gene disorders can be done using large extended family groups covering several generations. This method has been applied to major psychiatric disorders with results that have been difficult to replicate across families. Another type of linkage analysis is comparisons of affected relative pairs, in which both or neither sibling is affected. The most frequently used method is *sib-pair* analysis. If both members are affected they would show a greater than 50% sharing of markers in a region in which the gene related to the disease is located.

An example of this sib-pair method is the finding of a linkage on the X chromosone, inherited in men through the mother, with homosexuality (Hamer, Hu, Magnuson, Hu, & Pattatucci, 1993). Allele sharing for markers in a particular region of this chromosone was 67% for brothers who were both homosexual contrasted with only 22% for brothers of these men who were heterosexual. A biometric study found only modest heritability for homosexuality in males (52% concordance in identical and 22% in fraternal twins) (Bailey & Pillard, 1991) so that one cannot conclude that genetics alone can explain sexual preference. Homosexuality undoubtedly involves many genes and some kind of interaction or correlation with environmental factors as do most behavioral or personality traits. The method of *allelic association* is perhaps more applicable to the study of polygenetic traits in which the mode of transmission is unknown.

In studying continuously distributed personality traits, in contrast to disorders, investigators typically use some cutoff point on the distribution to define a high group, and another to define a low or moderate group. Association involves the comparison of the frequencies of particular alleles associated with a phenotype that could be membership in a diagnostic group or persons high or low on some personality trait. One starts with the phenotype and then compares the frequencies of different alleles of the same gene. The typical analysis involves a 2×2 frequency table with the two phenotype groups as one dimension and the presence or absence of the particular allele (or an alternative allele) as the other. The significance of the association is tested by chi-square. For instance, a study of the relationship between the alleles of the D4DR gene (characterized by different numbers of repeats of the base sequence) found that those who scored high on a scale of novelty seeking had a higher frequency of the long allele forms than the group scoring lower on this personality scale (Ebstein et al., 1996). In other words, the study showed an association between the longer forms of the gene and novelty seeking. Frequencies of alleles may vary among ethnic groups, so it is important that the criterion groups be homogeneous for ethnicity. Studies within families control the ethnicity factor, but other factors could distinguish experimental and control groups, such as age, gender, and associated behaviors such as drug use.

More detailed discussions of the methods used in molecular genetics can be found in several publications including: McGuffin, Owen, O'Donnovan,

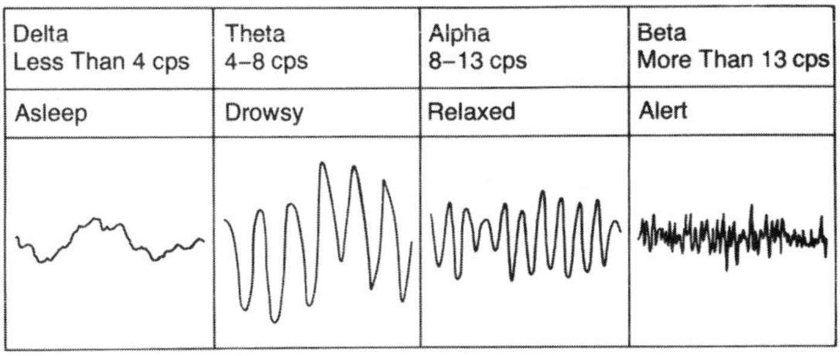

Delta Less Than 4 cps	Theta 4–8 cps	Alpha 8–13 cps	Beta More Than 13 cps
Asleep	Drowsy	Relaxed	Alert

Figure 2-2. From J. Hassett, 1978, *A primer of psychophysiology*, p. 104. San Francisco, CA: W. H. Freeman & Co. Copyright W. H. Freeman & Co. Reprinted by permission.

Thapar, and Gottesman (1994); Plomin, DeFries, McClearn, and Rutter (1997); and Rao and Gu (2002).

PSYCHOPHYSIOLOGICAL METHODS

Brain Physiology

The concept of cortical arousal or arousability has played an important role in theories of personality. Pavlov's (1927/1960) theory of individual differences was based on hypothetical traits of the central nervous system such as strength of cortical excitation and inhibition. Eysenck (1967) suggested that cortical arousal distinguished extraverts and introverts, the former being underaroused and the latter overaroused in an unstimulated state. Zuckerman (1969) originally made the construct of an *optimal level of arousal* (cortical) the basis of the trait of sensation seeking, although he later changed this to an *optimal level of catecholamine system activity* (Zuckerman, 1984). Strelau (1987) adapted Pavlov's typology based on traits of cortical activity as the basis for human temperament but more recently seems to have developed a theory of temperament with less of a debt to Pavlovian constructs (Strelau, 1998).

EEG

Before the invention of brain imaging methods, the most direct way to assess cortical arousal was the electroencephalogram (EEG). Raw EEG recordings are made by placing electrodes on the scalp and recording the potentials coming from the outer layer of the brain or the cortex.

Four basic wave patterns associated with different states of arousal are shown in Figure 2-2. The waves can be distinguished by frequency, synchronization, and amplitude. Beta waves are high frequency (13–30 cps), low amplitude, desynchronized waves found in excited states as during intense mental or physical activity, or high emotional arousal. Alpha waves are a regular rhythm of 8–13 cps of moderate amplitude occuring primarily in the occipital region during a relaxed but wakeful state. They are best obtained when the eyes are closed because visual stimulation tends to disrupt them. Persons differ in their characteristic frequency within the alpha range. Because amplitude varies inversely with frequency, it often is used as an inverse measure of arousal within the waking state. Theta waves are slower (4–8 cps) and of higher amplitude than alpha. They are associated with lower arousal, drowsiness, and are more frequent in the recordings of children. Delta waves are low frequency (less than 4 cps) and high amplitude that only occur in deep sleep. Over any extended period of time different shifts of wave forms appear. The computer can use band filters to analyze the EEG into time when each component wave is present over some specified period of time. This kind of analysis is called *spectrum analysis*. Genetic analyses have shown that characteristic individual spectrum activity is near totally genetically determined (Lykken, 1982).

The EEG recording varies in different parts of the cortex, and certain electrode locations are better than others for different purposes. Hemispheric differences in activity also exist and there are differences in the roles of the two hemispheres in cognition and emotion. In order to get a complete view of cortical activity it is necessary to obtain recordings from many sites in both hemispheres. Signals from all sites can be integrated by computers into a visual image of the changing activity of the cortex and computer processing enables investigators to quantify and analyze the data.

Averaged Evoked Potentials

The raw EEG can assess changes in arousal in response to a stimulus but only in a gross and slow manner. When a stimulus is presented there is a shift in the EEG from slower activity to faster, low voltage beta rhythms. The *cortical averaged evoked potential* (EP), or event-related brain potential, was developed to provide a clearer signal of the brain's response to a stimulus event. The same brief stimulus, visual, auditory, or somesthetic, is presented a number of times and the EEG is digitized at a fixed rate, time-locked to the stimulus delivery. By averaging the response across trials, the trial-to-trial "noise" is averaged out over a 500-millisecond (half-second) period immediately subsequent to the stimulus. A clear signal then emerges as shown in Figure 2-3. Characteristic peaks of positivity and negativity in the wave forms at different latencies are shown in the figure. The latencies of these peaks vary with the stimulus modality and intensity and recording sites.

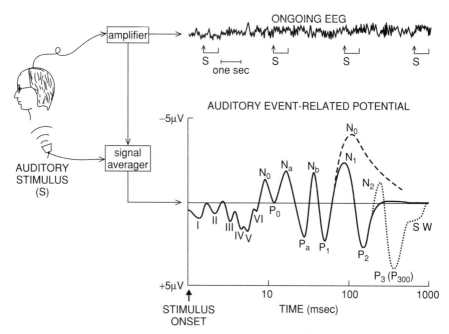

Figure 2-3. Amplitudes and latencies of EP components N1, P1, N2, and P2. Each of the two functions represents averaged responses to 100 light flashes on two different occasions. Positivity is downward. From J. L. Andreassi, 2000, *Psychophysiology, human behavior and physiological response.* 4th Edition (p. 95). Mahwah, NJ: Erlbaum. Copyright 2000 by Lawrence Erlbaum Associates. Reprinted by permission.

There also are some individual differences in the characteristic latencies for particular peaks, but generally the peaks fall close to the modal point. A negative peak (N1) for instance, usually occurs about 50 msec after stimulus presentation and a positive peak (P1) typically occurs at 100 msec post stimulus. This wave form (N1-P1) represents the first impact of the stimulus on at the cortical level and is sensitive to differences in stimulus intensity. Earlier wave forms occuring before 50 msec are of subcortical origins. For instance, early components (1–8 msec) of an auditory evoked response are produced at the brain stem. Subsequent waves reflect activity in the trapezoid body, pons, inferior colliculus, and thalamus. A negative peak at 80 to 90 msec in response to a tone and a positive peak at about 170 msec is called the N1-P2 complex and is generated at the auditory cortex in the temporal lobe.

The peak occuring about 300 msec after stimulus presentation (P300) is a response to the qualitative features of the stimulus and has been extensively studied in a task referred to as the "odd-ball" paradigm. Actually, the classical

P300 may occur anywhere from 300 to 900 msec post stimulus so that the EP range is extended to 1000 msec for this purpose. When one stimulus is presented frequently and an infrequent, or odd, stimulus is presented the response to the odd-ball stimulus at P300 is larger than the response to the frequently presented stimulus. The P300 has been utilized in a wide variety of areas, including orienting response, decision making, attention, signal detection, discrimination, and individual differences (personality, psychopathology, intelligence). For a summary of findings in these areas, see Andreassi (1989).

Contingent Negative Variation (CNV) is another kind of event-related potential, one involving slow waves often filtered out of the EEG. Walter, Cooper, Aldrich, McCallum, and Winter (1964), who discovered CNV, allowed these low frequency drifts in an experiment in which a warning stimulus (S1) was followed by an imperative stimulus (S2). The imperative stimulus (S2) was the signal for the subject to press a key. There is a slow increase in negativity at the vertex scalp location appearing just before the key press. Averaging the potential revealed that it was maximal over the frontal cortex. Unlike orienting responses measured by other techniques, it did not habituate over hundreds of trials, and was related to speed of reaction times. The CNV has been shown to occur in two waves: an orienting reaction to the initial stimulus (S1) and an *expectancy* response to S2. The latter also has been termed a "readiness for action." These two components have been shown to relate differentially to different personality traits.

The methods described thus far have been primarily useful in assessing psychophysiological reactions in the outer surface of the brain, or the cortex. The period before brain imaging is analogous to the time before the invention of diving equipment when exploration of the oceans was confined to the surface. The invention of brain-imaging methods has enabled investigators to study the brain at all levels. Many centers and pathways for emotional response are located in subcortical brain. Because emotional traits are an important component of personality, this advance in methodology opens new vistas in the psychobiology of personality.

Positron Emission Tomography (PET)

The PET method enables analysis of activity in brain structures at all levels. To push our aquatic metaphor deeper, it is equivalent to the bathysphere or submarine. The positron is emitted by unstable radio elements and is like an electron in mass and spin but possesses a positive rather than a negative charge. The most common method involves the injection of the subject with radioactive-tagged deoxyglucose (DG). DG is taken up by the brain over a period of 35 minutes. Structures of the brain that are most active during this period absorb the most glucose. The glucose emits positrons that decay into gamma rays at 180-degree angles. The subject's head rests in a PET scanner that detects the gamma rays. A computer analyzes the data from various "slices" of the brain cutting across structures at various depths. The computer then generates images in the form of little boxes corresponding to specific loci from which a particular group of emissions originate. The resolution of the cameras from 1980 to 1990 improved resolutions from 2 cm to 0.5 cm, but one system actually reached a 2.6 mm resolution, which approached the limits of the method. Some brain structures are too small to be detected by the less sensitive systems. A limitation of the method is that it can only reflect what has happened in the brain during the period of 30–35 minutes during the uptake of the tagged glucose. It cannot, therefore, measure response to specific stimuli, only to a total experience. Furthermore, there are individual differences in absolute glucose rates across all of the brain. Some control for this can be achieved by calculating a relative rate for each box divided by the mean rate for the entire slice.

Regional *cerebral blood flow* (CBF) is another kind of PET method. Blood flow is related to the activity of a particular brain area. One method involves the intravenous injection of water labeled with oxygen-15 and another has the subject inhale xenon-133 mixed with air through a face mask for 1 minute. The advantage of this method is that it allows measurement of brain activity over a 30- to 90-second period compared to the 30- to 35-minute period of the glucose method. The disadvantages are less specific localization of activity (only eight areas in each hemisphere) and the need to have an on-site cyclotron for the production of the radionuclides because of their short half-life.

PET may be used to visualize and measure receptor density for particular neurotransmitters in the brain (Schlyer, 1991; Wong & Young, 1991). There are two methods of accomplishing this. The first involves labeling the particular ligand of interest with a positron-emitting label and visualizing it directly from the PET image. Because many neurotransmitters have more than one type of receptor, and these receptor types are differentially distributed in different pathways and brain structures, it is important to be able to specify the state of specific receptors. The blocking experiments block one type of receptor while observing the uptake in another. These methods have been widely used in studies of psychopathology, both to investigate how therapeutic drugs work and perhaps illuminate etiology of the disorder. Only a few applications have been made to personality but one may anticipate more frequent use of these, and other imaging methods, as they become more widely available to investigators.

PERIPHERAL MEASURES OF AUTONOMIC NERVOUS SYSTEM ACTIVITY

There are two branches of the autonomic nervous system (ANS): the sympathetic (SNS) and parasympathetic (PNS). In general, the ANS regulates the internal environment of the body in a manner that meets the immediate demands of the situation and the maintenance of vital steady-state processes such as blood circulation, digestion, elimination, and temperature maintenance. The PNS maintains the steady state in the vital processes, whereas the SNS mobilizes the internal environment for sudden demands for action characterized as "fight or flight." The SNS accomplishes this by diverting blood flow from the central body areas to the periphery, brain, limbs, and musculature. Heart rate, blood flow and blood pressure are increased, along with respiratory rate. Increased sweating occurs particularly in the hands and feet. At the same time, processes involved in digestion, such as salivation, and elimination are inhibited (sphincter contraction). There generally is an inverse relationship between SNS and PNS, although the balance may shift rapidly in compensatory reactions of the PNS to surges of SNS activity.

The characteristic balance between the systems, combining different measures of each, might reflect a psychophysiological trait relevant to personality traits like neuroticism (Wenger, 1941; Wenger & Cullen, 1972). But most personality research has used specific measures, partly because measures in different systems, such as cardiovascular and electrodermal, are not correlated, or correlated very low, arguing against combination in any overall measure. Other problems are stimulus-response and individual-response specficity. Certain systems respond more than others to specific types of situations, and some individuals are more reactive in certain response systems compared to others. Therefore, we will focus on the more commonly used measures: the cardiovascular (heart rate, blood pressure), electrodermal (skin conductance), respiration, and muscle tension. In all of these, one also must distinguish between tonic (resting, unstimulated) levels and phasic (reactive to stimuli or situations) levels of physiological activity.

Electrodermal Activity

Activity in the sweat glands has been an important source of data for psychophysiologists because of their sensitivity to arousal by both external and internal stimuli. The ecrine sweat glands are located nearly everywhere in the skin but are most numerous in the palmar surfaces of the hands and the soles of the feet. They are less dense in the arms, legs, and trunk of the body. The ecrine glands in the forehead, neck, and back of the hands respond strongly to thermal stimuli and weakly to psychological or sensory stimuli, whereas those in the palms and fingers of the hand are primarily sensitive to psychological and sensory stimuli and weakly responsive to thermal stimuli. This is why the most usual site for the active electrode in psychological experiments is the palm or fingers of the hand. One of the signs of a state of fear is "sweaty palms." A clinician is alerted to anxiety in a patient on first shaking hands because of the wetness or "clammy" condition of the patient's hands. However, palmar sweating is not specific to fear as a trait or state but also occurs in phasic response to novel and or intense stimuli of any kind, such as erotic stimuli or sudden loud sounds.

Activity of the sweat glands in the palm may be measured by applying a constant current and measuring the variations in voltage across electrodes attached to the palmar surfaces. This technique measures skin resistance (SR), which is inversely related to skin conductance and arousal. Skin conductance (SC) is the reciprocal of SR but may be measured directly by applying a constant voltage and measuring variations in current. Whatever the method of recording, the favored data for analysis is SC because it yields data more adapted to parametric statistical analyses. Further normalization of the data is accomplished by log or square root transformations of SC.

Another method is assessment of skin potential (SP). SP is measured without the application of an external current and uses a unipolar electrode arrangement with one electrode attached to the active palmar or finger site and the other to a relatively indifferent site like the forearm. SP is measured by a sensitive DC amplifier. It measures the endosomatic variations in activity of the sweat glands.

Skin conductance level (SCL) is the tonic or baseline level of the SC over some specified period of time, whereas skin conductance response (SCR) is the phasic or maximal response reached in immediate reaction to a stimulus. Similar terminology is used for SP (SPL and SPR). The characteristics of the SCR are shown in Figure 2-4. The unit of conductance is the micromho (mho). The reaction occurs in two phases, a slow rise and a

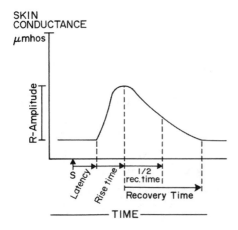

Figure 2-4. A skin conductance response. From M. Zuckerman, 1991, *Psychobiology of personality*. p. 259. Cambridge: Cambridge University Press.

recovery to the SCL baseline, which can be fast or slow. The characteristics of the response include the latency to the beginning of the rise, the rise time to peak, the amplitude of the rise, and the half recovery time or full recovery time from response peak to baseline.

SCRs may appear during a baseline period of recording when there are no apparent changes in the external environment. These are termed nonspecific or "spontaneous" SCRs and reflect fluctuations in arousal, sometimes due to internal stimuli (like exciting or apprehensive thoughts).

The SCR is a useful technique in experiments where stimuli are used to elicit response because of its sensitivity to both CNS and SNS responses. The ecrine sweat glands are directly innervated by SNS fibers. The CNS origins are in premotor cortex, limbic areas, and hypothalamus. Heritability of the SCL is moderately high (64%) and SCR in response to an intense tone is also high (59%), suggesting their potential usefulness as measures of individual differences (Lykken, Iacono, Haroian, McGue, & Bouchard, 1988).

Cardiovascular Activity

In ancient times, many philsophers considered the heart the seat of the emotions. It is easy to see why this was so in view of the associations of heart activity to felt emotions. We say that the heart "pounds" or "races" during states of fearful anticipation. The patient with panic disorder is acutely aware of his or her racing heart during a panic attack, and in the absence of any logical reason for the tachycardia, like having exercised, experiences an extreme state of fear. Blood pressure and blood flow changes are not as subjectively obvious, but when we see an angry person turning red in the

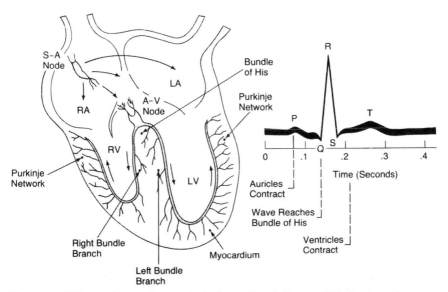

Figure 2-5. EKG wave form and events in the heart. From J. Hassett, 1978, *A primer of psychophysiology*, p. 57. San Francisco, CA: W. H. Freeman & Co. Copyright 1978 by W. H. Freeman & Co. Reprinted by permission.

face, an embarassed person blush, or a fearful person blanch (a compensatory PNS reaction), we associate these observations with emotion. The psychophysiologist has developed experimental methods for quantifying these qualitative changes.

The electrocardiogram is usually recorded from electrodes placed on the surface or sides of the chest or limbs of the body. A recording of pulse from a finger can be used for measuring heart rate (HR), but clearer recordings of heart action are obtained from chest recordings. The peaks within a single heart beat, shown in Figure 2-5 represent electrical events in the heart. The P wave is a function of the electrical currents generated just before contraction of the atria and the QRS wave is caused by the excitation presaging contraction of the ventricles. The T wave represents the repolarization of the ventricles.

HR is expressed as the number of beats, counted from the R peaks, over some specified period of time. Heart period (HP), or interbeat interval (IBI) is the time between one R wave and the next expressed in milliseconds. The longer the interval, the slower the HR. This measure can assess changes in HR from one beat to the next and therefore is useful in measuring reactions to stimuli over short periods of time. Another measure used is heart rate variability, measuring stability of HR during a baseline period or during a performance of some task.

The beat-to-beat changes in HR during the first 11 seconds after the presentation of a stimulus can show different patterns depending on the intensity and content characteristics of the stimulus (Graham, 1979). Low to moderate intensity stimuli with nonemotional content usually elicit an initial deceleration of HR over the first few seconds after the stimulus. Graham considered this an *orienting reflex* (OR) typically expressing interest or curiosity about the stimulus. As the stimulus is repeated the OR tends to diminish as the subject habituates to the stimulus. High intensity or painful stimuli, or stimuli with highly aversive significance usually elicit a *defensive reflex* (DR) expressed as an accelerating HR over the first seconds after the stimulus. DRs are slower to extinguish than ORs and may not extinguish at all.

The two patterns of response in relation to stimulus intensity are shown in Figure 2-6. According to Graham the OR is "input enhancing" reflecting attention to the stimulus as the first phase of information processing. The DR is said to be "output enhancing" reflecting a readiness for action (such as flight from an aversive stimulus). Lacey (1959) presented a similar interpretation with HR deceleration associated with stimulus "intake" (focused attention) and HR acceleration reflecting stimulus "rejection" or cognitive function excluding stimuli as distracting or aversive. The contrast between OR and DR patterns of HR indicates a relationship to personality, as will be discussed in later chapters.

Blood Pressure (BP) is a widely used measure of SNS arousal that varies with momentary environmental demands and also shows characteristic individual differences. BP is normally distributed in the population, but certain disease conditions and other factors, possibly including personality, can produce extremes of tonic levels called "hypertension."

There are three major classes of blood vessels: arteries, which conduct blood from the heart to the body; veins, which return the blood to the heart; and capillaries, smaller tubes that distribute the blood to the tissues of the body. All of these vessels except the capillaries are innervated by the SNS, which controls the degrees of constriction of the blood vessels. The PNS plays no role in controlling these vessels. The SNS control is exerted via a vasomotor center located in the lower pons and upper medulla, but the hypothalamus can also exert strong inhibitory or excitatory effects on the vasomotor center. Fluctuations in emotional state exert their effects through the hypothalamus. A normal level of sympathetic system tone keeps all blood vessels constricted to about half of maximum diameter.

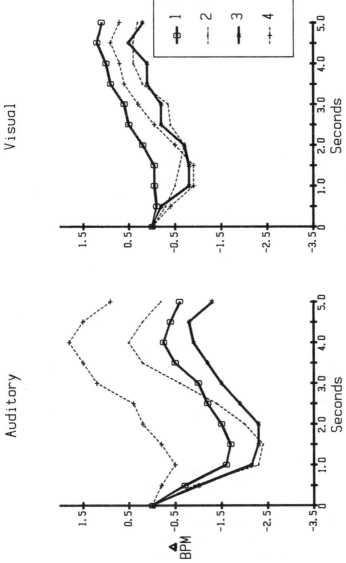

Figure 2-6. Two patterns of heart rate (HR) in relation to stimulus intensity. From "Sensation seeking and stimulus intensity as modulators of cortical, cardiovascular, and electrodermal response: A cross-modality study," by M. Zuckerman et al., 1988, *Personality and Individual Differences*, 9, fig. 2, p. 366. Copyright 1988 by Pergamon Press. Reprinted by permssion.

Increases in SNS activity further increase vasoconstriction producing elevations in BP. Vasodilation is effected through inhibition of normal tone. Thus, SNS state controls both constriction and dilation in a bipolar manner. Baroreceptors in the walls of the arteries provide a feedback system that slows HR when BP rises above normal levels. HR and BP thus tend to be inversely related during tonic changes but under conditions of high demand, as in exercise or during aversive stimulation, both may increase together.

The systolic BP reflects the pressure on arterial walls during the ventricular contraction of the heart whereas the diastolic reading is taken when the heart is relaxing between beats. The most widely used method for measuring BP in medical exams is a mercury manometer attached to a pressure cuff. The cuff is inflated well above the expected systolic BP, while the sounds in the brachial artery is monitored with a stethyscope. The cuff pressure is then gradually reduced until the first sounds are heard as the blood gets through the artery. The level indicated on the manometer at this time is the systolic BP. The pressure in the cuff is then further lowered until no pulse sounds are heard. The reading at this time is the diastolic pressure.

Laboratory methods are automated and some offer a semicontinuous reading of systolic and diastolic pressures on a beat-by-beat basis. Methods include a cuff inflated on a programmed schedule, a constant-cuff pressure system, and an ultrasound method using Doppler signals to identify the diastole and systole of the artery. These methods have been validated against actual intraarterial BP, the most direct but intrusive method for measuring BP.

Shifts in *blood volume* (BV) occur in various parts of the body as regulated by selected vasoconstriction or dilation of blood vessels. In general vasodilation occurs in the vessels leading to the head and limbs during high SNS activity, but vasoconstriction occurs in the skin, perhaps as an adaptive protection against loss of blood. BV is measured using various kinds of plethysmographic devices including hydraulic or pneumatic, electrical impedance, and photoelectric systems. Genital BV devices comprise the only specific measure of sexual arousal (Geer, 1975; Zuckerman, 1971). BV changes in the forehead show increases during orienting to novel or unexpected stimuli (orienting reflex) and decreases during painful or aversive stimuli (defensive reflex) (Sokolov, 1963). Individual differences as a function of phobic fearfulness have been demonstrated in forehead BV (Hare, 1973), suggesting the usefulness of this measure in personality research.

Twin studies of HR and BP have shown only moderate heritabilities, ranging from .40 to .60 for HR and about .40 for BP. These are about the same as those found for personality traits. Boomsma and Plomin (1986) concluded that genetic factors do not play a role in the limited connection between cardiac and personality trait measures.

Movement is accomplished by contractions of muscle fibres. But even before movement is observable, an increase in muscle tension can be recorded from electrodes placed on the skin just above the muscle. Just the thought of making a movement increases the tonic level of activity in the muscle fibres. There is a tonic level of activity in the muscles even during relaxation. The complaints of chronic fatigue by highly anxious persons could indicate a high level of muscle tension even during inactive states. The technique for measuring and recording electrical potentials associated with contraction of muscle fibres is called *electromyography* (EMG).

The EMG is recorded by bipolar electrode placement above the muscle of interest. Electrodes above the frontalis muscle of the forehead are frequently used to measure mental or nonspecific muscle tension. Another site often used is the forearm. The muscles controlling facial expressions are widely used in the study of emotion. Particular patterns of EMG activity have been shown to be related to specific emotional responses even in the absence of changes in overt facial expressions (Fridlund, Schwartz, & Fowler, 1984).

Problems in Psychophysiology

Psychologists have been attracted to psychophysiology because physiological processes can be studied without overly invasive procedures. Although some theories have attributed causal significance to these measures, it must be remembered that these are responses to some stimulus or situation and their significance may not be generalizable beyond that situation. Even the recording of tonic or baseline levels of activity involve the reaction to an unusual laboratory situation surrounded by strange instruments and strangers in white coats attaching electrodes to various parts of the body. This is not a neutral or relaxing situation for many persons. It is not surprising that tonic levels of physiological activity of any kind have not proven useful in personality studies.

The reaction to a single standard stimulus may be useless in terms of revealing patterns of response significant for personality. More often, the significant paradigms have involved the relationships between a stimulus dimension, such as intensity, and a response dimension such as heart rate or amplitude of cortical-evoked potentials.

For a more detailed presentation of psychophysiological methods, see Andreassi (1989).

NEUROPSYCHOLOGY

Neuropsychology may be described as the study of the connection between brain structure and function. Of necessity, the description of neuroanatomy and function will be brief. Any number of more recent volumes on psychobiology can be consulted. I assume that most readers of this volume will have some background in psychobiology even if only a single graduate course. Personality involves all of the brain and perhaps even some spinal motorneuronal reflexes as well (Pivik, Stelmack, & Bylsma, 1988). Individual differences in structure may affect physiology and behavior as well. I will focus on the brain structures and tracts that have been shown to be most relevant to individual differences. The autonomic system has already been discussed, but these responses begin in higher brain centers such as the amygdala, hypothalamus, and cortex.

It is important to avoid the mistake of the 19th-century phrenologists who assigned character traits to discrete areas of the brain as if the brain consisted of little compartments, one for each trait. It is true that there are certain structures important in particular functions, but these are usually parts of circuits involving other structures. It is important to understand the role of each structure in the complex system regulating the function. (Examples will be given later).

MacLean (1982) has discussed the brain from an evolutionary standpoint in his formulation of the *triune brain*. The human brain is the end product of an evolutionary pathway beginning in reptilian brain, and developing through the paleomammalian brain, to the primate brain, elaborated into the human brain. Evolution does not necessarily discard older mechanisms, replacing them with newer models, but frequently builds the new one on the old. This seems to be the case for the human brain which contains newer and older levels of development. It is as if a small basic house is constructed, and new rooms and floors are added to the basic nuclear house over periods of years. This is beautifully described by Konner (2002):

… our brains for better or for worse, contain our evolutionary history … when we see a potentially threatening stranger, we react with the brain stem we got from fish, the amygdala we got from reptiles, the hippocampus we got from early mammals, as well as the culturally informed and cognitively powerful new association cortex that is the legacy of human evolution. (p. 660)

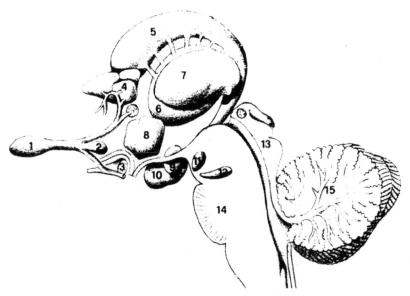

Figure 2-7. The "reptillian brain." 1. olfactory bulb; 2. olfactory tubercule; 3. optic chiasma; 4. septal nuclei; 5 caudate; 6 putamen and globus palladus; 7. thalamus; 8. hypothalamus; 9. mamillary body; 10. amygdala; 11. interpeduncular nucleus; 12. substantia nigra; 13. quadrigeminal bodies (tectum mesencephali); 14. pons; 15. cerebellum. From L. Valzelli, 1981, *Psychobiology of aggression and violence*, p. 34. New York: Raven Press. Copyright 1981 by Lippincott Williams & Wilkins. Reprinted by permission.

The "reptillian brain" consists of brain stem structures (pons, cerebellum, medulla) shown in Figure 2-7 and the striatal complex (caudate nucleus, putamen) shown in Figure 2-8. Although the brain of a lizard is less developed than that of a mammal, reptilian behaviors are similar to those seen in mammals, territoriality, aggression, dominance, greeting, grooming, and courtship. The difference is in the fixity of action patterns ("instinct"), or automatic reactions to releasers, in reptiles as contrasted with the plasticity of mammalian behavior and its susceptibility to change from learned experience.

The paleomammalian brain corresponds closely to what is called the *limbic system*, including hypothalamus, thalamus, hippocampus, septum, corpus callosum, and cingulate gyrus (Figure 2-9). These structures are involved in emotional, motivational, appetitive, aversive, and exploratory behavior, as well as learning and memory functions. All of these are important in personality differences.

The neomammalian brain consists of the cerebral hemisphere, which covers the reptilian and paleomammalian brains and is most highly

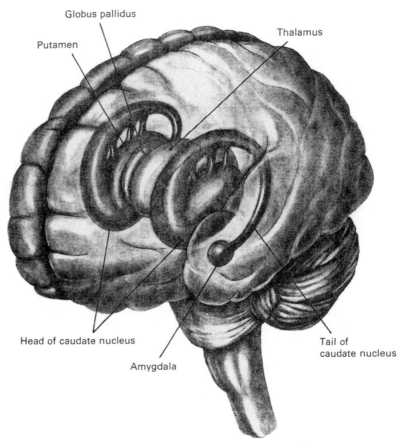

Globus pallidus

Thalamus

Putamen

Head of caudate nucleus

Tail of
caudate nucleus

Amygdala

Figure 2-8. The location of the basal ganglia in a human brain. From N. R. Carlson, 1986, *Physiology of behavior, 3rd edition,* p. 102. Boston, MA: Allyn and Bacon. Copyright 1986 by Pearson Education. Reprinted by permission.

developed (particularly the frontal lobes) in the primate and hominid branches of the mammalian tree (Figure 2-10). The development of language in the left hemisphere of the human brain accounts for much of the difference between humans and other mammals including apes. Language extends memory backward in time and anticipation extends it forward. The frontal lobes have an inhibitory role, which allows delay of reaction until cognitive processes can evaluate the situation and its projected consequences more carefully.

The cerebrum consists of two hemispheres, right and left. Figure 2-10 shows the left hemisphere with the primary lobes identified: frontal,

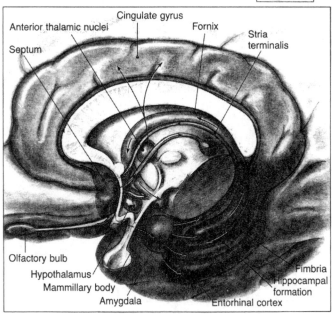

Figure 2-9. Schematic of the limbic system and its location in the brain (smaller schematic). From N. R. Carlson, 1986, *Physiology of behavior, 3rd edition,* p. 101. Boston, MA: Allyn and Bacon. Copyright 1986 by Pearson Education. Reprinted by permssion.

parietal, occipital, and temporal. The outer layer of the hemispheres, the *cerebral cortex*, contains the neurons involved in the higher mental functions, such as learning, memory, cognition, and speech. Underlying the cortex (gray matter) are the white matter neurons consisting of bundles that connect the cortex with the underlying limbic and brain stem structures and form interconnections among areas of the cortex and corresponding areas in the two hemispheres. The corpus callosum collects some of these bundles and underlies the cerebrum, connecting the two hemispheres. The primary lobes serve specific sensory analysis functions: vision in the occipital, audition in the temporal, somatosensory in the parietal postcentral gyrus. The primary area for control of movement is the precentral gyrus. Association areas around the primary sensory areas serve more detailed analysis of sensory input necessary for recognition or perception.

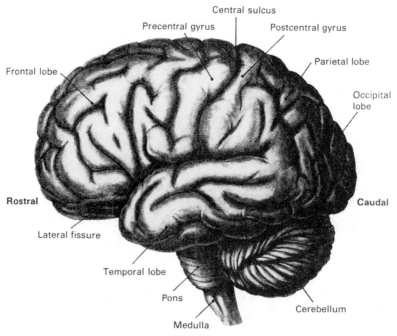

Central sulcus
Precentral gyrus   Postcentral gyrus
Frontal lobe   Parietal lobe
                                               Occipital lobe
Rostral   Caudal
Lateral fissure
Temporal lobe
Pons
                          Cerebellum
Medulla

Figure 2-10. A lateral exterior view of the left hemisphere of the brain. From N. R. Carlson, 1986, *Physiology of behavior, 3rd edition*. Boston, MA: Allyn and Bacon. Copyright 1986 by Pearson Education. Reprinted by permission.

The frontal lobe receives inputs from the other brain areas and integrates experience across the senses. This is the source of ideational and affective experience. It also serves the executive function, in the sense of planning and organizing behavior, drawing on memories of previous actions and their consequences and inhibiting impulsive action when necessary. For a detailed description of the anatomy, physiology, and neuropsychology of the prefrontal cortex, see Fuster (1997).

Most of our knowledge of brain function comes from experimental work with animals, destroying or stimulating particular structures. Until the recent development of brain-imaging methods, work with humans has been largely correlational, depending on cases of brain damage with imprecise locations until autopsy. From the 1930s through the 1950s, the technique of lobotomy was developed in the belief that the severing of the connections between the frontal lobes and the rest of the brain would cure schizophrenia. This hypothesis was not supported by research finally done after tens of thousands of patients were lobotomized throughout the world. Much of

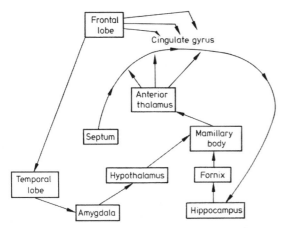

Figure 2-11. Diagrammatic representation of the Papez circuit. From "A survey of the effects of brain lesions upon personality," by G. E. Powell, 1981, in H. J. Eysenck (Ed.) *A model for personality*, p. 71. Heidelberg, Germany: Springer-Verlag. Copyright 1981 by Springer-Verlag. Reprinted by permission.

the earlier research was worthless because of the lack of control groups and the difficulty of separating the effects of chronic psychosis from those of the operation itself. However, the results of most of these studies as well as those of patients with frontal lobe damage produced by war wounds or accidents showed *decreased* anxiety and depression and increased impulsivity and general disinhibition. The latter are symptoms noted in the famous case of Phineas Gage, a worker whose frontal lobes were nearly destroyed by a tamping rod driven through his brain by an explosion (Damasio, Grabowski, Frank, Galaburda, & Damasio, 1994).

Lateralization refers to the fact that the two hemispheres have somewhat different functions in the human. Speech and language and an analytic, rational type of cognitive function are in the left hemisphere. The right hemisphere is important in visual-spatial perception, and a more global-holistic mode of cognitive analysis. Davidson (1992) has suggested that the right hemisphere is more involved in negative emotions (anxiety, depression, anger) and the left hemisphere is more concerned with positive emotionality.

The Papez (1937) circuit, shown in Figure 2-11, has been suggested to be the limbic circuit of emotional expression. The cingulate gyrus lies between the cerebral hemispheres and the lower brain areas, forming the upper arch of the limbic vault. It serves as the higher center of the limbic system, receiving information from the association areas of the cortex and passing it on to the hippocampal, amygdaloid, and hypothalamic areas, where emotional significance is assigned and emotional expression is organized in behavioral and physiological patterns of activation. Feedback branches connect back to the association cortex from the hippocampal formation and from the hypothalamus to the prefrontal cortex. For discussion of the role of the limbic system in behavior and emotions, see Adams, Victor, and Ropper (1997), Isaacson (1982), and LeDoux (1987).

A cingulotomy operation performed on patients with chronic anxiety and depression showed reduction in these negative emotions as well as HR and BP during both basal and stress periods (Mitchell-Heggs, Kelley, & Richardson, 1976; Laitenan & Vilki, 1973).

Davis (1986) suggested that the central nucleus of the amygdala is a major center for the perception and organization of response to fear and anxiety. Figure 2-12 shows the connections of the central nucleus of the amygdala to areas of the brain producing the characteristic behavioral, autonomic, and facial expressions of fear. Stimulation of the central nucleus of the amygdala in primates produces all of these responses.

The centromedial area of the amygdala seems to be the locus of a trigger for aggressive behavior (Valzelli, 1981). Patients who were episodically aggressive and uncontrolled were treated with unilateral or bilateral destruction of the amygdala and showed marked reduction of hostile and aggressive behavior (Heimburger, Whitlock, & Kalsbech, 1972; Mark, Sweet, & Ervin, 1972; Siegfried & Ben-Shmuel, 1972). Similar reductions of aggression were not seen after prefrontal lobotomies. For broader discussions of the role of the amygdala in emotions, see Aggleton and Mishkin (1986); Chozick (1986); and Davis, Hitchcock, and Rosen (1987).

The thalamus is a sensory relay station receiving signals from the primary sense organs and routing them to appropriate cortical lobes or to intermediate relay structures. The thalamus also has more diffuse projections to the cortex, which serve an arousal function in response to the stimulation from the sense organs. The thalamus has connections with other limbic structures mediating emotional reaction, like the amygdala. Sensory information at the thalamus that has not been fully processed at the cortical level can trigger a response in the amygdala before a person is fully conscious of the source of the emotional response. Conditioned stimuli for anxiety may work in this fashion.

The hypothalamus is seated near the base of the thalamus. The role of the hypothalamus in the homeostatic regulation of the autonomic nervous system has been previously discussed. Negative emotional reactions such as anxiety trigger responses in the sympathetic branch of the autonomic

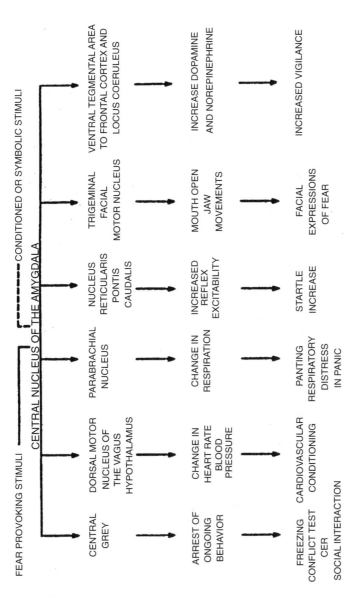

Figure 2-12. Connections of the central nucleus of the amygdala to a variety of target areas that are probably involved in the patterns of behaviors typically associated with fear. From "Anxiety and the amygdala: Pharmacological and anatomical analysis of the fear-potentiated startle paradigm" by M. Davis in J. M. Hitchcock and J. B. Rosen (Eds.), 1987, *The psychology of learning and motivation*, vol. 21, p. 293. New York: Academic Press. Copyright 1981 by Academic Press. Reprinted by permission.

system, preparing the organism for "fight or flight." The hypothalamus receives neural and hormonal signals of the internal state of the organism such as hunger, level of circulating sex hormones, heart rate, and water balance, and responds to these in a feedback fashion. The hypothalamus also stimulates the pituitary gland via releasing hormones and thus has ultimate control over the peripheral hormone glands. This function will be discussed in the section on psychopharmacology.

The reticular formation runs up through the brain stem from the medulla to the midbrain. It is stimulated by collaterals from sensory nerves as well as from the cerebellum, thalamus, and frontal, motor, and sensory areas of cortex.

It also has descending pathways that can act in a homeostatic function on lower sensory centers. The ascending connections to thalamus and cortex serve to regulate alertness. Thus, the system sometimes is called the "ascending reticular activation system." It also is a transmission center for pain. The reticular formation modulates extensor muscle tone and HR and BP. The descending system can reduce arousal in these systems in response to overarousal and it can attenuate pain. Thus, it serves an inhibitory protective function as well as an excitatory one within the nervous system. As we will see in later chapters, the relative strengths of the excitation and inhibition components of the system may furnish an explanation for a EP phenomenon called "augmenting-reducing," which is related to certain personality differences.

The focus on structures in the brain easily can lead to the fallacy of phrenology if one ignores that fact that these structures are nodal points for pathways, much like a train terminal is a place in which different lines converge and trains are switched from one line to another. The old methodology of lesioning entire structures like the amygdala can lead to erroneous conclusions, because more than one type of system is thereby interrupted. Despite these cautions, it is conceivable that the examination of the gross structure of the brain and its significant loci could reveal some kind of relationship to personality. Until the latter part of the 20th century, the brain could only be examined in autopsy, not a very useful method for studying personality relationships. The invention of the *computed tomographic* (CT) method of brain imaging in the 1970s and the *magnetic resonance imaging* (MRI) method in the 1980s allowed the examination of the brain in vivo.

These new methods have been widely utilized in neuropsychological studies of neurological and psychiatric disorders (Lim, Rosenbloom, & Pfefferbaum, 1995), but they have been little utilized in relation to personality. One might think that they are not applicable to the continuous normal dimensions of personality because they reveal qualitative differences. But, in actual fact, the differences found between schizophrenics, mood and anxiety disorders, and normals are based on quantitative differences in size of cerebral ventricles, whole brain, and structures such as the frontal lobes, hippocampus, amygdala, and cingulate gyrus. If such differences in structure reflect some of the behavioral and emotional differences between patients and normals, it is possible that the personality dimensions characterized by the same kinds of differences could be related to size of these structures. This "neophrenology," unlike the discredited older version, would at least be based on real brain structure not the shape of the skull. Because nearly all of this research is done on clinical groups and small numbers of normal controls, one would have to look into the relationships between personality dimensions within both groups to see if replicable relationships can be found.

CT scans resemble the conventional X-ray technique but allow the visualization of brain instead of just bony matter. A series of narrow, parallel beams of radiation are passed through the brain tissue onto sensitive scintillation crystals. The X-ray source and detectors are rotated around the head and the radiation absorption of each brain region is calculated on computer summing the readings passing through that region. The measurements are converted to digital form, which in turn is converted into a visual display showing relatively light or dark areas. The first applications of this method to schizophrenia showed enlarged ventricles (spaces filled with cerebrospinal fluid), suggesting loss of surrounding brain tissue in patients with schizophrenia.

The CT has largely been supplanted by the MRI method in the last decade. The MRI has a sharper resolution of image and the ability to view and measure specific structures in the brain (Lim et al., 1995). The physics is complicated but essentially uses the magnetic fields of brain nuclei which when exposed to a strong external magnetic field align themselves parallel or antiparallel with that field. The MRI uses tuned radiofrequency coils to detect the radio signals emitted as the nuclei return to equilibrium. Two-dimensional and three-dimensional images can be obtained. The image orientations may be manipulated to provide optimal views of different brain structures. Sizes of brain structures can be estimated as volume, area, length, and width, as well as shape. The three-dimensional images are "virtual reality."

Apart from artifacts produced by the method itself, interpretation of brain images for comparisons of individuals must be controlled for size (larger people have larger brains and therefore larger parts of brains).

Correction for brain size is complicated because different parts of the brain have different correlations with overall brain size. A regression approach rather than a simple ratio method is a better way to correct for brain size. Men are larger than women, so sex is a critical variable. Age is another variable that must be controlled, because cortical gray matter declines and cortical cerebrospinal fluid (in ventricles) increases with age.

A more recently developed functional MRI (fMRI) detects regional blood flow and enhanced oxygen content of blood. This method can be used to detect short intervals of activity and can be used like the PET method for measuring changes in brain activity induced by stimulation. It has an advantage over the PET because it can record changes over much shorter intervals, seconds rather than minutes, and therefore the reaction to more specific stimuli.

PSYCHOPHARMACOLOGICAL METHODS

Psychopharmacology refers to the action of drugs on mind and behavior and the broader term *neuropsychopharmacology* includes the action of drugs on the biochemistry and physiology of the brain as well as the endogenous actions of the natural biochemicals of the brain and nervous system. In actual practice, the term psychopharmacology is used for the science that includes both reactions to exogenous and endogenous chemical stimulation. Much of the impetus to the science occurred as a result of the introduction of psychotropic drugs in the 1950s. Progress since then has been summarized in volumes on each decade of progress; the most recent is the large tome edited by Bloom and Kupfer (1995).

Psychopharmacological research has accelerated over the last two decades, resulting in a paradigm shift in psychiatry from the psychodynamic to the psychobiological. Biosocial views of personality, such as that by Gardner Murphy (1947), were based on a minimum of biological knowledge, and that of Hans Eysenck (1967) two decades later was based largely on behavior genetics and psychophysiology rather than psychopharmacology. The advances in the latter science resulted in new theories of personality assigning a primary importance to individual differences in the biochemistry of the brain, particularly in regard to some of its basic neurotransmitters and hormones (Cloninger, 1987; Depue, 1995; Depue & Collins, 1999; Gray, 1982, 1987; Zuckerman, 1984, 1991).

Monoamine Systems

Neuronal transmission is mediated chemically by the release of *neurotransmitters* across the synapses, or gaps between neurons as illustrated in Figure 2-13. The neurotransmitter is synthesized in the cell body and

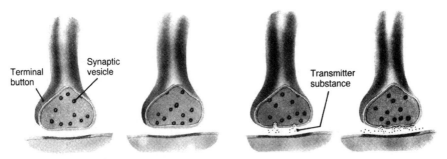

Figure 2-13. Release of neurotransmitters into the synaptic space. From N. R. Carlson, 1986, *Physiology of behavior,* Newton, MA: Allyn & Bacon. Copyright 1986 by Allyn and Bacon. Reprinted with permission.

transported down the axon in small sacs called *vesicles* to the terminals of the axon. When the axon of a cell fires, the vesicles spill the neurotransmitter into the synaptic space. The free transmitter attaches to *receptors* in the postsynaptic neuron, either exciting or inhibiting it. Specific neurotransmitters in neuronal systems are "keyed" to particular receptors. Some of the neurotransmitter may be catabolized in the synaptic space producing inactive metabolites, which are ultimately excreted from the body, whereas other parts are taken up again to be stored again in the presynaptic neuron. Any chemical that blocks this *reuptake* process may potentiate the sensitivity of the postsynaptic neuron by keeping more of the neurotransmitter in the synaptic space, furnishing "tinder" for the next impulse coming down the presynaptic neuron.

There are many types of neurotransmitters, but this book will focus primarily on the group called *monoamines* because of their importance in motivation, emotion, and personality. There are two major classes of monoamines: the indoleamine *serotonin,* and the *catholamines*, dopamine, norepinephrine, and epinephrine. Norepinephrine is sometimes referred to as noradrenaline and epinephrine as adrenaline. The adjectival forms are noradrenergic or adrenergic. Figure 2-14 illustrates the neurotransmission process using one of these monoamines, the noradrenergic neuron. Figure 2-15 shows the biosynthesis pathways of the monoamines, the enzymes involved in their synthesis and catabolism, and their metabolites.

Production of norepinephrine (NE) begins with the amino acid tyrosine, the source of which lies in certain foods. Tyrosine is converted to dihydroxyphenylalanine (DOPA or L-DOPA) by an enzyme called tyrosine hydroxylase. Another enzyme converts DOPA to dopamine (DA). In the dopamine neuron this is the end of the production process, but in the NE neuron another enzyme, dopamine ß-hydroxylase (DBH) converts DA into NE.

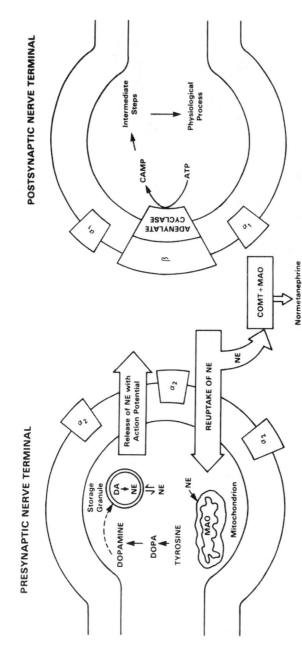

Figure 2-14. Illustration of a noradrenergic synapse. DA, dopamine; NE, norepinephrine; DOPA (dihydroxyphenylalanine, a precursor of the transmitters DA and NE. The enzymes monoamine oxidase (MAO) and catechol-O-methyltransferase (COMT) are involved in the degradation of NE; 3-methoxy-4-hydroxyphenlyglycol (MHPG) and vanillymandelic acid (VMA) are metabolites from the breakdown of NE. Alpha1, alpha2, and beta are receptor sites on the cell membrane. Adenosine triphosphate (ATP) is an energy source for the cell and a precursor to the "second messenger," cyclic adenosine monophosphate (cAMP). From "antidepressants and biochemical theories of depression" by E. T. McNeal and P. Cimbolic, 1986, *Psychological Bulletin*, 99, p. 363. Copyright by the American Psychological Association. Reprinted by permission.

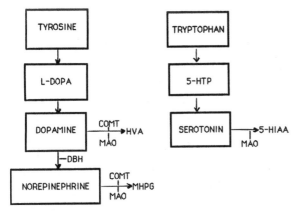

Figure 2-15. Biosynthesis and breakdown of the monoamines dopamine, norepineph-rine, and serotonin. From M. Zuckerman. *Psychobiology of personality, 1st edition.* Cambridge: Cambridge University Press.

If there is a deficit or inactivation of any of the enzymes involved in the production process, the final product of NE will be depleted.

Figure 2-15 shows the production and disposal process of all three monoamines including the final metabolites produced by the catabolic

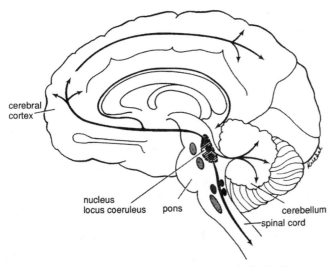

Figure 2-16. Noradrenergic projection systems in the brain. Shown are the major nor-adrenergic nuclei of the brain, the locus coeruleus (hatched), the lateral tegmental nu-clei (fine stipple). Epinephrine nuclei are shown in black. The projections from the locus coeruleus (described in the text) are markedly simplified and projections from the other nuclei are not shown. From 5.6. Hyman and E. J. Nestler, 1993, *The Molecular Foundations of Psychiatry.* © American Psychiatric Publishing, http://www.appi.org.

breakdown of the neurotransmitters by the enzymes *monoamine oxidase* (MAO) and *catechol-O-methyltransferase* (COMT). These inactive metabolic products, *homovanillic acid* (HVA) for DA, *3-methoxy-4-hydroxyphenylglycol* (MHPG) for NE, and *5-hydroxyindoleacetic acid* (5-HIAA) for serotonin, provide one method of gauging the activity of the neurotransmitters, which are their sources. They can be sampled from cerebrospinal fluid (CSF), blood, or urine. Measures from urine are not a good index of brain activity. MHPG in urine, for instance, reflects only an estimated 20% of brain NE activity. Plasma MHPG is not much better, with an estimated 30–65% originating in brain. One simply cannot determine with any certainty how much of the transmitter's metabolite is coming from the brain and how much has its origin in peripheral catecholamines (Heninger, 1999). Another limitation is that synthesis, release, and metabolism are not necessarily highly related. Differences in MAO level, for instance, could limit or enhance the amount of catabolism and metabolite present after activity of the neuronal system. CSF should be a better source of metabolites that index brain activity, because it is in direct contact with the brain, or at least the parts surrounding the cerebral ventricles. However, NE also is produced in the spinal column and there is a gradient between the ventricles and the lower lumbar region from which CSF is drawn. The CSF is not useful in most experiments that require two or more samples within a relatively short time period. One sample itself is an intrusive procedure and more than one is hardly thinkable. Use of metabolites as indices of brain monoamine activity is based on a faith that activity in the brain and peripheral nervous systems are somehow correlated and that activity among different parts of the brain is also correlated. These are tenuous assumptions (Owens & Ritchie, 1999).

The blood serum or plasma is widely used as the source for assays of drug or catecholamines using chromatographic techniques. However, the blood platelet has proven useful as a source for assays of serotonin. The platelet shares many characteristics with serotonin neurons including active transport for serotonin, serotonin receptors of the 2A type and MAO type B which is also obtained from platelets (Owens & Ritchie, 1999). The connection with MAO-B is interesting in view of the association of that enzyme with personality and a variety of clinical symptoms including depression and impulsive aggression. Swedish investigators have suggested that the numbers of serotonergic neurons are coregulated with MAO, and that CSF measures of the serotonin metabolite 5-HIAA are correlated with platelet MAO (Oreland et al., 1981).

During the last decade, there has been increased interest in the receptors for neurotransmitters as possible sources of individual differences and drug actions. In Figure 2-14, which shows adrenergic neurons, one can see two types of alpha receptors (1 and 2) and a beta receptor. The A1 and beta receptors have excitatory effects on the postsynaptic neuron. The presynaptic A2 is called an autoreceptor. It has a negative feedback effect, dampening activity when it detects excessive neurotransmitter in the synaptic cleft. Blocking an autoreceptor usually increases the excitatory effects on the system because of the absence of homeostatic regulation.

Dopamine has two major types and at least five subtypes of receptors (Seeman, 1995). Serotonin has at least seven major types and 17 subtypes of receptors (Glennon & Dukat, 1995). Each type of receptor has somewhat different neural actions and may mediate different types of behavior.

Radioactive ligand binding methods have been developed for most receptors. The two characteristics of receptors studied are the *affinity* and the *amount* and concentration of receptors in a given sample. Changes in receptor concentration are used to assess changes in the transmission of the system. Receptor numbers may increase when there is decreased neural transmission as a compensatory response to the lack of transmitter substance. But, if there are normal levels of the neurotransmitter, the number of receptors suggests increased neurotransmission. Affinity measures the potency of a drug at binding to the receptor, or how much of the drug it takes to occupy 50% or 100% of the receptors. It is not a characteristic that would be expected to reflect individual or group differences.

Neurotransmitters define neural pathways in the brain. These will be described briefly in what follows. (See also Figures 2-16 to 2-18.) Figure 2-16 shows the primary noradrenergic systems. The *dorsal tegmental* or *locus coeruleus (LC) complex* begins in the LC and ascends to the cerebellum, thalamus, hippocampus, amygdala, septum, hypothalamus, and virtually the entire forebrain and neocortex. Caudal projections descend the spinal cord. The LC is a small structure but is the source of nearly all of the NE innervation of the telencephelon. The neurons in the LC are inhibited during sleep and eating but activated by novel or threatening stimuli. The LC and its ascending system have been characterized as an alarm or vigilance system and studies have shown it to be involved in fear and anxiety in humans, other primates, and rats. It therefore may be relevant to the primary trait of neuroticism.

Two other systems are the *lateral tegmental*, beginning in nuclei in the medulla and pons, and the dorsal medullary group. The lateral tegmental group is involved in the regulation of cardiovascular and visceral functions via the hypothalamus. The *dorsal medullary* group provides inputs to the cranial parasympathetic functions that are inhibited during sympathetic system arousal.

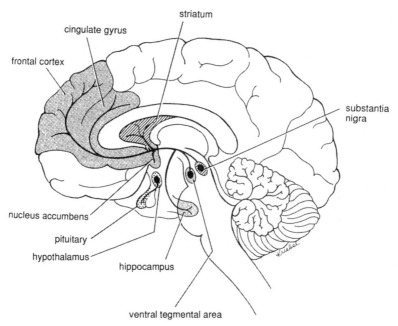

Figure 2-17. Dopaminergic projection systems in the brain. The major dopaminergic nuclei in the brain are the substantia nigra pars compactia (*hatched*), shown projecting to the striatum (also *hatched*; the ventral tegmental area (*fine stipple*) shown projecting to the frontal and cingulate cortex, nucleus accumbens, and other limbic structures (*fine stipple*), and the arcuate nucleus of the hypothalamus (*coarse stipple*), which provides dopaminergic regulation to the pituitary. From 5.6. Hyman and E. J. Nestler, 1993. *The Molecular Foundations of Psychiatry.* © American Psychiatric Publishing, http://www.appi.o.

Dopaminergic systems are shown in Figure 2-17. The *mesostriatal or nigrostriatal* system originates in the substantia nigra, the ventral tegmental area (VTA). It innervates the striatum (caudate/putamen) structures involved in motor control. Damage to this pathway is a cause of Parkinson's disease. The *mesolimbocortical* system originates primarily in the VTA and projects to the nucleus accumbens (NA), septum, amygdala, hippocampus, and frontal cortex. The pathway between the VTA and the NA, passing through the lateral hypothalamus, is called the *medial forebrain bundle* (MFB). The MFB is the area where the strongest rewarding effects of intracranial self-stimulation are found. When rats are allowed to self-stimulate by pressing a bar, they respond as if the stimulation were a strong positive reinforcement, continuing to press even ignoring other primary rewards. The stimulant drugs, such as cocaine and amphetamine, have their major effects in this pathway, particularly in the NA, and the morphine drugs, such as heroin, also act here, particularly at the VTA (Bozarth, 1987). This

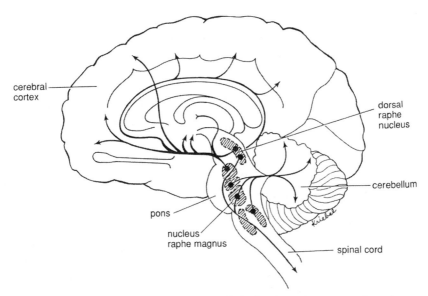

Figure 2-18. Serotonergic projection systems in the brain. The major serotonergic nuclei are the brainstem raphe nuclei (*hatched*). The nuclei are shown slightly enlarged and their diffuse projections (described in the text) are markedly simplified. From 5.6. Hyman and E. J. Nestler, 1993. *The Molecular Foundations of Psychiatry.* © American Psychiatric Publishing, http://www.appi.o.

area is conceptualized as mediating a primary reward function. It has been suggested to be involved in personality traits such as impulsivity, sensation seeking, and extraversion.

There are a number of other dopaminergic systems. One of some interest is the *mesopontine* system, which originates in the substantia nigra and the VTA areas and projects to the LC. This suggests a source of interaction between the dopaminergic and adrenergic systems. Stress can activate both systems.

Figure 2-18 shows serotonergic systems originating in the raphe nuclei. The *ventral ascending pathway* innervates many of the same limbic and striatal system loci as do the catecholamine systems and ascends to all parts of the neocortex, as does the noradrenergic system. The system originating in the medial raphe (MR) inputs largely to the hippocampus and septum, whereas the one originating in the dorsal raphe (DR) innervates the striatum and frontal cortex. Both systems are represented in the neocortex. The serotonergic systems tend to have inhibitory effects on emotions and approach behavior in animals, and low levels of serotonin in humans have been related to impulsive, aggressive behaviors and a lack of emotional control. Low levels also have been related to depression. A major class of antidepressants called *selective serotonin reuptake inhibitors* (SSRIs) potentiate the action of serotonin neurons. These drugs also have antianxiety effects in some kinds of anxiety disorders.

Amino Acid Neurotransmitters

Amino acids are organic molecules coded for by the DNA, which combine to form proteins. They are thus the very biological building elements of the organism. However, some of them also function as neurotransmitters. Glutamate and aspartate are excitatory transmitters in the brain and spinal cord. *Gamma-aminobutyric acid* (GABA) is an inhibitory transmitter. It is synthesized from the amino acid glutamate. Blocking its action can lead to convulsions. GABA is estimated to be present in nearly one third of all synapses and is especially concentrated in nerve terminals in cerebral cortex, hippocampus, subtantia nigra, cerebellum, and striatum. It is vital in inhibitory control mechanisms in the brain. The benzodiazipine (BZ) drugs, such as diazepam, act on receptors called by the same name. Although there are candidates for a neurotransmitter fitting these receptors, none have been definitively established. However, the BZ receptors are coupled with the GABA type A receptors and their distribution closely follows that for the GABA receptors. Some evidence suggests that the effects of BZ drugs, barbiturates, and alcohol on the BZ receptor are modulated by if not mediated by GABA at the type A receptor. This makes GABA and its receptors candidates for a substrate of trait anxiety or neuroticism. However, GABA interacts with the monoamines and is involved in a variety of behavioral mechanisms including those involved in activity, aggression, sexual behaviors, and feeding behaviors. Thus, it could be relevant to personality traits beyond neuroticism including those in which a lack of behavioral inhibition is the underlying mechanism.

Peptide Neurotransmitters and Hormones

Hormones, in contrast to neurotransmitters, are produced in glands and travel via the blood to distal parts of the nervous system, where they have their effects on receptors. In the last two decades, however, neuropharmacologists have discovered an intermediate type of neuroactive substances called peptides. Peptides are chains of two or more amino acids. Peptides function both as neurotransmitters and hormones, that is, they affect both adjacent neurons and distal ones. Examples are the hypothalamic releasing hormones. Figure 2-19 shows some of the pituitary-hormone systems. The pituitary is the master gland, secreting tropic hormones that have the

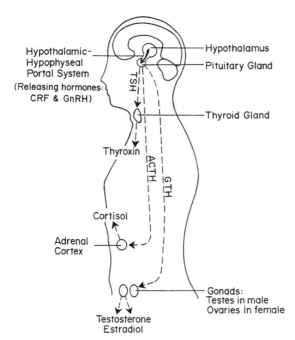

Figure 2-19. Hypothalamic pituitary-hormone systems. From M. Zuckerman, 1991, *Psychobiology of Personality, 1st edition.* New York: Cambridge University Press.

primary hormone glands as their targets and stimulate the release of hormones from those glands. Adrenocorticotropic hormone (ACTH) travels to the adrenal cortex releasing corticosteroid hormones including cortisol. Thyroid stimulating hormone (TSH) targets the thyroid gland, where it releases thyroxin. Gonadotropic hormone (GTH) travels to the gonads, where it releases testosterone from the testes in the male and estradiol from the ovaries in females.

The hypothalamus was known to mediate between higher brain centers and the pituitary gland and for years this control was thought to be mediated via neural control. In the late 1940s, it was discovered that blood vessels called the *hypothalamic-pituitary portal system* connected the two and that the stimulation from one to the other was chemically mediated. The mediating chemicals, discovered in the 1970s, proved to be peptides originating in the hypothalamus: thyrotropin-releasing hormone (TRH), corticotropin-releasing factor (CRF), and gonadotropin-releasing hormone (GnRH). The *hypothalamic-pituitary-adrenal cortex* (HYPAC) system is stress-reactive and of relevance to trait anxiety and depression or neuroticism. Apart from its stimulation of adrenocortical release of glucocorticoids, CRF acts on the other stress pathway in the autonomic nervous system increasing release of epinephrine and norepinephrine, and increasing heart rate and blood pressure. Corticosteroids released during stress activate the serotonergic system and increase the activity of the GABAa-benzodiazepine receptors providing a counterregulation or dampening of the effects of stress.

Opiate receptors were found in the brain, and in the 1970s peptides in the brain were discovered that had opiate-like sedative effects. These endogenous opiates were called *endorphins*. The amino acid sequences of two of these were identified and were called *Met-enkephalin* and *Leu-enkephalin*. Many peptides coexist with other neurotransmitters in their neurons where they modify or regulate their actions. Enkephalin, for instance, coexists with NE in the locus coeruleus and therefore may regulate arousal in this dorsal ascending NE system. Enkephalin also is found in serotonergic and GABA neurons. Enkephalin also is moderated by the dopaminergic input from the substantia nigra. Dopamine receptor antagonists increase expression of enkephalon. The idea that neurons only contain one specific neurotransmitter is giving way to the finding that most contain two or more. The complex interactions between brain systems begin at the neuronal-receptor level and should be a caution against simple systems that identify one personality or behavioral trait with one neurotransmitter.

Individual differences in the presence of these natural opiates may help in understanding the vulnerabilities to abuse of the manufactured opiates and the personality factors that may be involved in such vulnerabilities.

Two other peptides made in the hypothalamus and secreted from the pituitary are of potential importance in personality. Vasopressin as a hormone increases blood pressure and when secreted into the hypothalamic-pituitary portal increases the response to stress. As a neurotransmitter in the brain, it has been shown to be involved in learning and memory and circadian rhythms. Oxytocin in female animals increases sexual receptivity and pair-bonding and maternal behavior after the delivery of offspring. It has been suggested that this peptide could be involved in the sociability core of the trait of extraversion, although the first correlational studies with humans revealed little to support this hypothesis (Londen et al., 1997).

Substance P (SP) was isolated in the 1930s but defined as a peptide 40 years later. It is a sensory transmitter in the peripheral nervous system, of particular importance in pain, and a neuroregulator peptide in the CNS. In rats, it leads to behavioral excitation with locomotor activation perhaps related to stimulation of central dopamine systems. Dopamine antagonists increase levels of SP. It also may be involved in female sexual behavior.

Cholecystokinin (CCK), like SP, was first found in the gut but later dis-covered in the brain as a peptide. Studies of humans as well as animals show that CCK plays an important role in anxiety. It is a potent provoker for panic attacks in nearly all patients with panic disorders (Bradwejn, Koszycki, & Covetoux-de-Terte, 1992). It interacts with dopamine to produce hyperactivity.

Only a limited selection of the 50 or more neurotransmitters have been discussed in this section. The ones selected were on the basis of some work linking them to personality, behavioral traits relevant to personal-ity, or psychopathology. Other neurotransmitters, or different forms of the ones treated in this chapter, may become prominent in future research. Psychopharmacology is a rapidly changing science. The molecular mecha-nisms have received much more attention in recent decades and this trend will probably continue.

SUMMARY

Important advances have been made in the methods of neurobiology during the last decade, but the application of these innovations to the field of personality has been slow. Personality is the stepchild of psychiatry when it comes to psychobiology. This situation may change as the importance of preexisting personality in psychopathology becomes more obvious.

In the area of genetics interest is shifting from the calculations of heri-tabilities from family, twin, and adoption studies to molecular genetics. It is difficult to find a personality trait that does not have a substantial degree of heritability. But environment, at least the nonshared environment, remains at least equally important. What remains to be established is how environ-ment interacts with genetic predisposition at different stages of develop-ment. Molecular genetics attempts to go beyond the biometric methods to identify the particular genes involved in personality traits. All personality traits are polygenic and many involve more than simple additive genetic mechanisms. The current methods of molecular genetics depend on find-ing genes with major effects. As we will see, completely replicable results are rare.

The relatively inexpensive DNA analysis combined with the method of allelic association should lead to an increased research in the genetics of personality. The recent decoding of the human genome will help, but the functional properties of genes in the structure and physiology of the nervous system must be elucidated before we can select candidate genes for analysis.

At mid-century, most of the theories of personality were based on the Pavlovian idea of differences in excitation or inhibition of the cortex, or theories of arousal. Little was known about the role of limbic system circuits in motivation and emotion. The psychophysiological methods available for testing hypotheses derived from arousal theories were the EEG for theories of extraversion and peripheral autonomic meaures, like heart rate and skin conductance, as possible trait indicators for neuroticism. The inconclusive and negative findings were extensively treated in the previous edition (Zuckerman, 1991). The cortical evoked potential, a measure of reactivity, fared somewhat better. In the 1980s, the first studies appeared using brain-imaging methods (PET, CBF) to study personality. These methods promise to answer questions regarding the role of subcortical as well as cortical systems in personality. However, the methods are still not generally available. They are used primarily for psychiatric studies that usually do not include personality measures.

The new brain-imaging methods also have revolutionized neuropsychology. Before these methods were developed, the study of the functions of brain circuits and nuclei depended on experimental studies with other species and the imprecise observations of humans with brain damage.

It is now possible to measure structures in the human brain in vivo (MRI) and to observe the changes in different areas of brain during stimulation (PET and fMRI). Again, the benefits for personality study are only trickling down from cognitive and psychiatric studies.

Of all the areas of psychobiology the greatest advances and changes in the last decades have occurred in neuropsychopharmacology. In the 1960s, there were supposed to be only about six transmitters in the nervous system, three of which were norepinephrine, dopamine, and serotonin. GABA was also one of them. There also was interest in the enzymes regulating the monoamines such as MAO and COMT. Hormones have been a matter of interest even further back.

But it was the great variety of peptides discovered in the 1970s and later that increased the range of neurotransmitters of potential importance in psychiatry and, more recently, personality.

The first studies focused largely on the monoamine neurotransmitters and their enzymes. The catechoamine [norepinephrine] hypothesis of depression and mania (Schildkraut, 1965), the dopamine hypothesis for schizophrenia (Matthysse, 1973), and the specification of a noradrenergic system as the substrate for panic (Redmond, 1987), and anxiety, state, and trait (Gray, 1982) account for the early interest in the catecholamines. The first psychiatric studies of the monoamines used their metabolites in CSF, plasma, and urine in correlational studies of psychopathology and personality. The methodological impreciseness of metabolite levels has been discussed. The enzyme MAO was found to have replicable relationships with traits such as sociability and sensation seeking, but correlative work using the monoamine metabolites has yielded few stable findings in personality. Discovery of a variety of receptors for each of the monoamines has turned interest in this direction. Some of the unreliability of the findings with the metabolites has been a function of looking at these systems as unitary, when in actual fact each receptor may have a different function in the brain and affect behavior in different ways.

Each neurotransmitter comprises complex feedback systems with enzymes involved in production and catabolic degradation, receptors that are excitatory and inhibitory, peptides that also affect transmission, and neurotransmitters such as GABA that interact with other transmitters to inhibit or enhance transmission. Looking at the level of the metabolite of a single neurotransmitter now seems almost naive. Personality and psychopathology theories and research need to catch up with the complexities of molecular neurobiology.

There is a kind of methodological problem that cuts across several of the psychobiological areas. Many theories, such as the arousal theories of the 1950s and 1960s and the neurotransmitter-based theories of the 1970s, suggest stable, characteristic traits of the nervous system that reliably differ among individuals and at extreme levels produce psychopathology. Baseline psychophysiological or pharmacological measures have not proven useful for reasons discussed. It is measures of system reactivity, such as cortical-evoked potentials or neurotransmitter responses to drug challenges that often reveal meaningful differences between individuals. This makes sense. Individuals are distinguished by how they adapt to social-environmental stimulation, or upsets in the equilibrium of internal systems, rather than their physiological levels during unreactive periods.

CHAPTER 3

Extraversion/Sociability

This chapter begins with a review of some of the definitions of the trait of extraversion found in Chapter 1. Eysenck (1947, 1967) traced the history of the introversion-extraversion construct back to Galen's 2nd-century types. These types were based on the "humors" of the body: phlegmatic, sanguine, melancholic, and choleric. The ancient Greeks regarded these as pure types rather than bipolar traits. In the 19th century, psychiatrists described the types in terms of psychopathologies: schizophrenic versus manic-depressive (Kraepelin, 1899) and psychasthenia versus hysteria (Janet, 1907), regarding the abnormal manifestations as the extremes of normal personality types. Jung (1933) used the terms introversion and extraverson to describe what he believed to be the major dimension of personality: an orientation to the external world of people and objects versus a primary direction of interest and motive to the internal world. He described extreme types, but he recognized that "the normal man is, by definition, influenced as much from within as without," implying a continuum or normal dimension of personality. Freud (1920), in contrast to Jung, regarded introversion as a precursor of neurosis. The association between introversion and neuroticism was reflected in some of the early American questionnaires that showed high correlations between introversion and neuroticism. The idea of a normal introvert was not widely accepted in the extraverted American culture.

Eysenck's construct was closer to Jung's, in that he regarded introversion-extraversion as a normal dimension independent of and uncorrelated with the major dimension of neuroticism. Eysenck used the statistical method of factor analysis to define dimensions of personality. Cattell (1957), also using factor analysis, found a broad, higher-order factor quite similar to Eysenck's introversion-extraversion, which Cattel renamed "Exvia-Invia."

Extraversion (E) is a major factor in nearly every major system of personality classification, but it is defined somewhat differently in terms of its subtraits. In the original questionnaire, Eysenck defined E trait in terms of items measuring two factors: sociability and impulsivity. This dual nature of E was challenged, however, as described in Chapter 1. In the later test (EPQ) that introduced the Psychoticism dimension, the impulsivity items shifted from the E to the P dimension, leaving primarily sociability and some activity items in the E scale. Despite the limitation of content in the 3-factor scale, Eysenck conceived of E as a collection of narrower traits: sociability, liveliness, activity, assertiveness, sensation seeking, carefreeness, dominance, surgency, and venturesomeness (Eysenck & Eysenck, 1985).

Cattell (1957) conceived of Exvia-Invia (E-I) as a collection of three narrower traits:

1. *Cyclothymia* describes a mild, good-natured sociability with cooperativeness, trustfulness, soft-heartedness, and warm-heartedness.
2. *Surgency* includes dominance, assertiveness, high activity, with strong positive affect or joyousness, and an energetic, manicy type of sociability, manifested in wit, humor, and talkativeness.
3. *Parmia* represents an adventurous, impulsive type of E, with a strong interest in sex. Persons high on this subtrait are adventurous, responsive, frank and outspoken. This resembles the disinhibition subtrait of sensation seeking (Zuckerman, 1979, 1994).

Goldberg's (1994) E factor, based on ratings using trait-relevant adjectives, is closer to the surgency type of E including terms such as talkative, bold, and assertive. Terms suggestive of the cyclothymic type of E – such as warm, helpful, kind, sympathetic, and helpful – are classified in the agreeable factor. Costa and McCrae's (1992) questionnaire version of the Big-Five is a mixture of the two types of E, including warmth, sociability, and positive emotion, as well as assertiveness, excitement seeking, and activity.

Zuckerman's (2002, Zuckerman et al., 1993) E factor, also based on questionnaire items, is largely sociability or intolerance of isolation. Sensation seeking and impulsivity form their own factor, and activity is another factor.

The sociability and surgency E factors are distinguished in some systems such as Depue and Collins (1999), who describe two related factors: interpersonal engagement (sociability and warmth) and agentic E (dominance and exhibitionism). Hogan (1982) also distinguishes sociability and surgency.

Does the particular definition of E in terms of subordinate traits make a difference? Despite the high correlations between E in different systems (Zuckerman et al., 1993), some of the behavioral and psychobiological studies show different relationships for the subtraits of E. Part of the answer may lie in the genetical analyses of the traits. If there is a shared genetic factor underlying component traits, then their grouping on the basis of phenomenological similarities may be justified.

The approach temperament is the first manifestation of E in infants. This initially involved the reactions to novel stimuli of any kind; later, it is more specific to reactions to strange adults or children. Its opposite is inhibition. At a later stage of infancy, sociability can be distinguished from mere approach, in terms of the preference for solitary or social activity. Extraversion and agreeableness are the personality traits that are the most consistent over time (Roberts & DelVecchio, 2000). However, depression may cause a temporary reduction in sociability, and this is what may have led Freud and others to assume that introversion is associated with neurosis. In the normal range, E is strongly associated with positive affect of the surgent type but more weakly and negatively associated with depression (Zuckerman, Joireman, Kraft, & Kuhlman, 1999). E is strongly related to expectations of reward and sensitivity to signals of reward. Extraverts, compared to introverts, have more happy reactions to pleasant situations (Lucas & Diener, 2001), and respond to pleasant mood induction with more positive affect (Rusting & Larsen, 1997). In summary, extraverts are more optimistic and usually happier people than introverts.

GENETICS

Twin Studies

Table 3-1 summarizes the results on studies of adolescent or adult twins tested using questionnaires or other self-report methods. Eaves, Eysenck, and Martin (1989) summarized the twin findings in 36 studies done before 1976. Median correlations of seven studies (nine-groups) done between 1976 and 1988, and newer studies or later results, with increased ns, published between 1996 and 2001 are presented in Table 3-1. The heritabilities based on Falconer's (1981) simple subtraction method are presented along with the values from model-testing methods. The latter method tests the significance of models including broad heritability,

Table 3-1. Adolescent or Adult Twins: Correlations and Heritabilities on Extraversion

			Correlations		Heritabilities	
Study	Population	Test/Subjects	MZ r	DZ r	Fal.h²	Mo.h²
Eaves et al. 1989	36 studies before 1976	EPI	.53	.24	.58	.52
Zuckerman 1991	7 studies, 1976–1988	Various countries, ages	.54	.19	.54	–
Jang et al. 1996	Canadian	NEO-PI-R	.55	.23	.55	.53
Rieman et al. 1997	German	NEO	.56	.28	.56	.56
Loehlin & Martin (2001)	Australian	EPQ short				
		Males-young	.52	.23	.58	Total:
		middle	.51	.24	.54	.47
		old	.57	.20	.57	
		Females-young	.42	.15	.54	
		middle	.35	.20	.30	
		old	.46	.10	.46	
Saudino et al. 1999	Russian	EPI-short	.61	.13	.61	.59
Loehlin et al. 1998	American	self-ratings	.47	.01	.47	Total: .57
		CPI	.60	.30	.60	
		ACL	.39	−.06	.39	

Note: Since the heritability cannot exceed the correlation for MZ twins, the h² is given as the MZ r. when the formula (2 × MZ r = DZ r) result exceeds the MZ r.
Fal. h² = heritability from Falconer formula, Mo.h² = heritability from model testing; NEO = Neuroticism, Extraversion, Openness Questionnaire; EPQ = Eysenck Personality Questionnaire; EPI = Eysenck Personality Inventory; CPI = California Personality Inventory; ACL = Gough's Adjective Check List.

shared environment (SE), and nonshared environment (NSE), or various combinations of these in explaining the twin data. If one or more of these is shown to be unnecessary, it is excluded and the variance is divided among the remaining factors. Other models allow for the differentiation of additive and nonadditive types of genetic mechanisms. One can get some rough idea of the presence of nonadditive mechanisms from the relationship between the correlations of monozygotic (identical, MZ) and dizygotic (fraternal, DZ) twins. If the genetic mechanism is an additive one, we expect the MZ correlation to be about twice the correlation between DZ twins. To the extent that the correlation is much lower than this 2 to 1 ratio, there is a possible indication of nonadditive mechanisms such as Mendelian dominance or epistatic ones.

A glance at Table 3-1 shows that most of the correlations for MZ twins are between .45 and .60, whereas the correlations for DZ twins are lower and more variable. However, the majority of them fall between .15 and .30, or about half of the values for the MZ twins, suggesting primarily an additive type of genetic mechanism. Some of the exceptions are those using nonquestionnaire methods such as adjective rating tests. The heritabilites, whether by the Falconer subtraction method or derived from model fitting methods, are mostly in the .5 to .6 range.

DZ correlations exceeding half of the MZ correlations might indicate the influence of shared environment. This is found in only 1 of the 14 groups. Actually, the model fitting methods show no significant effect for SE in any of these studies. These data suggest that we do not learn to be extraverted or introverted within the family. If we happen to resemble our parents on this trait it is most likely because of their genes rather than their examples or reinforcements. However, our peer environments may have some influence on the trait and identical twins may have some influence on each other. In a large-scale Finnish twin study, the resemblance of twins depended on the frequency of their contact and their age of separation (Rose, Koskenvuo, Kaprio, Sarna, & Langinvainio, 1988). A longitudinal analysis, however, showed that for E the decreased social contact observed in identical twins leading more separate lives may be a consequence rather than a cause of their lack of similarity in the trait (Kaprio, Koskenvue, & Rose, 1990). Those twins who were more similar in E to begin with were likely to spend more time together when they came to the age of independence from the parental home.

Is the heritability of the broad E trait a function of the same genes as the narrower traits that make up E? The Canadian and German studies both used the NEO-PI-R in which E is the sum of six narrower traits: warmth, gregariousness (sociability), assertiveness, activity, excitement seeking, and positive emotions (Jang, McCrae, Angleitner, Riemann, & Livesley, 1998). The best-fitting model included only genetic and nonshared environment effects. The heritability of the broad E trait was .50. Heritabilities for the facet scores range from .38 to .46. However, each scale also showed specific genetic variance after the common heritable portion was removed, ranging from .23 (warmth) to .36 (excitement seeking). This suggests that components of a trait have a biological basis that is partially independent of the supertrait. They share some genes with each other, accounting in part for

Table 3-2. Twin Correlations and Heritabilites for Extraversion Based on Three Methods

Method	MZ r	DZ r	h^2	se^2	nse^2
video-based ratings	.59	.23	.62	.00	.38
self-report ratings	.45	.41	.06	.38	.56
average peer ratings	.42	.13	.41	.00	.52

Note: Data from Borkenau, Rieman, Angleitner, & Spinath (2001).
h^2 = proportion of variance due to genetics; se^2 = proportion of variance due to shared environment; nse^2 = proportion of variance due to nonshared environment.

their intercorrelation, but they also are affected by genes that are specific to themselves.

All of the studies in this table used self-report methods and in all but the Loehlin et al. (1998) studies the self-reports were based on questionnaires. To what extent are the results a function of self-report as opposed to peer ratings or observer ratings of actual behavior? German investigators studied twins using all three methods (Borkenau, Reiman, Angleitner, & Spinath, 2001). The observation ratings were made by judges observing videotapes recording behaviors of one twin of each pair in 1 of 15 different settings. The results are shown in Table 3-2.

The results show dramatic differences in heritabilities and shared environment effects using the three methods. Self-reports in this study showed little heritability and moderate shared environment effects, the video-based ratings show a strong heritability (.62) and no shared environment effects, and the averaged peer ratings show moderate heritability (.41) and no shared environment. The results with self ratings were an anomaly compared to all previous studies and perhaps a chance finding based on an unusually high correlation among fraternal twins. However, the results using observer ratings and peer reports are quite comparable with the previous results using questionnaire self-reports shown in Table 3-1. The fact that the video observations were based on behavior in a limited number of situations on a single day make their results particularly interesting.

Studies contrasting twins who have been adopted and raised in different families with those raised in their family of biological origin offer a more stringent test of shared environment relationships. The resemblance of identical twins separated from birth and raised in different families only can be based on the influence of the genetic factor. The influence of shared environment is indicated by any positive difference between twins raised in the same family and those raised in different families. Studies including

Table 3-3. Correlations on Extraversion of Twins Raised Together and Apart

Study/Test	Country	MZ-T	MZ-A	DZ-T	DZ-A
Shields (1962)/MPI	UK	.42	.61	–	–
Pederson et al. (1988)/EPI Short form	Sweden	.54	.30	.06	.04
Langinvainio et al. (1984)/EPI short form	Finland	.33	.38	.13	.12
Bouchard (1993) /MPQ	USA	.53	.40	.16	−.13
/CPI		.56	.60	.22	.04
Bouchard & Hur (1998)/MBI	USA	–	.60	–	.02

Note: MPI = Maudsley Personality Inventory; EPI = Eysenck Personality Inventory; MPQ = Multidimensional Personality Questionnaire; CPI = California Personality Inventory; MBI = Myer-Briggs Inventory.

separated twins have been done in four countries: Britain (Shields, 1962), America (Bouchard, Lykken, McGue, Segal, & Tellegen, 1990), Sweden (Pederson, Plomin, McClearn, & Friberg, 1988), and Finland (Langinvainio, Kaprio, Koskenvuo, & Lönnqvist, 1984). The earliest separation of twins occurred in the American study with a median time of separation at 3 months. The Swedish study had the largest *n*s for separated twins, more than twice as many as in the other studies. The American study used three different instruments for measuring E, the Multidimensional Personality Questionnaire (MPQ), California Personality Inventory (CPI), and the Myer-Briggs Type Indicator (MBTI), a test based on Jungian type theory. The results of the four studies are shown in Table 3-3.

Looking first at the correlations between identical (MZ) twins raised apart for most of their childhood, the broad heritabilities – as indicated by the correlations themselves – range from high (.60–.61) in Bouchard's results with the CPI and MBTI and Shield's results using a questionnaire similar to Eysenck's Personality Inventory (EPI), to moderate (.30–.40) in the remaining studies. The fraternal (DZ) twins raised apart, however, correlated close to zero in all studies, and those raised together, in contrast to most previous studies (Table 3-1), showed correlations that were much less than half of the MZ correlations. These results are suggestive of a nonadditive type of genetic mechanism. E. Loehlin's analysis of the data from all four studies reveals a large broad heritability of .43, but most of it would be due to a nonadditive genetic mechanism, most likely epistasis. Loehlin also found that unequal twin environments, as represented by the amount of twin contact as adults, was required to explain the data.

Loehlin's (1992) analysis shows a smaller but reliable effect of shared environment of .12; however, a glance at Table 3-3 shows that this result

Table 3-4. Correlations on Extraversion between Children and Biological and Adoptive Parents

Study/test	Father-Biol. Child	Mother-Biol. Child	Father-Adoptive Child	Mother-Adoptive Child	Biol. Related Siblings	Adopt. Related Siblings
Loehlin et al. (1985) Zuckerman (1991) median of 7 E-type Scales	.20	.15	.07	.03	.38	.08
Loehlin et al. (1985)/CPI-E	.20	−.03	.03	.00	.13	−.13
Scarr et al. (1981) EPI	.21	.04	.05	−.03	.06	.07
Eaves et al. (1989)/EPQ	.21	.21	−.03	−.02	.25	−.11

Note: The first row contains the data from Loehlin et al. based on medians of seven extraversion-type scales from Zuckerman (1991). The remainder of the table is adapted from Genes and environment in personality development, Table 2.4, p. 32, by J. C. Loehlin (1992). Newbury Park, CA: Sage Publications. Reprinted by permission.

is not consistent from study to study in terms of a positive discrepancy between raised together and separated twins.

Nontwin Adoption Studies

Studies involving familial relationships, other than twins, are concerned only with the additive-type of genetic mechanism, or narrow heritability. Adoption studies contrast the correlations between children and parents or between siblings who are related biologically with those who are exposed only to environmental influences. Table 3-4 summarizes the results in some of the major studies of this type. The table contains three kinds of correlations: (1) between adopted children and their biological parents who did not raise them and their natural siblings; (2) between adopted children and their adoptive parents who raised them or stepsiblings. Although tested as adolescents or adults, the subjects had been adopted soon after birth and raised by their adoptive parents.

The Texas adoption study (Loehlin, Willerman, & Horn, 1985) used a mixture of adolescent and young adult subjects from adoptive families. In the previous edition of this book (Zuckerman, 1991), I presented the data summarized from scales of the CPI and the TTS representing the extraversion dimension (sociable, dominance, social presence, active, capacity for status). Results for different scales varied so I calculated the median correlations for the seven scales, and these are shown in Table 3-4. The median correlations between children and biological parents (father .20, mother .15) can be contrasted with the near-zero correlations with the adoptive parents. Similarly, the correlation with the biological siblings of .38 is in contrast to near-zero correlations between biologically unrelated siblings.

The Minnesota study (Scarr, Webber, Weinberg, & Wittig, 1981, and un-published data from Loehlin, 1992) found a correlation of .21 between chil-dren and their biological father, but only a near-zero correlation with the biological mother. Neither biologically related children nor siblings showed any significant correlations.

The British study (Eaves, Eysenck, & Martin, 1989) found correlations of .21 between children and biological fathers and mothers, but near-zero correlations with adoptive parents. Biologically related siblings correlated .25 on E in contrast to adoptively related children who only correlated −.11.

Except for the anomalies of nonsignificant correlations between chil-dren and their biological mothers and between biologically related siblings in the Minnesota study, the results are consistent with an additive genetic influence with no effect of shared (adoptive) environment. Loehlin (1992) calculated a heritability of .35 for the three studies combined with no ef-fect of shared environment. The remainder, of course, is the variance due to nonshared environment and errors of measurement. The heritability is somewhat lower than that derived from twin studies, but this could be due to the differences in age between children and parents and between siblings in the nontwin studies, as well as the effect of epistasis.

Twins become less similar as they become older, perhaps due to a de-crease in the effect of shared environment (Loehlin, 1992). The effects of heredity may therefore not be as apparent in children and shared environ-mental effects may be stronger at younger ages when family environment is more predominant in the life of the child. The Colorado adoption project studied biological and adoptive correlations of adopted children involved in a longitudinal study from age 1 to age 7 using sociability ratings of the chil-dren by their parents and sociability scores on the EASI self-report question-naire for parents (Plomin, Coon, Carey, DeFries, & Fulker, 1991). Table 3-5 shows the correlations between the ratings of the adopted children at the seven ages with the EASI sociability scores of their biological and adop-tive parents and correlations between parents and children in nonadoptive families.

Only 1 of 14 correlations between adoptive children and their biologi-cal parents was significant for any age, clearly a chance result. The results are different for the adoptive parents, particularly between ages 5 and 7,

Table 3-5. Parent-Offspring Correlations on Sociability for EASI
Temperaments for Biological, Adoptive, and Nonadoptive Parents

Age	Biological		Adoptive		Nonadoptive	
	Mother	Father	Mother	Father	Mother	Father
1	.07	−.15	.12*	.16*	.28*	.11
2	.09	−.02	.10	.18*	.19*	.12*
3	.13*	.09	.10	.15*	.11	.05
4	.08	−.14	.09	.07	−.01	−.07
5	.08	−.12	.24*	.21*	.07	.01
6	.08	−.02	.23*	.17*	.15*	.00
7	.03	.12	.18*	.12	.23*	.05
1–7 mean	.12*	−.05	.18*	.16*	.22*	.08

* $p < .05$
Source: Plomin, Coon, Carey, DeFries, & Fulker (1991) Tables 1 and 2, pp. 69–
70. Copyright 1991 by Duke University Press. Reprinted by permission.

where five of the six correlations with adoptive mothers and fathers were significant. There is also evidence of significant correlations with adoptive fathers between ages 1 and 3. Curiously, the correlations between children and adoptive parents are the same or even higher than the correlations between children and parents in nonadoptive families. Correlations of siblings were nonsignificant for both adoptive and nonadoptive siblings. The results yielded nonsignificant heritability for sociability. Some weak but significant effects of shared parental environment were found.

The results from this study are in marked contrast to those of twins at average age 5 using ratings of sociability by the parents (Buss & Plomin, 1984) where correlations on sociability of .53 for identical and −.03 for fraternal twins were found. The results are similar in the lack of correlation of fraternal twins and nonadoptive siblings but different in the strong correlation for identical twins. Could the difference be in an epistatic genetic mechanism, only operating in identical twins, or in a parental rating bias (seeing identical twins as more similar in behavior than they actually are)?

Dramatically different results, particularly on the role of shared environment in the trait of sociability, were obtained from a study of genetically unrelated siblings reared in the same family (Loehlin, Neiderheiser, & Reiss, 2003). The twin and sibling correlations were much higher than in previous studies and, unlike previous studies of genetically unrelated siblings, the correlation in this study was significantly different from zero, although not as high as that for genetically related siblings (.52–.55).

The measure of sociability was a composite of behavior checklists filled out by the adolescents and ratings of them by both parents. The broad heritability based on both twin and nontwin samples was .56 with the proportion for shared environment of .32. For nonshared environment and measurement error, it was only .12. The narrow heritability, excluding the monozygotic twins, was .44 with proportions due to shared environment of .37 and nonshared environment of .19. A model combining both additive and nonadditive genetic effects yielded a predominantly additive effect (.44) compared to the nonadditive effect (.08), and a combined heritability of .52, a shared environment effect of .36, and a nonshared environment effect of .12.

The heritabilities obtained in this study were about the same as those in other studies (see Table 3-1), but the effect of shared environment relative to nonshared environment was quite different. Could this be due to the influence of parental ratings used in the composite measure? Perhaps parents see siblings as more similar regardless of their genetic relatedness, although this tendency was not seen in other studies. The results are a challenging anomaly.

Genetics of Temperament in Infancy and Early Childhood

Scales designed to assess temperament in infancy do not usually include a measure of sociability because that trait is not directly observable, but they do include traits such as approach-avoidance and activity that some would classify as early expressions of the extraverted personality. Torgerson (1985) used parental ratings of the traits in the set of temperament categories developed by Thomas and Chess (1977) in comparisons of identical and fraternal twins. Neither approach nor activity showed significant heritability ratios at 2 months of age, but both did at 9 months and 6 years of age. The correlations of both traits for identical twins (.93 and .94) were significantly higher than those for fraternal twins (.14 and .45), yielding heritabilities close to unity. These values are suspiciously high suggesting an undue parental bias in seeing their identical twins as similar in behavior.

Matheny (1980) used the Bayley's (1969) Scales of Infant Development, based on observations and ratings by experts in the laboratory. One of their factors is called *Affect-Extraversion* and another is called *Activity*. Infants were observed at periods from 3 to 24 months. The results on these two traits are shown in Table 3-6. The differences between correlations on sociability for identical and fraternal twins were significant at 6, 12, and 24 months, whereas those for activity were only significant at 18 and 24 months.

Table 3-6. Correlations on Affect-Extraversion and Activity
Ratings of Infant Twins

Age (months)	Affect-Extraversion		Activity	
	MZ *r*	DZ *r*	MZ *r*	DZ *r*
3	.18	.26	.30	.33
6	.55*	.10	.24	.11
9	.35	.33	.25	.22
12	.43*	.07	.33	.28
18	.49	.37	.43*	.14
24	.53*	.03	.58*	.14

* MZ twin correlation significantly ($p < .05$) higher than DZ twin correlation.
Source: Matheny (1980), from Table 7, p. 1164. Copyright 1980 Society for Research in Child Development. Reprinted with permission.

The investigators in the Colorado adoption study combined their data on adoptive and nonadoptive siblings with the Matheny data to obtain estimates of heritability at 1 and 2 years of age (Braungart, Plomin, DeFries, & Fulker, 1992). For the 12-month-old infants, the heritability was 35%, and at 24 months it was 48%. All of the genetic effect was of the nonadditive type. For activity, the heritable variance was 38% at 1 year and 57% at 2 years of age. Neither trait showed any influence of shared environment exceeding 1% at 1 year, but at 2 years the affect-extraversion factor increased to 4%.

Later, the investigators reported the data on sociability and activity using ratings of 7-year-old adopted and nonadopted siblings made by teachers and testers during a 5-hour session in the laboratory (Schmitz, Saudino, Plomin, Fulker, & DeFries, 1996). Correlations between the two sets of ratings were significant but low (.26, .19). Sibling correlations on sociability based on teacher ratings were low and insignificant for both adopted and nonadopted siblings. Tester ratings of sociability for adopted siblings also were close to zero ($-.06$) but were significant (.32) for nonadoptive siblings, yielding a heritability of .64. For activity, the correlations of nonadoptive siblings were higher for both teacher and tester ratings, yielding heritabilities of .74 for the former and .39 for the latter. Shared environment was not a significant factor for either trait.

Goldsmith and Gottesman (1981) used laboratory ratings by psychologists for twins at ages of 8 months, 4 years, and 7 years. Ratings of activity level and activity versus passivity correlated significantly higher in identical than in fraternal twins at 8 months and at 7 years of age. Ratings of person interest at 8 months were not significantly higher in identical than in fraternal twins, although one of them did show a difference at 4 years of age.

Genetic effects on activity show up in early infancy but those for sociability only emerge later. This may be because of the greater exposure to social stimuli inside and outside of the family in later infancy and early childhood. The magnitude of heritability in early childhood is about equivalent to that for extraversion in adolescents and adults. A large-scale Finnish population study of twins found that heritability of extraversion decreased from late adolescence to the later 20s and tended to stabilize thereafter (Viken, Rose, Kaprio, & Koskenvuo, 1994). New environmental influences, however, emerged at all ages.

Nonshared, but not shared, environmental influences on extraversion are strong in most studies and equal to or even surpassing genetic influences. This may account for the curious finding of increases in E scores of American college students between 1966 and 1993 (Twenge, 2001). The increase is not trivial, amouting to nearly a standard deviation over 20 to 25 years. American culture has changed during these decades with more children exposed at earlier ages to peer social environments in day care and preschool, an emphasis on social skills in the workplace, and permissiveness of self-expression and assertiveness in women as well as in men (Whyte, 1956). Although all members of a family are exposed to these cultural changes, they may have different effects on siblings within the family.

Molecular Genetics

The first findings of specific genes associated with normal personality traits concerned novelty or sensation seeking rather than extraversion (Ebstein et al., 1996). The first replication (Benjamin et al., 1996), however, used Costa and McCrae's (1992) NEO-PI-R test in addition the Tridimensional Personality Questionnaire (Cloninger et al.'s 1994). Two dimensions of the NEO are related to novelty seeking: extraversion and conscientiousness. The NEO also measures subtraits or facets for each of these two broad traits. These facets also were examined in the study.

The gene selected for examination was the D4 dopamine receptor (D4DR) gene. Different forms (polymorphisms) of the gene are characterized by varying number of repeats of the base sequence. The number of repeats varies from two to eight in Western populations but the most frequent alleles are the four and seven repeats. The longer forms are found more frequently in those scoring high on the Novelty Seeking scale. These results will be addressed later in this book.

Benjamin et al. (1996) did replicate the differences on the novelty seeking scale, but they also found differences on the extraversion scale and several of its facets including warmth, excitement seeking, and positive emotions. On all of these subtraits, those who had the long form of the D4DR had higher scores. Differences were not found on other E facets: gregariousness, assertiveness, and activity. It is interesting that the differences were found on emotional and not behavioral subtraits of E. Strobel, Wehr, Michel, and Brocke (1999) also found that those with the longer (seven repeat) form of the gene had higher scores on the NEO extraversion scale. They used a short form of the NEO, which did not allow scoring for facet components of E.

Persson et al. (2000) attempted to replicate these findings using the NEO in a Swedish population without success. As usual with a failure of replication, we do not know if the first finding was in error or if population differences alone or in interaction with age and gender accounted for the different findings (Benjamin's study used American and Strobel's used German subjects).

Summary

Studies of twins raised together in the same household show heritabilities ranging from about .4 to .6 with some variation due to the instruments used and gender of subjects. Generally, the results can be encompassed within a model of additive genetic variance with no effect for shared environment. The environmental effect is almost entirely due to nonshared environment. However, there was one notable exception in the study by Loehlin et al. (2003), in which shared environment effects were prominent and even stronger than nonshared environment ones.

Studies of separated and adopted twins also show heritabilities in the same range, but in these the main type of genetic mechanism seems to be a nonadditive one, primarily because of the lack of any correlation between separated fraternal twins. There was no consistent effect of shared environment in these studies.

Studies of parent-child and sibling relationships, depending solely on additive type genetic mechanisms, yield lower heritabilities than those calculated for twins, perhaps due to the total absence of nonadditive mechanisms. The correlations between adopted, nonbiologically related, parents and children, and siblings are quite low in most studies, but so are the correlations between biologically related relatives.

Studies of temperament in infants and young children, largely based on laboratory observations of sociability, affect, and activity, show heritabilities for extraversion nearly equivalent to the results for adolescents and adults. As with studies of adults, there is little evidence for shared environment effects; most of the environmental effects are of the nonshared type.

Molecular genetic studies have shown some influence of a dopamine receptor gene (D4DR) in extraversion, particularly in its emotionally expressive manifestations, but these results failed to replicate in another study.

PSYCHOPHYSIOLOGY

Eysenck's (1957) earlier theory of the biological basis of extraversion combined constructs from the learning theory of Clark Hull (1943) and the brain models of Ivan Pavlov (1927/1960). Hull's construct of *reactive inhibition* (inhibition built up by stimulus repetition) and Pavlov's constructs of *cortical excitation and inhibition* as the basis for temperament were the basis for Eysenck's model. Extraverts were said to be less reactive to cortical excitation and more likely to develop reactive inhibition than introverts. As a consequence of these differences in cortical physiology, introverts more readily developed strong conditioned responses and were slower to extinguish them in the absence of reinforcement. Extraverts, however, were harder to condition and their conditioned responses were less stable. As a consequence, they were more likely to be impulsive and unable to learn much from punishment.

Eysenck made no distinction between positively reinforced conditioning (reward) and aversive conditioning (punishment). In this respect, his theory differs from that of Jeffrey Gray (1971), which proposes that extraverts are more susceptible to conditioning by reward and introverts are more influenced by punishment.

In the 1960s, Eysenck (1967) changed his model of extraversion to one based on the idea of *optimal levels of stimulation and arousal*. Hebb (1955) based his construct of an optimal level of arousal (Figure 3-1) on the newly discovered reticular activation system (RAS, Lindsley, Bowden, & Magoun, 1949; Moruzzi & Magoun, 1949). The RAS in its ascending branch aroused the cortex when activated by stimulation from any of the senses including the proprioceptive ones. The cortex, in turn, regulated the level of stimulation from the RAS by a descending branch, closing channels for incoming stimulation. Eysenck suggested that extraverts and introverts differ in the sensitivity of arousal and inhibition thresholds (see Figure 3-2). Introverts are aroused by low intensities of stimulation and more likely to shut down cortical arousal at high intensities of stimulation. Extraverts are less

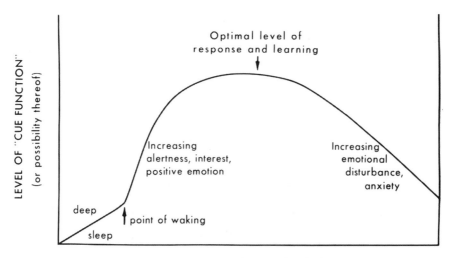

Figure 3-1. The relationship between cue function (efficiency of performance) and level of arousal function (nonspecific cortical arousal by RAS). From "Drives and the C. N. S. (conceptual nervous system)" by D. O. Hebb, 1955, *Psychological Review, 62.* Copyright 1955 by American Psychological Association. Reprinted by permission.

responsive to low intensities of stimulation but more able to respond effectively and affectively (positive) to high intensities of stimulation. Hebb's theory (Figure 3-1) is that there are optimal levels of arousal for different tasks (cue function) and that below or above this optimal level affect was more negative and performance less efficient. Imagine two overlapping inverted "U" curves with the extravert curve pushed more to the right (higher intensity) and the introvert curve to the left (lower intensity); this is Eysenck's construct of differences between extraverts and introverts in optimal levels of arousal.

A similar explanation was independently derived for the trait of sensation seeking (Zuckerman, 1969), as will be described later. This was no problem for Eysenck because he regarded sensation seeking as a subtrait of extraversion. As a consequence of their higher optimal levels of arousal, extraverts needed more intense stimulation to feel good and function more efficiently.

The simplest prediction from Eysenck's theory was that in a waking state with low levels of ambient stimulation, introverts would be more cortically aroused than extraverts.

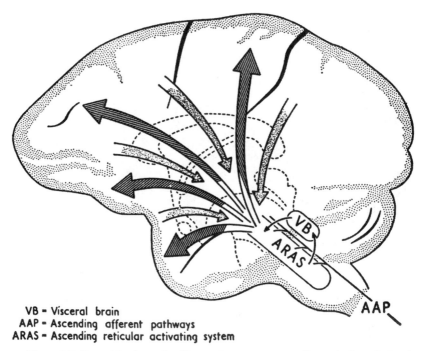

VB = Visceral brain
AAP = Ascending afferent pathways
ARAS = Ascending reticular activating system

Figure 3-2. Eysenck's schematic of interactions among ascending reticulocortical activating system, visceral brain (limbic systems), and cortex. From H. J. Eysenck, 1967, *The biological basis of personality*, Fig. 80, p. 231. Springfield, IL: Charles C. Thomas. Copyright 1967 by Charles C. Thomas. Reprinted by permission.

Cortical Arousal

Before the development of the brain imaging methods, the EEG provided the most direct measure of cortical arousal, as described in Chapter 2. Studies done before the 1990s were described in the first edition of this book (Zuckerman, 1991). Most studies used the EEG spectrum analysis or focused on the characteristics of the alpha rhythm. The outcomes of these studies in relation to Eysenck's hypothesis were reviewed by Gale (1983), Gale and Edwards (1986), and O'Gorman (1984). Both reviews were inconclusive, with some supporting Eysenck's hypothesis (extraverts lower in cortical arousal), some showing no differences, and some showing results in the direction opposite to the hypothesis (extraverts higher in cortical arousal). Gale attempted to explain the results in terms of the procedures that produced more or less stimulation or activity. Zuckerman (1991) noticed that in the studies in which both reviewers agreed on the outcome in relation to the hypothesis, studies using women or a mixture of the genders tended to support the hypothesis, whereas those using exclusively men did not.

Table 3-7. EEG Studies of Cortical Brain Activation

Study-Author	Subjects (sex)	Tests	Conditions	Results
Matthews & Amelang (1993)	181 (M & F)	EPI, EPQ, EIS (impulsivity)	eyes closed, visual fixation, cog	Delta correlated .16 with E and Imp. No relation to sociability
Stenberg (1992)	40 (M & F)	EPI, KSPF actor E, Imp, SS	relaxed & pos,. neg. imagery	More posterior theta in high E-Impulsive-SS
Schmidt (1999)	40 (F)	Shyness & Sy scales	eyes open & closed	Shyness assoc. with right frontal alpha, sy with left frontal alpha
Tran et al. (2001)	50 (M & F)	16PF, E factor	eyes open & closed	High amplitude alpha all frontal sites with E, dom, imp., & boldness
Fink et al. (2002)	60 (M & F)	NEO E & IQ test	eyes closed & during cog. tests	At rest: low IQ E lower arousal; during task high IQ E lower arousal
Ivashenko et al. (1999)	69 (M)	EPI	eyes closed & open, cog tasks	More act. in E, L hemisphere, temporal lobe
Knyazev et al. (2002)	49 (M & F)	EPI, G-W Pers. Questionnaire	eyes closed & open	Neg. r between E & high freq. EEG; pos. r with low freq. Bands

Table 3-7 summarizes some of the more recent studies testing the arousal hypothesis using EEG analyses. The study by Matthews and Amelang (1993) was the largest one among the new studies and it was specifically designed to test the Eysenck hypothesis of lower arousal in extraverts and/or impulsives. It also used a range of conditions from least arousing (eyes closed, resting) to highly arousing cognitive tasks in order to examine the post hoc hypothesis of Gale suggesting that the predicted relationship with extraversion would only emerge in moderately arousing conditions.

Both extraversion and impulsivity (but not sociability) correlated low but significantly ($r = .16$) with delta slow wave activity, weakly confirming the hypothesis. The correlation with E was only significant in the least arousing condition (eyes closed), but the correlations in the medium and high arousing conditions were not that different. Correlations did not vary much between men and women. Thus, the main reason for the lack of consistency in prior studies was probably because of a lack of power in detecting the weak relationship rather than the specific conditions of EEG recording or the gender of the subjects.

Two Russian studies found different results, one supporting and the other not supporting the Eysenck hypothesis of lower arousal in extraverts. One study found *more* EEG activation in the left hemisphere in extraverts than in introverts regardless of arousal state (Ivashenko, Berus, Zhuravlev, & Myamlin, 1999). The other study reported E to be negatively correlated with high frequency EEG in the temporal lobe in an eyes-open condition, and positive correlations with low frequency EEG, supporting the hypothesis (Knyazev, Slobodoskaya, & Wilson, 2002).

The remaining studies also tended to support the hypothesis, but only when qualified by interactions with other traits such as shyness or intelligence. Stenberg's (1992) study used a personality factor combining E with impulsivity and sensation seeking and found more posterior theta slow wave activity in those high on the factor. Schmidt (1999) found an interaction between shyness and sociability. Tran, Craig, and McIssac (2001) found that extraverts characterized by impulsivity had more high amplitude alpha (lower arousal) in the frontal sites. Fink et al. (2002) did not find a main effect of E on EEG measured arousal but instead reported an interaction with intelligence.

The EEG studies show only a weak relationship between arousal and extraversion. Although extraversion, as a higher-order trait, may be related to arousal, it may be only the more surgent-type components of E, such as impulsivity, which account for this relationship.

Arousal theorists had high hopes for the new research using the Positron Emission Tomography (PET) method for measuring brain arousal. A glance at the results column of Table 3-8 reveals the same inconsistencies of findings that plagued the EEG research. One source of inconsistency can be seen in the second column of the table showing the ns involved in the studies ranging from 17 to 33. These numbers are too small for reliable results unless the relationships are remarkably strong, which they are not. Another problem is that given the number of brain areas analyzed the number of chance relationships is high. Most investigators do not correct for the number of comparisons. The tests used include Eysenck's EPI and EPQ and the NEO. This is probably not a major source of error because measures of

Table 3-8. Brain Imaging (PET) Studies (1984–1999)

Study-Author	Subjects (sex)	Tests	Method, Conditions	Results
Mathew et al. (1984)	33 (F)	EPI	CBF-resting	E neg. correlated with CBF in all brain areas.
Haier et al. (1987)	18 pts with Generalized Anxiety Disorder (M & F),	EPQ	glucose uptake, active task (CPT)	E pos. correlated with uptake in frontal and temporal gyri, L & R putamen, R caudate, cingulate, hippocampal, and parahippocampal.
Stenberg et al. (1990)	37 (M & F)	EPI	CBF resting	higher CBF in R & L anterior temporal lobes.
Stenberg et al. (1993)	17 (M & F)	EPI & KSP	CBF resting	higher CBF in introverts in temporal lobes.
Ebmeier et al. (1994)	33	EPQ	TcE. uptake resting	E pos. correlated with uptake in cingulate. No relation to temporal or frontal lobe uptake.
Fischer et al. (1997)	30 (F)	NEO-PI-R	CBF resting	higher CBF in introverts in caudate, putamen, secondary visual cortex. No diff. in frontal or temporal lobes, or cingulate, thalamus, hypothalamus.
Johnson et al. (1999)	18 (M & F)	NEO	CBF resting	E neg. correlated with CBF in R frontal cortex, insular cortex, putamen, Rtemporal cortex, thalamus, hippocampus. E pos. correlated with CBF in anterior cingulate, temporal lobes (R & L), L amygdala, pulvinar nucleus. No relation with whole brain BF.

extraversion from the three are highly correlated. Most investigators have used the Xenon inhalation method of measuring cerebral blood flow (CBF), although some have used injection of tagged substances such as glucose. Most measurements have been made under resting conditions or during presentation of bland videotapes and some have added various kinds of cognitive tasks. However, most of the data comes from measurements during the resting condition.

The first study by Mathew, Weinman, and Barr (1984) supported Eysenck's arousal hypothesis for extraversion, because E was negatively correlated with CBF in all brain areas; introverts showed greater brain activation. All of their subjects were female, recalling the tendency to obtain positive results in the EEG studies using female subjects. Stenberg, Wendt, and Risberg (1993) used subjects of both genders but found that the overall negative correlation between E and cortical arousal was a function of the high correlation among females. The correlation for males was close to zero.

The greater arousal of introverts, as measured by CBF in the temporal lobes, was found in both studies by Stenberg and his group (Stenberg, Risberg, Warkentin, & Rosen, 1990; Stenberg et al., 1993), and by Johnson et al. (1999), but not by Ebmeier et al. (1994) or by Fischer, Wik, and Fredrikson (1997). Haier, Skolski, Katz, and Buchsbaum (1987) actually found positive correlations between E and glucose uptake in temporal and frontal lobes, but these were found in a condition in which subjects were engaged in a challenging task, the continuous performance test (CPT). Another complication is that all of the subjects in this condition were patients with Generalized Anxiety Disorder (GAD). There were few significant correlations between E and brain areas in either the patient or a control group during the resting, no-task condition.

Eysenck's prediction of lower arousal in extraverts was limited to the cerebrum and the brain stem reticular activating system. Activation of limbic brain was supposedly related only to Neuroticism. But many of the imaging studies found significant relationships between E and limbic brain areas, including the putamen and caudate or striate areas (Fischer et al., 1997; Johnson et al., 1999; Mathew et al., 1984); and the cingulate gyrus (Haier et al., 1987; Ebmeier et al., 1994; Johnson et al., 1999). The introverts showed more activity in the striate areas, whereas the extraverts had more blood flow in the cingulum. The striate areas are largely dopaminergic. The cingulum is the major pathway between the frontal cortex and the limbic system and theoretically associated with neuroticism and anxiety rather than extraversion (Zuckerman, 1991).

The results of the PET studies are neither consistent nor immediately reconcilable with existing theories. Why should E be more specifically associated with striate and cingulum arousal and introversion with temporal lobe arousal? Why should women demonstrate the predicted relationship between cerebral arousal and E more clearly than men? Perhaps the answer lies in reactions of the brain to challenge rather than its resting levels. The PET methodology is not ideal for this purpose, because it can only measure brain activity over an extended period of time during which the uptake is taking place. In contrast, evoked potentials (EPs) derived from the EEG show the immediate reaction of the cortex and some subcortical areas to stimuli of different intensities or significances.

Arousability: Evoked Potentials

Studies of the relationship of EPs to extraversion were reviewed by Stelmack (1990) and Zuckerman (1991). The findings relating cortical auditory evoked potentials (AEPs) to E yielded some findings of negative relationships between E and AEPs (introverts more reactive), but a number of failures to replicate, which could not be attributed to differences in stimulus intensities or frequencies. But other promising EP paradigms were beginning to be explored. The P300 is a later component of the EP related to attentional processes and unexpectedness of the stimulus event. The "odd-ball" paradigm uses the response to an infrequent stimulus to assess the strength of the P300 (P3). Investigators using some variant of this paradigm found that introverts have higher amplitudes of the P3 than extraverts (Daruna, Karrer, & Rosen, 1985; Ditraglia & Polich, 1991; Wilson & Languis, 1990).

Most of the work through the 1980s concerned cortical evoked potentials. However, Stelmack and Wilson (1982) studied the relationship between E and the brain stem auditory evoked potential (BAEP), measured from the earlier components of the AEP) and found relationships between E and latencies of the BAEP wave V. Introverts had faster and extraverts slower reactions. Pivik, Stelmack and Bylama (1988) went even further down the nervous system to reflex reactions in the leg and found that extraverts showed reduced motoneuronal excitability. Taken together with the findings relating E to activity in subcortical brain areas, already discussed, we might conclude that extraversion is a function of more than cortical thresholds for excitation and inhibition, but is a general characteristic of the entire nervous system.

Table 3-9 shows subsequent EP studies of extraversion. Stenberg (1994) used a visual evoked potential (VEP) and Guerra, O'Donnell, Nestor, Gainski, and McCarley (2001) an auditory evoked potential (AEP), and both studies

Table 3-9. Evoked Potential Studies of Arousability (1993–2002)

Study-Author	Subjects (sex)	Tests	Method, Conditions	Results
Stenberg (1994)	40 (M & F) L, Med, Hi E	EPI	VEP during a visual target task	E pos. related to AEP amp. for P3. Correlation higher with impulsivity than sociability.
Guerra et al. (2001)	18 (M)	NEO	AEP target tones 97dB, also novel S	E pos. correlated with AEP amp. for P3, target stimuli, frontal leads.. not parietal leads.
Brocke et al. (1997)	18, extreme scores on E	EPI	VEP task with white noise at 3 intensities	At 40 dB VEP P3 amp. introverts > extraverts; at 60 dB VEP P3 extraverts> introverts. At 0 dB no difference between groups.
Buckingham (2002)	56 (F) four groups, extremes of E and N	EPQ	AEP & VEP For AEP: 30, 50, 70 db, long ISI	No main effects of E or N but AEP P1N1 amp. higher in high I-N group than in hiE lowN. Steeper slopes in hi I-N group. No differences for VEP.
Robinson (2001)	93 (M & F) 4 groups, E X N	EPQ	AEP, 85 dB within delta, theta, alpha freqs	E not correlated with any AEP scores, but AEP index of inhibition lower in hiE-hiN than in lowE-hiN.
Stelmack et al. (1993)	28 (F)	EPQ, extremes E	BAEP, 80, 85, 90 dB, waking and sleep	latency for wave V faster in introverts than extraverts for all six conditions but short of significance.
Cox-Fuenzalida (2001)	78 (M & F)	EPI, EPQ	BAEP 70 dB	EPQ & EPI E pos. correlated with BAEP wave V latency (rs .23–.27). Sociability but not impulsivity correlated with EP.
Bartussek et al. (1993)	20 extremes on E	EPI	AEP tones signifying winning or losing in a gambling task	Es larger P2 amp. to tones associated with winning than tones associated with losing. Is larger P2 to tones associated with losing. Similar results for N2 at frontal sites.
Bartussek et al. (1996)	Exp. 1: 48: four groups EXN Exp. 2: 24: four groups EXN	EPI EPQ	VEP words pos.& neg, emotional VEP slides pos. & neg.emotional	Is more VEP amp. to neg. & neutral than to pos.words. Es more VEP amp. to neg. & pos. than to neutral words. Is same VEP amp to neg., pos., & neutral slides. Es more VEP to neg. & pos. than to neutral slides.
De Pascalis et al. (1996)	65 (F)	EPQ, Imp, Gray-Wilson Pers. Quest.	VEP. Words "win," "lose" after trials	No relation of VEP 3 to E P6 amp to win or lose related to Approach.

found a positive relationship between E and P3 amplitudes. This would seem to contradict the Eysenck hypothesis of more arousability in introverts, but another aspect of the theory suggests that intense stimuli or stimuli sufficiently varied may elicit a stronger response from extraverts. Guerra et al. (2001) used a very intense auditory stimulus (97dB) that could elicit transmarginal inhibition in introverts. Stenberg's study used a high rate of events, more varied stimuli, and required more processing of the odd-ball task, all of which prevented the lapse of attention characteristic of extraverts in the ordinary odd-ball paradigm.

The study by Brocke, Tasche, and Beauducel (1997) further illustrates the way intensity of stimulation may influence the relationship between EP amplitudes and extraversion. Using different intensities of white noise as background to a VEP, they found that at zero dB there was no difference between introverts and extraverts, at 40 dB introverts had larger amplitude VEPs than extraverts, but at 60 dB the extraverts had larger VEPs. Previous research had indicated that the lower level of white noise was optimal for introverts, whereas the higher level was favored by extraverts. The findings support an optimal level of arousal theory of introversion-extraversion.

It has been maintained by some that the causal dimension of influence lies between extraversion and neuroticism rather than simply along the extraversion dimension (e.g., Gray, 1982). Eysenck (1967) interpreted the four classical temperaments in terms of four different combinations of E and N scores: sanguine (high E low N), phlegmatic (low E low N), choleric (high E high N), and melancholic (low E high N).

Buckingham (2002) found that the major differences in AEP at P1N1 was between the melancholic (low E high N) and the sanguine (high E low N) types. The melancholic, or introverted neurotic, type had higher P1N1 amplitudes averaged across the three stimulus intensities than the sanguine, or stable extravert, type. The melancholic type also had a steeper slope of the AEP-stimulus intensity relationship. This kind of function has been called "augmenting-reducing" and will be further elaborated in the chapter on impulsivity and sensation seeking. The problem with this finding is that the stimulus intensity range of 30–70 dB was too narrow to detect true differences in augmenting or reducing, which usually occur in the 80–110 dB range (Zuckerman, 1990). Zuckerman, Murtaugh, and Siegel (1974) found no relationship between E and the augmenting-reducing function for the VEP. Buckingham found no relationships at all between E or temperament types and the VEP.

Robinson (2001) also used Pavlovian types based on E and N, but he predicted differences between the melancholic (low E low N) and the choleric (high E high N) types, rather than the sanguine type. He also used a different kind of AEP index, contrasting AEPs within different bands of EEG arousal, delta, theta, and alpha. An index of cortical inhibition was lower in the choleric than in the melancholic type, as predicted. E as a single dimension was unrelated to any of the AEP indices.

Eysenck (1967) hypothesized that extraversion was related to "differential thresholds in the various parts of the ascending reticular activating system [ARAS]" so it would be consistent with the theory to find differences in arousability between introverts and extraverts at levels of brain below the cerebrum and limbic system. AEP components of latencies between 3 and 10 msec are thought to arise from the brain stem nuclei between the cochlear nucleus and the inferior colliculus. Stelmack and Wilson (1982) found that extraverts had longer latencies than introverts for waves I and V of the BAEP representing the extremes of this pathway. The inferior colliculus is the part of the auditory pathway that transects the ARAS. The difference in the wave emanating from the auditory nerve (cochlear nucleus) is consistent with higher auditory sensitivities in introverts, and the difference in both of these structures could account for the differences found in amplitudes of later components of the AEP such as the N1-P2.

Stelmack, Campbell, and Bell (1993) replicated these findings in a later experiment although not reaching the same level of significance of the differences. Another study using a larger number of subjects did replicate the finding with E correlating with BAEP wave V latency (Cox-Fuenzalida, Gilliland, & Swickert, 2001). The correlations were low, ranging from .23 to .27, but significant because of the larger number of subjects than in previous studies. As with other findings on the arousal hypothesis, there is weak support for the theory relating arousal to extraversion.

Eysenck's theory accomodates the role of stimulus intensity but not stimulus significance in terms of association with reward and punishment. Some investigators have used the EP paradigm to test Gray's (1982, 1987) theory that claims a special sensitivity to punishment in highly anxious (introverted neurotic) subjects compared to strong sensitivities to reward in highly impulsive (extraverted neurotics) subjects. The theory also predicts differences between extraverts and introverts, as major groups, in sensitivities to signals of reward and punishment.

Bartussek, Diedrich, Naumann, and Collet (1993) tested Gray's theory using the AEP at P2 and N2 with tones associated with winning or losing in a gambling task. In support of the theory, extraverts had larger P2 AEP amplitudes to tones associated with winning, whereas introverts had larger P2 to tones associated with losing. Similar results were obtained for the N2 component but at frontal sites only. In a later experiment, however, Bartussek and his colleagues found that extraverts, using the VEP with emotionally positive, negative, and neutral words and pictures, showed higher amplitude P3 VEP amplitudes to negative *and* positive stimuli than to neutral stimuli (Bartussek, Becker, Diedrich, & Naumann, 1996). Introverts gave responses more in conformance with theory, with higher amplitudes VEPs to negative and neutral than to positive stimuli. If the P3 measures interest, one could conclude that the extraverts were more interested in highly emotional stimuli, whether positive or negative.

DePascalis and colleagues (De Pascalis, Fiore, & Sparita, 1996) used measures of E, Impulsivity and Approach tendency from the Gray-Wilson (Wilson, Barrett, & Gray, 1989) personality questionnaire. They measured VEPs in response to the words "win" and "lose" associated respectively with rewarded or punished performance outcomes. There was no relation of E to the VEP P3, but high scorers on the Approach scale had higher VEP P6 amplitudes in response to "win" than to "lose." Although the approach scale is theoretically a measure of Gray's dimension of impulsivity that also should be related to E, E and approach were not significantly correlated in this study. Approach did correlate with an impulsivity scale.

The results of the EP research have mixed outcomes. Eysenck's theory predicts higher arousability of introverts than extraverts but allows for some shift in the relationship at higher intensities of stimulation. The research shows that the relationship of cortical arousal to extraversion depends on stimulus intensity and an interaction of extraversion and neuroticism. There is evidence that the differences in arousability between introverts and extraverts is not limited to cortical reactivity but extends down to the brain stem (inferior colliculus). Actually, differences may even be found in the peripheral nervous system in a spinal motor-neuronal reflex in the leg (Pivik, Stelmack, & Bylsma, 1988). Studies using the AEP and VEP to test Gray's theory of differential sensitivities to stimuli associated with reward or punishment have not given consistent results. The most positive findings were in a study using the AEP by Bartussek et al. (1993). Perhaps the VEP is less useful in testing the theory because it may be harder to determine what is rewarding or punishing in terms of emotional reactions. What are meant to be unpleasant stimuli can be more rewarding to impulsive extraverts or high sensation seekers simply because they are more interesting and arousing (Rawlings, 2003; Zaleski, 1984; Zuckerman & Litle, 1986).

PSYCHOPHARMACOLOGY

Monoamines

In the 1970s and 1980s, several theorists, working from studies of nonhuman species, proposed that dopaminergic systems in the brain served to energize or activate behavior directed toward primary biological rewards such as search, exploration, and foraging (Crow, 1977; Gray 1987; Panksepp, 1982; Stein, 1978). Some of these investigators suggested that dopamine mediates human positive emotions such as hope, desire, and joy (Panksepp, 1982) characteristic of extraverts, and others suggested a more direct connection of the dopaminergic approach system to novelty or sensation seeking in both humans and animals (Bardo, Donohew, & Harrington, 1996; Cloninger et al., 1993; Le Moal, 1995; Zuckerman, 1984, 1991).

Dominance is a salient trait in primates and is regarded as an aspect of agentic extraversion in humans. Dominant monkeys in social groups had higher concentrations of HVA (the metabolite of dopamine) in their CSF than subordinate monkeys (Kaplan, Manuck, Fontenot, & Mann, 2002). Male, but not female, monkeys had lower concentrations of 5-HIAA (the serotonin metabolite) in CSF than subordinates. Gray's (1987) model proposes that dopamine mediates the trait of impulsivity (high E, P, and N).

DePue and Collins (1999) have a broader view of E consisting of two factors: *affiliation*, or interpersonal engagement, agreeableness, and warmth, and *agency*, or dominance, exhibitionism, and achievement motivation. This distinction has been made by others. Agency is often called *surgency* and affiliation is called *sociability*. Depue and Collins regard impulsivity and sensation seeking as constituting an emergent factor, rather than a primary one, and representing a combination of the primary traits of extraversion and constraint. Constraint is a factor in the system of Tellegen (1985), consisting of scales for control, harm avoidance, and traditionalism.

Depue and Collins suggest that dopamine is primarily associated with extraversion, particularly its agentic form, and that the lines of biological influence, in general, are along the orthogonal dimensions of extraversion and constraint rather than what they regard as the "emergent" dimension of impulsive sensation seeking or the third dimension of Psychoticism, or Unsocialized Impulsive Sensation Seeking. Corr (1999), Gray (1999), MacDonald (1999), and Pickering (1999) disagree and regard impulsive sensation seeking, including psychoticism and aggression, as the primary dimension associated with dopaminergic activity. Zuckerman (1991, 1995) actually suggests that dopamine is related to the approach motive inherent in extraversion *and* impulsive sensation seeking. What is the evidence from human studies?

The previous edition of this book (Zuckerman, 1991) presented studies in which the monoamine metabolites obtained from cerebrospinal fluid (CSF) plasma, and urine had been correlated with personality traits in normals (Ballenger et al., 1983; Limson et al., 1991; Schalling, Asberg, & Edman, 1984, unpublished). None of the correlations between E from the EPQ and metabolites of dopamine (HVA), norepinephrine (MHPG), and serotonin (5-HIAA) were significant in normal controls or patients. King et al. (1986), however, found a positive correlation between CSF dopamine levels and E from the EPI in depressed patients, and Lindström (1985) reported a positive correlation between nurses' ratings of social interest and the dopamine metabolite HVA in a group of drug-free schizophrenics.

Lowered CSF HVA is associated with psychomotor slowing in brain diseases such as Alzheimer's and Parkinson's disease as well as in depression, and CSF HVA is elevated in mania. The reason for this association is probably due to the origin of most of the CSF HVA. This dopamine metabolite is mostly derived from the caudate nucleus because of its size and proximity to the periventricular location (Willner, 1995). The primary dopamine tract that is theoretically associated with extraversion is the mesolimbic, including the nucleus accumbens and frontal cortex. This tract, however, contributes little to the metabolite accumulating in the brain's ventricular space and eventually the spinal cord from which it is extracted.

Parkinson's disease is caused by a severe diminishing of dopamine cells in the nigrostriatal tract and striatum (putamen and caudate). There is a long preclinical phase during which changes in personality are often noted. Depression is common, some of which may be due to reactions to the increasing motor impairment, and sometimes to cognitive loss and dementia (Korczyn, 1995). However, depression is more common in Parkinson's disease than in other chronic diseases sometimes involving even more physical impairment or threat of imminent death (Dakof & Mendelsohn, 1986). This finding raises the possibility that the depression and personality changes may result from the dopaminergic deficiency as well as disease reactive factors.

An interesting study of personality change in patients with Parkinson's disease compared their self and spousal ratings of their current status with the way they were before the development of the illness (Mendelsohn, Dakof, & Skaff, 1995). A healthy community control group matched in age was used as a control for the normal effects of aging. The mean duration of illness in the patients was 10 years.

In addition to expected self- and spouse-rated increases in neuroticism, abasement, and succorance (dependency), and decreases in self-confidence and personal adjustment, there also were decreases in extraversion, affiliation, dominance, achievement, and exhibitionism. There also were significant losses in other Big-Five dimensions, including agreeableness, conscientiousness, and openness. The community group also showed before-now changes in all Big-Five variables except agreeableness, but the changes were less pronounced. Dopaminergic neurons are reduced with age in normals but not as severely as in patients with Parkinson's disease. It is difficult to say how much of the changes in personality are due to the reactions to and limitations produced by the disease and the direct effects of dopamine loss on personality. It would be interesting to correlate the dopamine and personality changes.

Commenting on the role of disease in personality change, McCrae and Costa (2003) said: "Diseases of the heart or liver or lungs have substantial effects on people's lives, but they do not have permanent effects on personality. Diseases of the brain, however, often do" (p. 132).

As was the case for psychophysiological measures, activity in a resting unstimulated state seldom has any relationship to personality. However, studies that use drugs that are agonists or antagonists to the neurotransmitter and measure effects on the transmitter or behavioral effects have provided some more interesting findings.

Rammsayer, Netter, and Vogel (1993) used a drug that blocked dopamine synthesis. They found no difference between introverts and extraverts in dopaminergic activity or reactivity to the blocking agent. However, the treatment markedly impaired reaction times in introverts but not in extraverts. Rammsayer (1998) used a drug that selectively blocked D2 receptors and inhibited dopamine neurons and again found detrimental effects in introverts but not in extraverts.

Depue and his associates (Depue, Luciana, Arbisi, Collins, & Leon, 1994) used a potent agonist for dopamine at D2 receptor sites and measured the prolactin index of dopamine response and the activation of eye-blink response, another putative measure of dopamine reaction. The personality test used was the MPQ which has three factors: (1) positive emotionality (PEM, extraversion); (2) constraint (C); and (3) negative emotionality (NEM, neuroticism). Depue seemed to feel that the primary line of biological determinism ran between the PEM and C dimensions and therefore selected only 11 subjects who were high on PEM and low on C, or low on both traits. Within this small, highly selected sample, PEM correlated significantly and positively with the prolactin and eye-blink indices of dopaminergic reaction. C and NEM did not correlate with these indices. There were no relationships to baseline measures.

PET methodology has been used to study the density of D2 receptors in the brain. Farde, Gustavson, and Jönsson (1997) found a correlation between D2 receptor density and a scale of "detachment"; those scoring high on this scale had a low density of these receptors. Detachment involves the tendency to avoid involvement with other people, coldness, and social aloofness; however, it is not the same as normal introversion, because it involves the lack of any intimate friends and an indifference to people not found in normal introverts. It is suggestive of the type of schizoid tendencies involved in schizotypic personality or some types of schizophrenia.

In a follow-up study, Depue (1995) used a larger, unselected sample and included a prolactin measure of serotonergic as well as dopaminergic reaction. They included Eysenck's E, N, and P scales as well as the MPQ factor scores. The correlation of dopamine (prolactin) reaction with PEM was again significant, but the correlations with C, NEM and E, N, and P scales were not significant. The serotonergic response was not correlated significantly with any of these scales. Other relationships were found with measures of NEM, aggression, impulsivity, and sensation seeking; these will be discussed in later chapters.

Monoamine Oxidase (MAO)

MAO-type B is an enzyme involved in the catabolic deamination of monoamines, particularly dopamine (Murphy, Aulack, Garrick, & Sutherland, 1987). MAO can be assayed from blood platelets in humans, although its relationship to brain MAO is unclear and the assumption that it must be related to MAO, at least in some brain areas, is based on the many behavioral and trait correlates of platelet MAO.

A correlative study of MAO-B performed on monkeys living in a colony in a natural environment showed that monkeys with low MAO were more sociable, playful, dominant, aggressive, and sexually active, whereas monkeys with high MAO levels were more inactive, submissive, and socially isolated (Redmond, Murphy, & Baulu, 1979). It is not too anthropomorphic to describe them as Depue and Collin's (1999) did: "agentic extraversion." In humans, MAO-B has been frequently correlated (negatively) with sensation seeking but less consistently with extraversion (Zuckerman, 1991). Depue (1995), however, did find a significant negative correlation between PEM and MAO. On a more behavioral measure of sociability, the low MAO types in a normal population exceeded the high MAO types in self-reported time spent in social activities (Coursey, Buchsbaum, & Murphy, 1979). They also reported more risky activities such as smoking, drug use, and criminal behavior, suggesting a combination of extraversion with low constraint and high sensation seeking.

Testosterone

Both men and women produce testosterone, but men produce 10 times as much as women. Plasma testosterone is highly heritable in young adult males and moderately heritable in females (Harris, Vernon, & Boomsma, 1998). Testosterone in rats has reward effects in the nucleus accumbens, the major site of dopaminergic mediated reward. A dopamine blocker eliminates the rewarding effects of testosterone in rats suggesting that these effects are mediated through an interaction with dopamine in the mesolimbic system (Packard, Schroeder, & Gerianne, 1998).

Testosterone may account for some of the gender differences on personality traits. Although women are higher than men on sociability, warmth, and positive emotions, men are higher on the agentic type that includes assertiveness and excitement seeking (Costa, Terracino, & McCrae, 2001). These differences are found across cultures. Daitzman and Zuckerman (1980) found that testosterone in young males was correlated with extraversion, sociability, sensation seeking, social presence, dominance, and activity, and inversely correlated with introversion and socialization. Windle (1994) reported that testosterone was correlated with a scale of "behavioral activation" including "boldness, sociability, pleasure-seeking and rebelliousness." Dabbs (2000) found that testosterone is associated with a type of extraversion defined by high energy and activity and low responsibility. All findings indicate that testosterone in males influences a dimension that falls between extraversion and low constraint or high impulsive sensation seeking. This dimension might be described as agentic extraversion, except that it includes the irresponsibility, impulsivity, and sensation seeking that are not part of extraversion proper.

As mentioned in Chapter 2, there has been interest in the role of two peptides, oxytocin and vasopressin, as mediating social attachment (Insel, 1997). Nearly all of this research is based on animal experiments and natural observations. These peptides are made in the hypothalamus and secreted from the pituitary gland. They are found only in mammals. In certain species of voles, they serve the function of pair-bonding, parental nuturance, and infant attachment. There have not been enough studies of humans to say whether or not these peptides may play a role in sociability.

NEUROPSYCHOLOGY

The term "neuropsychology" is used in Gray's (1991) sense of the role of the brain in human or animal behavior or psychological processes, rather than in the description of the study of the psychological effects of brain damage in humans. Much of our knowledge of neuropsychology comes from the experimental study of other species, primarily rats, rather than the imprecise correlational studies of human brain damage and psychological and behavioral sequelae.

Eysenck (1967) localized the neurological substrate of extraversion in the physiological reactivity of the cortex and reticular activating system (RAS). This hypothesis led to the extensive research on cortical arousal and arousability described earlier in this chapter. Gray (1982, 1987, 1991), and most of those who followed him, worked on the assumption that extraversion was identified with the approach mechanism, sensitivity to stimuli associated with reward, and activity in pursuit of reward. In the area of emotions, extraversion is said to be associated with positive emotionality. The question, then, is what brain loci and tracts govern the behavioral and emotional tendencies?

A prime candidate for this function is the *mesolimbic dopamine system* beginning in the ventral tegmental area (VTA) and projecting to the nucleus accumbens (NA), other limbic areas including the amygdala, septum, and olfactory tubercle, and several forebrain areas, including lateral and medial prefrontal cortex (see Figures 2-17 and 3-3). The reason for the choice of this system as a prime candidate for extraversion is its identification as an area of primary reinforcement as indicated by studies of electrical brain self-stimulation. The VTA and NA also have been identified as the primary sites of action of drugs taken by humans to induce states of pleasurable arousal (Bozarth, 1987). Another dopaminergic pathway, the *nigrostriatal system*, also has been suggested as a substrate for extraversion. This system originates in the substantia nigra (A9) and projects to the neostriatum, including the putamen and caudate nucleus. Because this sytem is involved in the initiation and regulation of activity, and because the subtantia nigra and caudate also support brain stimulation (Stellar & Stellar, 1985), it is possible that this system is involved in the exploration and active pursuit of reward. I also have suggested that these systems may be involved in the trait of sensation seeking (Zuckerman, 1984, 1991, 1994).

Gray (1991) has elaborated on an interactive system in which the caudate encodes the motor program necessary to reach the potentially rewarding stimuli, the septo-hippocampal system checks the outcome of each motor

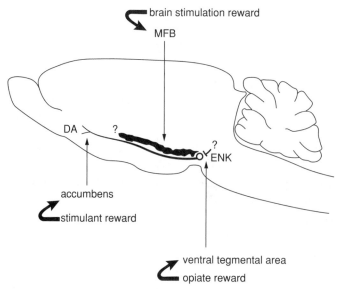

Figure 3-3. Proposed reward circuitry (Bozarth). Nucleus accumbens is the target of psychomotor stimulant reward and ventral tegmentum initiates reward action of opiates. The ventral tegmentum action of opiates probably involves enkaphalinergic system (ENK) whose anatomical location is not yet identified. Brain stimulation reward activates descending mylenated fibers within the medial forebrain system (MFB), which transsynaptically activate the ascending dopamine (DA) system. From "Ventral tegmental reward system," by M. A. Bozarth, 1987, in J. Engel et al. (Eds.), *Brain reward systems and abuse* (p. 13). New York: Raven Press. Copyright 1987 by Lippincott Williams & Wikins. Reprinted by permission.

step, and the prefrontal cortex coordinates the entire system. Apart from drugs, a source of intrinsic elation for humans, the mesolimbic dopamine system evolved in all species to provide the ultimate reinforcement (pleasure) for basic biological pursuits, particularly food and sex.

Depue and Collins (1999) outline a similar system with emphasis on other specific areas such as the basolateral complex of the amygdala, in stimulus reinforcement conditioning, and the medial orbital prefrontal area 13, involved in the integration of associations of reinforcement with both stimuli and responses.

Frith and Frith (2001) have used functional imaging studies in the exploration of "the biological basis of social interaction." These researchers stress what they called "mentalizing" or the capacity to make judgments about the mental states of others as a necessary basis for real social interactions. Autistic children who lack this ability often cannot engage in meaningful interactions with others, even those closest to them. Frith and Frith's experiments are brain-imaging studies in which subjects perform simple tasks requiring the judgment of mental states in others such as pain, emotions, and thoughts. During such tasks, changes are found in the most anterior part of the anterior cingulate cortex. The same area is activated when subjects judge their own mental states. This suggests that the area could serve the function of empathy. Cells in this area are selectively involved in stimulus recognition as well as in affective properties of painful stimuli (Hutchinson, 1999).

The cingulum is the major pathway between the frontal cortex and the limbic system. The most anterior part is activated by tasks with an emotional content; the next area is activated by complex decision and decision tasks. The sites activated by the emotional recognition tasks fall between these two. Three of the imaging studies discussed earlier showed a relationship between activation of the cingulate and extraversion (Ebmeier et al., 1994; Haier et al., 1987; Johnson et al., 1999). However, reports on the effects of cingulotomies in human patients showed reductions on the EPI scale for neuroticism but no change on the scale for extraversion (Laitinan & Vilki, 1973; Mitchell-Heggs, Kelly, & Richardson, 1976).

Many brain areas are involved in the ability to recognize and react to emotional expressions in others (Preston & de Waal, 2002). But is empathy a necessary precondition for extraversion or sociability? It would certainly seem so for autistic children. But a lack of genuine empathy in antisocial personalities seems compatible with a high degree of extraversion. In agentic extraversion, the need to dominate others may not be accompanied by a high degree of empathy with them. The manipulative psychopath may be capable of recognizing emotional reactions in others and even use this ability to control them but may not experience any empathy with their feelings.

It is obvious that the psychopharmacology or neuropsychology of extraversion depends on how broadly or narrowly this trait is defined and what subtraits are included in the definition. In the past, impulsivity was part of extraversion, as defined by Eysenck, but realignment of the subtraits after the introduction of the third dimension – psychoticism – made it less salient compared to sociability. Analysis of some of the literature has suggested that biological traits, and even conditioning (Eysenck & Levey, 1972), are more closely related to impulsivity than to sociability. Gray (1987) places the main biological line of influence in impulsivity, defined as both high E and P.

SUMMARY

Extraversion is defined in broad and narrow senses. The most narrow is largely limited to sociability. The broad definition can include many different subtraits such as assertiveness, warmth, positive emotions, activity, and traits others regard as other major dimensions of personality, such as sensation seeking and activity (Zuckerman et al., 1988, 1991). Although correlations between narrow and broadly defined traits are high, the psychobiological correlates may be limited to one or another of the subtraits and not to the others. The tendency to approach novel objects or strange persons and general activity may be the temperamental origin of extraversion in infants and young children, although other factors such as fearfulness and sensation seeking also may be influences in these behavioral traits.

Heritabilities of extraversion depend on the type of study (twin vs. siblings or child-parent), definition of extraversion, age (young children vs. adults) and method of observation (self-report questionnaires, parental, peer, observer ratings, or behavioral indices). Studies of twins raised together show heritabilities of .4 to .6 with no effect of shared environment and the remainder due to nonshared environment and errors of measurement. Adults show higher heritabilities than young children. Nontwin adoption studies yield lower heritabilities than twin studies. Heritabilities derived from behavioral observations are just as high as those based on self-report methods. Heritabilities of subtraits are due in part to a shared genetic factor, but they also show some specific genetic influences not shared with other subtraits. Siblings raised in the same family but biologically unrelated and adoptive parents and their adopted children show no correlation on extraversion, supporting the conclusion that shared environment has little or no effect on this trait. Studies of protypical temperament traits related to extraversion, such as approach, positive affect, and activity, show significant heritabilities at the ages at which they are clearly observable. One study showed a relation of some of the subtraits associated with extraversion, warmth, positive emotions, excitement seeking, and presence of one form of the D4 dopamine receptor gene, but this was not replicated.

Much of the research on the physiological basis of extraversion has been stimulated by Eysenck's theory that extraverts are less cortically aroused than introverts. EEG studies, even recent ones, have shown a very weak but significant relationship between EEG indices of arousal during nonstimulated or weakly stimulated conditions and extraversion, particularly the surgent type. The hypothesis has been confirmed in some, but not all, studies using new brain imaging methods, particularly for activation in the temporal lobes, but also for subcortical areas such as the striate areas and the cingulum.

Studies of arousability, using cortical evoked potentials (EP), tend to show more arousability for introverts than extraverts at low intensities of stimulation but often a reversal at higher intensities, where extraverts show higher EP amplitudes. The EP differences have been found with subcortical sites such as the brainstem EP, and even in spinal motorneuronal reflexes. Some studies show an interaction of extraversion and neuroticism in influencing the cortical EP response. Other studies show an influence of stimulus significance. These latter studies are compatible with Gray's theory about sensitivities to stimuli associated with reward or punishment as characteristics of extraversion and neuroticism.

Eysenck never got far beyond psychophysiology in his theory of extraversion, but "bottom-up" theorists such as Gray and others have suggested that the neurotransmitter dopamine is involved in extraversion, particularly of the surgent or "agentic" type. Studies simply correlating levels of the dopamine metabolite with extraversion have not shown any significant associations. Studies stimulating the dopaminergic systems, however, have shown some relationships between extraversion and dopamine as indicated by dopamine influenced behavior, such as reaction time and eye-blink responses. It is arguable, however, where the major influence of dopaminergic reactivity lies among the major trait dimensions.

Monoamine oxidase type B (MAO-B) is selectively involved in the deamination or regulation of dopamine, in contrast to MAO-type A, which metabolizes all three monoamines. Many behavioral and psychopathological correlates of MAO-B obtained from blood platelets have been found in primates and humans. Among these is sociability, as judged from behavioral rather than self-report trait measures. Sociable monkeys and people tend to have lower MAO levels than unsociable types. This could indicate a dysregulation of the dopaminergic system with higher reactivity to strong stimuli. They also engage in many types of risky behaviors associated with sensation seeking. The hormone testosterone also has been associated with extraversion of the surgent type and sensation seeking.

Phrenology was a pseudoscience of the 19th century that attempted to localize character traits in different areas of the brain. Modern neuropsychology differs in several respects from this older "science." Above all, it is based largely on experimental studies of brain ablation and stimulation performed on other species, and less precise correlational studies of human brain damage. It also stresses the important role of the subcortical limbic systems in the motivational and emotional mechanisms involved in personality. The ascending dopamine mediated systems, in particular, have been assigned a primary role in exploration, approach behavior, positive emotionality, activity, and novelty seeking. Other areas, such as parts of the amygdala, the cingulum, and the prefrontal cortex, have been suggested as loci within the tracts governing approach behavior. Interactions with other areas regulating inhibition, such as the septal-hippocampal one, interact with approach pathways so that behavior is an outcome of the relative strengths of both systems. At one extreme, with a strong approach system and a weak inhibitory one, you have impulsivity. At the other extreme, with a weak approach and a strong inhibitory system, you have anxiety.

Progress has been made in trying to define the psychobiology of extraversion since the last version of this story (Zuckerman, 1991). This has been largely due to advances in methodology, such as brain imaging methods and new ways to assess neurotransmitter reactivity other than through imprecise metabolic methods. However, there is still a weakness in the story. The main theories are still largely derived from research on other species, primarily the rat. Rats are not particularly sociable creatures compared to primates and therefore not the ideal model to assess extraversion. The extrapolation from these models to human extraversion is difficult and much depends on the type of extraversion. The surgent or agentic extraversion is based on traits more common in rats, such as dominance and exploration. The rat model is more appropriate for the next trait to be discussed (neuroticism). Neuroticism forms a tight factor defined primarily by the negative affects of anxiety and depression. Fear or anxiety has been studied widely in comparative research (e.g., Gray, 1982). Although the stimuli (or cognitions) eliciting anxiety may be quite different in humans and animals, it is likely that this evolved emotional mechanism is quite similar in its response systems in the brain, peripheral autonomic system, and endocrine glands.

CHAPTER 4

Neuroticism

The concept of neuroticism as a temperament can be traced back to the ancient Greek physicians Hippocrates and Galen. Their descriptions of the melancholic temperament included symptoms of depression and anxiety and social withdrawal. Both attributed the disorder to both an organic basis (an excess of black bile) and to an environmental one. Hippocrates said that melancholia could be precipitated by loss of love or conflict and guilt, whereas Galen, anticipating Freud by 18 centuries, suggested it could be due to blocked sexual outlet. In his early theory, Freud also ascribed pure anxiety states (panic disorder) to the tension generated by sexual frustration.

Freud regarded neurosis on a continuum lying between neurotic character and psychosis, depending on the extent of regression due to conflict between ego and id impulses. The concept of neurosis as a disorder suggested that it could be a temporary condition rather than a basic personality dimension. Freud included hysteria among the psychoneuroses, attributing differences between it and disorders such as anxiety and obsessive-compulsive to different levels of psychosexual fixation.

During the 19th century, a number of psychiatrists, including Jung, distinguished between "psychasthenic" and hysterical disorders on the basis of a second dimension of personality, extraversion-introversion. Eysenck (1947), whose early research used mental patients as subjects, regarded the "dysthymic" (anxious and depressed) types as introverted neurotics, and the hysteric and psychopathic types as extraverted neurotics. He defined neuroticism as a basic dimension of personality that could be regarded as going from extreme emotional stability at one end to emotional instability at the other. His explanations included genetic and physiological causes resulting in a special susceptibility to conditioning rather than traumatic childhood experiences or conflicts over sex and aggression.

Based on his theory, Eysenck developed scales designed to measure neuroticism and extraversion as *independent* dimensions of personality. The trait definition of neuroticism includes: anxiety, depression, guilt, low self-esteem, tension, irrationality, shyness, moodiness, and unstable emotionality (Eysenck & Eysenck, 1985).

Nearly every other system of personality classification has included a dimension of neuroticism, even though it may be called something else. Costa and McCrae's (1992) Big-Five measure of neuroticism includes facet scales for anxiety, angry hostility, depression, self-consciousness, impulsiveness, and vulnerability. Tellegen's (1985) negative emotionality includes: stress reaction, alienation, and aggression. Cloninger's (1987) harm avoidance is a mixture of neuroticism and extraversion with facets of worry versus optimism, fear of uncertainty versus confidence, shyness versus gregariousness, and fatiguability versus vigor. Despite differences in the makeup of subscales for the neuroticism factor, they tend to intercorrelate very highly and all have a tight factor structure (Zuckerman et al., 1993). The core of the factor is the negative emotions of anxiety and depression. In fact, scales of trait anxiety and neuroticism correlate as highly as their reliabilities allow. The inclusion of anger or hostility is more problematic since in some five-factor models, this kind of emotion tends to load more highly on a dimension of aggression (Zuckerman et al., 1999).

Temperament scales for infants and young children usually include a factor of negative emotionality, for example, quality of mood or difficult temperament (Thomas & Chess, 1977); negative emotionality (Rothbart et al., 1994); emotionality (Buss & Plomin, 1975, 1984); emotional reactivity (Strelau & Zawadzki, 1993); social fearfulness (Goldsmith & Campos, 1986); and inhibited temperament (Kagan, 1989). Longitudinal studies have shown that such scales of neuroticism at early ages predict adolescent and adult anxiety and unipolar mood disorders or other evidence of the persistence of the temperamental predisposition (e.g., Caspi, Moffitt, Newman, & Silva, 1996; Chess & Thomas, 1984; Kagan, 1994; Kagan & Moss, 1962).

Neuroticism scores can vary considerably during certain stressful periods of life. This is not surprising given the high correlation between measures of the negative affects of anxiety and depression and neuroticism. How then can neuroticism be regarded as a reliable trait measure? The answer lies in the trait-state relationship that I reviewed in the first edition of this book (Zuckerman, 1991). Measurement of state anxiety or depression on a single day is not very reliable or predictable from the trait measure, but when state measures are aggregated over more days they become reliable and trait measures are highly predictive of the average level of state measures (Epstein, 1979; Zuckerman, 1976). If the measure of neuroticism was totally unreliable then we could not hope to find much heritability as an influence. Remember that in calculation of heritability the error variance is included with the specific environmental influence as a residual term.

GENETICS

The studies reviewed in the subsequent tables are the same as those used for extraversion in the preceding chapter. This makes the comparisons between the genetics of extraversion and neuroticism more equivalent. In most cases, both traits were assessed from the same test instruments.

Table 4-1 shows the results on large studies of twins raised together. The results are remarkably uniform considering that the studies were done in many countries with subjects of different ages and using different methods. Identical twin correlations range from .36 to .53 but most are in the .4–.5 range. Fraternal twin correlations range from .06 to .25 with most in the .17 to .25 range. Heritabilities by either method are generally in the .4–.5 range. These heritabilities are somewhat lower than those for extraversion which are mostly in the .5–.6 range. There is only one subgroup (older males in the Loehlin and Martin [2001] study) in which the correlation for fraternal twins exceeded half the correlation for identical twins, probably an unreliable result because of the low ns in this group. Thus, there is little evidence of shared environment and most of the results in studies that use modeling assessments bear this out. Nearly all studies show that additive genetic mechanisms are sufficient to account for the data, but Rieman et al. (1997) found that peer ratings yielded a MZ correlation of .41 and a DZ correlation of .01, which could be accounted for by nonadditive mechanisms.

The joint Canadian and German twin study analyzed the genetic factors among the facets of each of the Big-Five factors (Jang, Livesley, Angleitner, Riemann, & Vernon, 2002). Within the broad factor of neuroticism, described as "distress," there were two genetic factors. One included all the facets except angry-hostility and impulsivity, whereas the other consisted mainly of angry-hostility. In the alternative five-factor model (Zuckerman, 1991), angry-hostility constitutes an aggressive-hostility factor, distinct from neuroticism, and impulsivity is part of the impulsive sensation seeking factor.

Anxiety and depression are highly correlated factors within the broader N factor. In the realm of psychopathology there is a great deal of "comorbidity" between mood and anxiety disorders (Zuckerman, 1999). Eley (1997) attempted to answer the question of how much of the correlation between depression and anxiety is due to genetic factors. The answer from a twin study of children and adolescents is 80%, with the rest due to shared environment.

Table 4-1. Adolescent or adult twins: correlations and heritabilities on neuroticism

Study	Population	Test/Subjects	Correlations		Heritability	
			MZ r	DZ r	Fal.h^2	Mo.h^2
Eaves et al. 1989	22 Studies before 1976	EPI	.44	.22	.44	.42
Zuckerman (1991)	7 studies 1976–1988	various nations, ages	.46	.22	.46	–
Jang et al. (1996)	Canadian	NEO-PI-R	.41	.18	.46	.41
Rieman et al. (1997)	German	NEO	.53	.13	.53	.52
Loehlin & Martin (2001)	Australian	Sex/Age				
		Males-Young	.36	.18	.36	
		Middle	.38	.02	.39	
		Old	.27	.24	.06	Total: .40
		Female Young	.37	.11	.37	
		Middle	.44	.25	.38	
		Old	.44	.19	.44	
Saudino et al. (1999)	Russian	EPI-Short	.48	.23	.48	.49
Loehlin et al. (1998)	American					
		self-ratings	.43	.17	.43	overall .58
		CPI	.53	.25	.53	
		ACL	.44	.06	.44	

Note: Because the heritability cannot exceed the correlation for MZ twins the h^2 is given as the MZ r when the formula ($2 \times$ MZ r – DZ r) result exceeds the MZ r.

Fal h^2 = heritability from the Falconer formula. Mo. h^2 = heritability from model testing; NEO = Neuroticism, Extraversion, Openness Questionnaire. EPQ = Eysenck Personality Questionnaire; EPI = Eysenck Personality Inventory; CPI = California Personality Inventory; ACL = Gough's Adjective Check List.

Table 4-2. Twin correlations and heritabilities for emotional stability based on three methods

Method	MZ r	DZ r	h^2	se^2	nse^2
video-based ratings	.61	.38	.62	.00	.38
self-report ratings	.40	.26	.27	.12	.61
average peer ratings	.38	.02	.33	.00	.67

Note: Data from Borkenau, Rieman, Angleitner, & Spinath (2001)
h^2 = proportion of variance due to genetics; se^2 = proportion of variance due to shared environment; nse^2 = proportion of variance due to nonshared environment.

Table 4-2 shows the results from the study by Borkenau et al. (2001), which used three different methods to assess emotional stability: video-based ratings, self-reports, and average peer ratings. The video-based observational ratings yielded the highest heritability, .62, the averaged peer ratings were next highest (.33) and the self ratings were lowest (.27). The video-based ratings and the averaged peer ratings showed no evidence of an influence from shared environment, but the self-report showed a small but significant influence (12%) compared to the much larger influence of nonshared environment. The results clearly refute the claim that heritability of personality traits is unique to self-ratings. In fact, the highly reliable ratings based on actual behavior recorded during a single day across multiple settings showed a considerably higher heritability than the self ratings.

Table 4-3 shows the results from the four studies comparing twins raised together and apart. If we took the results from the MZ twins raised apart as the heritabilities there are two diverse findings. In the studies by Bouchard

Table 4-3. Correlations of neuroticism of twins raised together (T) and apart (A)

Study/Test	Country	MZ-T	MZ-A	DZ-T	DZ-A
Shields (1962)/MPI	UK	.38	.53	–	–
Pederson et al. (1988)/ EPI short form	Sweden	.41	.25	.24	.28
Langinvainio et al. (1984) EPI short form	Finland	.32	.25	.10	.11
Bouchard (1993)/MPQ/ CPI	USA	.46	.53	.17	.41
		.50	.55	.05	.16

Note: MPI = Maudsley Personality Inventory; EPI = Eysenck Personality Inventory; MPQ = Multidimensional Personality Questionnaire; CPI = California Personality Inventory. Adapted from table 3.7, p 54 in *Genes and Environment In Personality, Development*, J. C. Loehlin (1992) Newbury Park, CA: Sage, reprinted by permission.

Table 4-4. Correlations on neuroticism of children and biological and adoptive parents

Study/Test	Father-Biol. child	Mother-Biol. child	Father-adoptive child	Mother-adoptive child	Biol. related siblings	Adoptive related siblings
Loehlin et al. (1985) CPI-N	−.13	.01	.16	−.03	−.12	.09
Scarr et al. (1981) EPI-N	.14	.21	−.09	.12	.28	.05
Eaves et al. (1989) EPQ-N	.10	.13	.21	−.03	.04	.23

The table is adapted from *Genes and environment in personality development*, Table 3.5, p. 53, by J. C. Loehlin (1992) Newbury Park: CA: Sage. Reprinted by permission.

(1993) and Shields (1962), there were significant heritabilities (.53 to .55). But in the Scandinavian studies the correlations for MZ twins reared apart were only .25 and lower than those for twins reared together, indicating some influence of shared environment. However, these differences were not found in the DZ twins raised together and apart. The findings are heterogeneous and could be because of the types of scales used in the studies. The Scandinavian studies used shorter scales with less reliability than the British and American studies.

Table 4-4 shows the correlations for parent-child and siblings comparing those with the biological parents and siblings, with those from the adoptive relationships. As with the adoptive twin studies, the results are significantly heterogeneous from study to study. Most correlations are quite low for all types of relationships. In two of the studies (Loehlin et al., 1985; Eaves et al., 1989), the correlations between children and adopted fathers are somewhat higher than those for children and their biological fathers, possibly indicating some effect of shared environment. But among siblings, one study (Scarr et al., 1981) shows a higher correlation for biologically related siblings as contrasted with that for adoptively related siblings, whereas another (Eaves et al., 1989) shows the reverse. Differences were negligible in the third study (Loehlin et al.). Low negative correlations in these studies should be regarded as non-significant deviations from zero.

Table 4-5 shows the correlations of biologically and adoptively related parents and children from the study by Plomin et al. (1991). In this study, there were practically no significant correlations between children and their

Table 4-5. Parent-offspring correlations on emotionality for EASI temperaments for biological, adoptive and nonadoptive parents

Age	Biological		Adoptive		Nonadoptive	
	Mother	Father	Mother	Father	Mother	Father
1	.04	−.11	.13*	.10	.03	.15*
2	.01	−.02	.18*	.04	.05	.09
3	−.04	.10	.18*	.03	.08	.06
4	−.04	.03	.14*	−.03	.11	.03
5	.03	−.02	.06	.11	.01	.14*
6	.02	−.04	.12	.00	−.14	.13
7	.17*	.08	.14*	−.05	−.01	.12
1–7 mean	.02	.00	.17*	.05	.09	.11*

Source: Plomin, Coon, Carey, DeFries, & Fulker (1991), Tables 1 and 2, pp. 69–70. Copyright 1991 by Duke University Press. Reprinted by permission.

biological parents between the ages of 1 and 7. Children did show some low but significant correlations in emotionality with their adopted mothers at ages 1 to 4 and at age 7. There were no correlations with their adopted fathers. In nonadoptive family relationships, combining both social and genetic influences, the only significant correlations found were between children and their fathers.

Sibling correlations were inconsistent. Nonadoptive siblings had a significant correlation at 1 year of age and adoptive siblings had one at 4 years of age. All other correlations were nonsignificant. The correlations of adoptive siblings increased steadily from 1 year to 4 years of age. Sibling influences might be expected to increase with age during early childhood.

In the study by Scarr et al. (1981), the mid-parent correlation with biologically related children was only .25 on EPI N and the sibling correlation was only .28. These correlations reflect the total narrow (additive) heritability. The mid-parent correlations with adoptive parents were close to zero.

What is surprising in these studies is the low correlations between children and parents in nonadoption families in which the biological and social influences are combined. This is not uncommon in other studies, such as that by Ahearn, Johnson, McClearn and Vandenberg (1982), comparing adolescent children and their parents. Correlations between parents and children on the EPI N scale were .12 for child and father, .11 for child and mother, and .07 for siblings. Although all of these correlations were significant because of the large *n*, they were quite low.

Table 4-6 shows the correlations of twins on temperament scales on four studies of children ages 6 to 10. Torgersen (1985) used ratings of mood, based

Table 4-6. Correlations of temperament ratings relevant to neuroticism in twins 5–10 years of age

Study/Temperament Scale	Age of Twins	MZ r	DZ r	h^2
Torgerson (1985)/Mood	6	.37	−.06	.37
Goldsmith & Gottesman (1981)/ Fearful-Inhibited	7	.36	.21	.30
Buss & Plomin (1984)/ Emotionality	5	.63	.12	.63
Matheny & Dolan (1980)/ Emotionality	7–10	.45	−.11	.45

on interviews with parents, from the Thomas and Chess (1977) system; Goldsmith and Gottesman (1981) employed the fearful-inhibited scale from the Bayley (1969) Infant Behavior Record; and Buss and Plomin (1984) and Matheny and Dolan (1980) used parental ratings on the emotionality scale developed by Buss and Plomin (1975). Heritabilities were in the .37 to .63 range, but three of the four were in the .37 to .45 range.

Molecular Genetics

The search for a gene involved in trait anxiety or neuroticism has concentrated largely on a serotonin transporter gene. Serotonin is a neurotransmitter highly involved in the regulation of emotion in the brains of humans, primates and other mammals. It also regulates the activity of several other neurotransmitter systems.

Selective serotonin reuptake inhibitors (SSRIs), which potentiate serotonergic activity, have therapeutic value for both depressive disorders (Montgomery, 1995) and certain types of anxiety disorders including panic, obsessive-compulsive, and mixed anxiety and depressive disorders (Shader & Greenblatt, 1995). A major theory of depression suggests that low serotonergic activity is either a proximate cause or a vulnerability factor in these disorders (Maes & Meltzer, 1995). Serotonin regulates many of the vital functions affected by depression including appetite, sleep, activity, and sexual function. Serotonin deficits are found in those who have committed impulsive and violent suicides or homicides, driven by uncontrolled dysphoric anger or desperation (Åsberg, Träskman & Thorén, 1976; Mann, 1995; New, Goodman, Mitropoulou, & Siever, 2002).

The action of serotonin (5-hydroxytryptamine or 5-HT) is terminated by the 5-HT transporter (5-HTT) that facilitates the reuptake process. Reuptake inhibitors block uptake by binding to the transporter protein. 5-HTT is the prime modulator of the serotonergic system.

Human 5-HTT is governed by a single gene with both long and short variants. Transcriptional activity of the gene is modulated at a gene-linked region close on the chromosone (5-HTTLPR). The latter is found only in humans and simian primates. The majority of alleles contain either 14 (short) or 16 (long) repeat sequences. The population genotypes are distributed 32% long/long, 49% long/short, and 19% short/short (Lesch et al., 1996). Cells homozygous for the long form (l/l) produce higher concentrations of 5-HTT messenger RNA (mRNA) than cells homozygous for the short form (s/s) or heterozygous (s/l). As a consequence, 5-HT uptake is two times higher in cells containing the l/l form than in either of the other two types (s/s, s/l). A PET study showed that the short form is associated with lower 5HTT genotype expression and function (Heinz et al., 1999).

Bennett et al. (2001) studied the expression of the genotype in rhesus monkeys from two groups: those reared with their peer and those reared with their mothers. The peer-reared show many behavioral abnormalities not shown by the mother-reared infants. The peer-reared monkeys with the long homozygous form of the genotype showed an increased CSF 5-HIAA, whereas those with the short alleles exhibited a decrease in the serotonin metabolite. Among the mother-reared monkeys, there was little effect of the genotype difference. The expression of the genotype seems to depend on prolonged early experience. It is reassuring to find that mother care does make a difference in view of the current trend among nondynamic psychologists to minimize its importance.

Lesch et al. (1996) compared the subjects with the different forms of the 5-HTTLPR genotype on the five factors of the NEO-PI-R. Subjects with either one (s/l) or two (s/s) copies of the short form had higher levels of Neuroticism than those homozygous for the long form (l/l). Those with either short form did not differ on N. A dominant-recessive influence was suggested by the biological and psychological distributions with the short form dominant. The result for N was confirmed by a within family sibling-analysis. Those facets of N showing the significant effect were: anxiety, angry-hostility, and impulsiveness. Results were similar using Cattell's 16PF inventory anxiety factor and Cloninger's TPQ harm-avoidance scale, both of which also showed a significant association with the 5-HTTLPR genotype.

There were no differences between the genotypes on the Extraversion, Conscientiousness, or Openness factors of the NEO, but Agreeableness was also higher in those homozygous for the long form of the 5-HTTLPR; this was a weaker effect and only significant in the combined group.

The transporter polymorphism accounted for only 3–4% of the total variance of N and 7–9% of the genetic variance, suggesting that perhaps 10 to 15 other genes might be involved.

The seminal findings from the Lesch et al. study set off another great gene hunt. Positive findings in the field of molecular genetics usually trigger a spate of replication attempts. Lesch and his colleagues (Lesch, Greenberg, Higley, Bennett, & Murphy, 2002) reviewed 19 subsequent studies.

The research group was quite successful in replicating its own results in a second study, but in 12 of the 18 remaining studies other investigators could not obtain significant results. Lesch et al. (2002) suggest that most of these studies used smaller numbers of subjects and therefore had weaker power to detect the differences. But of the two other large studies neither found significant relationships using the association method and one found results only for the within family design and with only two of the subscales for N and not for the total N score.

A large-scale study (634 subjects) contrasted subjects with the long and short forms of the 5-HTTLPR using both Cloninger's TCI and Costa and McCrea's NEO to assess personality traits (Hamer, Greenberg, Sabol, & Murphy, 1999). The gene variants were not associated with the TCI harm avoidance or any of its facets but were significantly associated with reward dependence, self-directiveness, and cooperativeness. Those with the homozygous long form were higher on these traits than those with the short form of the gene. On the NEO, however, the genotype was related to neuroticism and agreeableness. Neuroticism was higher and agreeableness was lower in those with the short-form genotype. But these correlations and variance accounted for were very low. The results suggest less a clean-cut correspondence between the genotype and N or HA specifically than a relationship with neurotic or anxious hostility (low agreeableness and cooperativeness).

A recent large study found that both the short allele of the 5-HTTLPR *and* a GABA(A) receptor variant (Pro385 Ser) were associated with neuroticism, as measured by the NEO-N, and its subscales for anxiety, hostility, and depression (Sen et al., 2004). The longer allele was associated with agreeableness and alcohol use. The connection between serotonin and GABA is interesting in view of the fact that most serotonin axons in the brain connect with cortical GABAnergic interneurons.

There is a curious disconnection between the results from these studies and those from the clinical literature. Most studies of depression and the therapeutic effects of SSRIs, as well as a study giving an SSRI to healthy normals (Knutson et al., 1998), suggest that *low* levels of serotonin are associated with anxiety. In the genetic studies, however, it is *low* levels of uptake, and high levels of activity, which are associated with anxiety.

A study of rhesus monkeys produced an interesting interaction (Bennett et al., 2001). In monkeys who were mother-reared, there was no difference in levels of the serotonin metabolite 5-HIAA in CSF. But in monkeys reared in the more deleterious mother-absent condition those with the shorter allele had lower CSF 5-HIAA levels than those with the longer alleles.

Another study by this group showed that infant monkeys with the short form were more distressed during an examination regardless of rearing condition (Champoux et al., 2002). These results were similar to an association between genotype and negative emotionality found in human infants (Ebstein & Auerbach, 2002). Monkeys with the short form showed a deficit in orienting to a novel stimulus (a Mickey Mouse face), but this difference was only found in the peer-reared group and not in the mother-reared group. In human infants the short form also was associated with distress when presented with sudden or novel stimuli, particularly when they also lacked the long form of the DRD4 allele.

It seems that the transporter gene is most strongly and consistently related to certain types of N, those involving anger, hostility, and impulsiveness, and lack of agreeableness. Jang et al. (2001) found that 10% of the covariance between N and agreeableness was attributable to the serotonin transporter genotype, and this was largely due to the angry-hostility and impulsivity components of the N factor.

Experimental affect differences between the homozygous long form group and those subjects with the short forms (either s/s or s/l) were demonstrated by Hariri et al. (2002). The subjects were exposed to fearful or angry faces in the context of an emotional recognition task, while the brain was imaged using the fMRI. This kind of emotional processing has been shown to affect the amygdala, specifically the right amygdala. The subjects with the short forms of the gene showed significantly greater activation of the right amygdala during presentation of the emotional stimuli. Actually, no distinction is made between the responses to fearful and angry stimuli in the report. The two genotype groups did not differ on anxiety-related traits on the TPI. A similar experiment using the fMRI found "robust activation" of the amygdala and medial prefrontal cortex associated with aversiveness of slides (Phan et al., 2003).

The gene controlling the enzyme tyrosine hydroxlase, involved in the biosynthesis of the catecholamines (dopamine, norepinephrine, and epinephrine) also has been related to neuroticism and other traits. The TCAT repeat polymorphism has five main alleles T6, T7, T8, T9, and T10, numbers representing the number of repeats of the base sequence. The T8 allele has been associated with CSF levels of MHPG, the norepinephrine metabolite (Jönsson et al., 1996). Clinical studies of the T8 allele have shown increased prevalence of those with T8 among groups often showing high levels of anxiety and depression, suicide attempters, and adjustment disorders. Persson et al. (2000) found an association between the T8 allele and and the Neuroticism factor in the NEO-PI-R and with two of the six facets of the factor: angry-hostility and vulnerability.

Summary

The broad heritabilities for neuroticism based on twin studies lie mostly in the .4 to .5 range, somewhat lower than those for extraversion. There is practically no evidence of an influence of shared environment; non-shared environment is the most powerful influence. This latter influence could be the events and influences that occur outside of the home. Of course, these events also are influenced by genetics (Chipeur, Plomin, Pederson, McClearn, & Nesselroade, 1993). Children choose their own interactions and activities outside of the home, in part, as a function of their temperaments.

There is practically no evidence for nonadditive genetic factors, unlike extraversion, where there was some. Neuroticism has been defined in broad and narrow ways. Analyses of the subfactors in neuroticism in the NEO suggests the presence of two different genetic factors: angry-hostility versus everything else, such as anxiety and depression, except impulsivity. There is the possibility that some of the traits within the broad factor combine different factors based on their genetics. If we are to "carve nature at its joints," we should start with the genetic definition of factors rather than the phenotype.

The methods of assessment can influence the heritabilities. Peer ratings and behavioral observations yield as high heritabilites as do self-report methods, but different quantitative results are obtained from different self-report methods.

Narrow heritabilities obtained from parent-child or sibling correlations are not as high as those obtained from twin studies. The results of nontwin adoption studies have various heterogenous results. In general, there is little or weak correlation of children with either biological or adoptive parents. In some studies, the adopted parents' correlations with children are significant and those with the biological parents are not, but in other studies the reverse is true. Age may interact in complex ways with the findings. Shared environment may be more important at earlier ages where the family is the major influence, but genetics may become more important as the child begins to be subjected to more extra-family influences and makes more choices as to who may influence her. Heritabilities based on temperament ratings of children by their parents yield heritabilities in the same range as those for adolescents and adults based on questionnaires.

Molecular genetic studies have found a major gene, that for the serotonin transporter, involved in neuroticism and trait anxiety. Replications of the initial study, however, have not been universally successful. Still, clinical and neuropsychological studies suggest a role for serotonin, and its regulating factors, like those that affect uptake, in a trait of neuroticism or a subtype of neuroticism (in some classifications) such as angry-hostility.

Another gene, that controlling the enzyme tyrosine hydroxylase, has been associated with neuroticism. This gene affects the production of the catecholamines and seems to have some relationship with norepinephrine in particular. The angry-hostility and depression types of neuroticism and vulnerability to stress seem to be central to the relationship with the gene.

One of the promises of molecular genetics is that it will point to the crucial biological interactions underlying traits. From the early genetic studies of neuroticism, we can see hints of the neuropsychological processes, such as emotion processing in the amygdala, and pharmacological factors, such as serotonin and norepinephrine, which may explain what we inherit that predisposes toward neuroticism or emotional stability. The results have significance for the disorders based on this dimension of personality.

PSYCHOPHYSIOLOGY

Cortical Arousal

Eysenck's theory (1967) of cortical arousal was primarily centered around extraversion; however, neuroticism was assumed to affect cortical arousal through collaterals between the limbic systems concerned with emotions and the reticular activating system that regulates cortical arousal. In other words, neuroticism may interact positively with introversion to augment the cortical arousal or arousability typical of the latter trait. Some investigators chose to confine their studies to E, ignoring or controlling N in the process. Those who analyzed both E and N sometimes found an independent effect of N or an interaction between the two traits. In a spectrum analysis one would expect to find an excess of fast-wave beta activity in those high on N, because this type of activity is associated with tension and fear, or a lack of alpha activity associated with more relaxed states.

Table 4-7 shows the effects of N in studies where it was assessed. Matthews and Amelang (1993) found a low but significant correlation ($r = .16$) between beta and the N scale from the EPQ and no interaction between E and N. Ivashenko et al. (1999) found that high N was associated with a higher frequency in the beta range during conditions of quiet wakefulness. Knyazev, Slobodskaya, and Wilson (2002) also found that N type scales correlated with beta and high frequency beta (gamma) in frontal areas and greater relative right hemisphere activation. Stenberg (1992) reported that trait anxiety was associated with more beta activity in temporal lobes during negative emotionally arousing conditions but also more right frontal theta activity under all conditions. Schmidt (1999) found shyness (a trait combining high N and low E) was related to relatively greater right frontal EEG activity relative to left frontal activity, but Tran et al. (2001) found no differences in EEG activity at frontal sites.

A study of infant temperament starting with infants at 4 months and following them to 11 years of age used classification of infants and young children as reactive (shy, timid, fearful) in response to unfamiliar events or strangers, or nonreactive. At 11 years of age, the reactives showed greater EEG activation in right frontal and parietal areas than in left hemisphere areas (Fox, 1991; Kagan & Snidman, 1999; McManis et al., 2002).

There is a weak but significant relationship between N and EEG fast wave activity, particularly at frontal and temporal lobe sites, during conditions of negative emotion arousal. Several studies suggest stronger activation of right hemisphere cortical areas in those high on neuroticism.

The theories of Gray (1982), Costa and McCrae (1992), Tellegen (1985), and Zuckerman (1991) identify the neuroticism trait primarily with negative emotions. A number of studies have shown that extraversion is primarily related to positive affect and neuroticism to negative affect.

Davidson (1992, 2002) theorizes that right hemisphere is more activated during negative emotions relative to left hemisphere activation in positive emotions. He suggests that positive affect is linked to an approach system and negative affect to a withdrawal system. Davidson (2002) summarized a number of studies supporting the lateralization theory concerning right hemisphere asymmetry and negative emotionality. In human infants those with greater right-sided activation are observed to be more behaviorally inhibited.

Groups demonstrating stable assymetrical EEG patterns of activation (right or left) were shown to differ in positive- and negative-affect traits (Tomarker, Davidson, Wheeler, & Doss, 1992). Those who had stable asymmetrical left mid-frontal EEG reported higher levels of general positive

Table 4-7. Neuroticism and EEG studies of brain activation

Study-Author(s)	Subjects (sex)	Tests	Conditions	Results
Matthews & Amelang (1993)	181 M & F	EPI, EPQ	Eyes closed, visual fixation	EPQ N sig. correlation with beta ($r = .16$). No interaction with E.
Stenberg (1992)	40 M & F	EPI, KSP Anxiety-N factor	relaxed, eyes open, closed, pos. & neg. imagery	High anxious Ss more right frontal theta all cond's. More temporal beta in neg. imagery condition.
Schmidt (1999)	40 F	Shyness (social anx)	Eyes closed & open	High shy relatively greater right frontal activity.
Tran et al. (2001)	50 M & F	16PF Anxiety factor	eyes closed & open	No differences in frontal sites.
Ivashenko et al. (1999)	69 M	EPI, STAI	eyes closed & open, cog. test	High N higher frequency of beta, particularly in right temporal area.
Knyazev et al. (2002)	49 M & F	EPI, STAI, Gray-Wilson Personality Questionnaire	eyes closed & open	High freq. beta pos. r with trait anxiety, N, BIS in frontal areas, and neg. r with theta & delta in temporal areas. N r with greater right hemisphere activation.

affect, whereas those showing stable right-sided activation reported more general negative affect.

Given the high relationship between affect and personality traits (Zuckerman et al., 1999), it might be assumed that neuroticism would be associated with asymmetrical right-hemisphere activation and extraversion with relatively greater left-hemisphere activation. This would be consistent with studies of monkeys with right-frontal EEG activity who exhibit more fear-related behaviors such as freezing and defensive hostility (Kalin, Larsen, Shelton, & Davidson, 1998).

Theories of brain sources of emotional traits such as anxiety have implicated limbic structures such as amygdala, hippocampus, and cingulate gyrus so that brain-imaging studies that are capable of assessing activity in subcortical centers could reveal more about the source of N in the brain. Most investigators using PET or CBF methods found few correlations between N and cortical, limbic, or brain stem areas during resting or cognitively stressing conditions (Fischer et al., 1997; Haier et al., 1987; Mathew et al., 1984). Stenberg et al. (1993) found significant correlations between N related scales and CBF activation in the temporal lobe during resting conditions but no significant correlation with the EPI N scale itself.

Using the fMRI response to negative and positive emotionally provoking pictures, Canli et al. (2001) found that N was associated with greater activation by negative stimuli relative to positive stimuli in left frontal and temporal cortical regions. Surprisingly, there were no significant relationships with limbic loci like the amygdala, and cingulate gyrus. The latter along with right temporal and frontal lobe activity were associated with extraversion. These findings are opposite to what would be expected from the lateralization hypothesis. However, other studies have found activation of the amygdala by negative emotion provoking stimuli (Dolan & Morris, 2000; Hariri et al., 2002; Phan et al., 2003). Both studies also found changes in prefrontal cortex. Hariri et al. (2002) found that activity in the *right* prefrontal cortex and the anterior cingulate cortex were correlated negatively with activity in the amygdala during the presentation of fearful stimuli, suggesting an attenuation of emotional reactions in the amygdala by the higher centers. Increased activation also was found in temporal cortex and parahippocampal gyri during presentation of negative emotion provoking stimuli. Skin conductance response varied directly with activation in the amygdala.

Slides of monkeys with threatening facial expressions elicit disturbed behavior in monkeys reared in social isolation from other monkeys suggesting an innate fear evoking mechanism (Sackett, 1966). Dolan and Morris (2000) found that pictures of fearful human facial expressions elicited CBF activation of the left amygdala.

Reiman and his colleagues, using PET brain imaging, found increases in activation in the anterior insular cortex in response to distressing cognitive stimuli, anticipatory anxiety, and lactate provoked panic reactions (Reiman, Lane, Ahern, Schwartz, & Davidson, 2000). Response to phobic stimuli included insular cortex along with the anterior cingulate and medial prefrontal cortex, thalamus, caudate, and hippocampal formation. Activation of some of the same areas was elicited during a social anxiety situation.

It is interesting that some EEG and brain-imaging studies have shown relationships between N and temporal lobe activity. Brain-imaging studies of panic attacks in patients with anxiety disorders have revealed an involvement of the parahippocampal gyrus that lies under the temporal lobe as well as the anterior end of the temporal lobe itself (Reiman, 1990). The insular cortex is another paralimbic region sensitive to anxiety provoking conditions. Perhaps N represents a vulnerability to panic attacks based on the sensitivity of these areas to emotionally provoking stimuli.

Arousability: Evoked Potentials

Most studies of the evoked potential (EP) have studied extraversion and ignored neuroticism. Guerra et al. (2001) found significant negative correlations between N and the P300 recorded from all frontal lobe leads in response to novel stimuli but not to infrequent target stimuli. Novel stimuli were not tones but auditory stimuli from the natural environment or computer generated. Responses to these represent a cortical *orienting reaction*. Apparently, the high N subjects had a weaker OR than emotionally stable subjects.

Robinson (2001) found some low positive correlations between N and amplitudes of P200 and P300 EPs. Brocke et al. (1997) noted no main effects for N for the auditory EP but a higher amplitude AEP in an introverted-neurotic (low E-high N) group than in an extraverted-stable group (high E-low N). They also found a steeper slope of the relationship between AEP amplitudes and stimulus intensities in the introverted neurotic group. No effects of E or N were found for the visual evoked potential.

De Pascalis et al. (1996) set up his experiment as a test of Gray's (1982) theory of sensitization of high-trait anxiety persons to visually presented words associated with winning or losing money. High N subjects showed larger N800 peak amplitudes to stimuli associated with losing compared to words associated with winning. The results tend to support Gray's theory of neuroticism, although the N800 is a late component, the significance of which is not clear. It is interesting, however, that infants classified as high-reactive (shy and fearful in response to unfamiliar events or people) by Kagan (1994) showed larger brain stem evoked potentials in response to auditory stimuli, and a larger negative amplitude wave form between 400 and 1000 msec in response to discrepant stimuli when they reached age 11.

The EP findings are not consistent. The positive findings tend to indicate that the high N subjects' responses depend on stimulus characteristics (novelty or associations) or interactions with extraversion. The influence of stimulus intensity has been more widely explored in studies using peripheral autonomic measures of arousal.

Autonomic Arousal

Eysenck's (1967) earlier theory suggested that a source of neuroticism was overactivation of the sympathetic branch of the autonomic nervous system as reflected in tonic levels of heart rate, skin conductance, blood pressure and other indicators of arousal. These also were indicators of arousal in brain limbic centers associated with emotionality. This hypothesis also was based on an extrapolation from clinical anxiety disorders, some of which show elevated levels of peripheral sympathetic system activity (Zuckerman, 1991, 1999). Studies of subjects high on N in the general nonclinical population, however, have failed to support any correlation between N and peripheral autonomic measures of arousal (Fahrenberg, 1987; Hodges, 1976; Myrtek, 1984; Naveteur & Baque, 1987).

It might be argued that although neuroticism might not predict resting levels, it should predict levels of response to stressful situations. However, two large studies refute this hypothesis. Myrtek (1984) used over 700 subjects, a variety of cardiovascular and respiratory measures and tested subjects in conditions of rest, hyperventilation, performance stress tests, and a cold-pressure pain test. Factor analysis was used to combine variables in order to remove some of the method error variance. Correlations between personality variables, including the N scale, and either single physiological or factor scores and personality were minimal and few could be replicated across different samples. The general conclusion was that there was no evidence of systematic variation between personality traits and cardiovascular or respiratory measures in any of the situations from rest to stress.

Fahrenberg's (1987) studies included conditions of rest, mental arithmetic, stressful interview, blood taking, preparing a speech, and the cold-pressor test. Physiological variables included: heart rate, finger pulse volume, electrodermal activity, respiration, eye blink, muscle tension, and EEG alpha. Again, the conclusion was that the null hypothesis (chance) could account best for the entire pattern of findings.

Neuroticism could conceivably be related to more basic physiological reactions to simple properties of stimulation such as intensity and novelty. In Chapter 2, I discussed two types of reactions: the *orienting reflex* (OR), a reflection of reaction to novelty of stimuli, and the *defensive reflex* (DR), a reaction to intensity or painfulness of stimuli. A third type of reaction, the *startle reflex* (SR), also may play a role in neuroticism. Graham (1979) described the characteristics in terms of changes in heart rate (HR) and effect on ongoing behavior. The OR enhances attention to the stimulus, the DR enhances preparation for action, but the SR merely interupts or inhibits ongoing behavior. It also results in a flexor reaction that has been regarded as protective, for example, eye blink to protect the eyes. The OR typically results in a prolonged HR deceleration, the DR in a long-latency HR acceleration, and the SR in a short latency HR acceleration. N might be predicted to be inversely related to the OR, and positively related to the DR and SR.

The OR is elicited by novel stimuli of low to moderate intensity and it habituates rapidly on repetition of the stimulus. Orlebeke and Feij (1979) reviewed 16 studies relating OR amplitude to trait measures of N, anxiety, or ego strength. In half of the studies there was no significant difference between high and low N or anxiety groups. The other results were almost equally divided between those in which one group or the other was higher. The conclusion is that N is unrelated to strength of the OR.

Richards and Eves (1991) used a very strong auditory stimulus (110 dB) to elicit DRs (and SRs?). Subjects were classified as accelerators and nonaccelerators (there were few decelerators) on the basis of their short- and long-latency acceleration patterns. There was no difference in baseline HR between these groups. The accelerators showed a greater short latency HR acceleration (1–4 sec.), followed by a deceleration (4–20 sec.), and a greater long latency acceleration (20–30 sec.) than the group labeled nonaccelerators. The short acceleration pattern could represent a SR or a DR, whereas the long one is certainly a DR.

These two response groups were compared on the EPQ and the Strelau Temperament Inventory (STI), based on Pavlovian concepts. The accelerators were low on E and high on N, and lower on Strength of Excitation (SE) and Mobility (M) from the STI. The accelerators tended to be introverted neurotics, the type most arousable by aversive stimuli according to Eysenck's and Gray's theories. SE and M correlate positively with E and negatively with N so the results on both tests are compatible (Strelau, 1983). SE is also theoretically related to the construct "strength of the nervous system" and those with weak nervous systems are particularly susceptible to defensive arousal by strong stimulation (Strelau, 1983, 1998). Unlike the lack of correlation between N and resting HR found in previously cited studies, HR did correlate significantly with N ($r = .25$) and E ($r = -.24$) during the HR baseline in this study.

The SR in humans is often measured by the amplitude of the eye-blink reflex measured by EMG in response to a sudden, intense auditory stimulus. The magnitude of the SR may be modulated by simultaneously presented visual stimuli. Negative stimuli usually result in an augmented SR whereas positive stimuli tend to attenuate the SR relative to neutral stimuli (Vrana, Spence, & Lang, 1988).

Corr et al. (1995) used this method to test Gray's theory that anxiety represents a sensitivity to anxiety provoking stimuli and impulsivity a sensitivity to positive emotional stimuli. Slides known to elicit positive and negative emotions were used with a 100 db auditory white noise used as an unconditioned stimulus for the SR. The auditory stimuli were presented during presentation of positive, neutral, and negative slides. Tests include the N scale from the EPQ and the Harm Avoidance (HA) scale from Cloninger's TPQ. As noted earlier, the HA scale is positively related to N and negatively related to E, and thus represents introverted neuroticism which is close to Gray's construct of trait anxiety than the N scale.

HA did not show a main effect across all types of slides but did show an interaction with the valence of the slides on amplitude of the SR. High HA subjects had an augmented SR during unpleasant slides relative to reactions to neutral and positive slides. Low HA subjects showed an attenuated SR during the unpleasant slides relative to reactions to the neutral and unpleasant slides. N did not show this kind of modulation of the SR.

A replication of this study, using only the HA scale, again found the significant interaction between slide valence and HA. High HA subjects had augmented SRs during the presentation of unpleasant slides, although there was no attenuating effect of pleasant slides (Corr, Kumari, Wilson, Checkley, & Gray, 1997). This time, however, there also was a significant main effect for HA: high HA subjects had greater amplitude SRs across all conditions.

The use of slides did not differentiate between anxiety provoking and other types of unpleasant stimuli, for instance, mutilation pictures that elicit disgust rather than fear. The research group used clips from horror films that were known to elicit anxiety reactions, and others that had been rated as "disgusting" (Wilson, Kumari, Gray, & Corr, 2000). They used the N rather than the HA scale. There was no main effect for N but a significant interaction between film valence and N. High N subjects showed greater SRs to the fearful films but low N subjects had greater SRs to the disgusting films. Apparently, neuroticism is specifically related to elicited anxiety rather than the broad category of negative affect.

Children (average age 12) of adults with anxiety disorders (high-risk children) show an increased startle eye-blink reflex and stronger SCRs, particularly under threat conditons, than offspring of normal controls (Merikangas, Avenevolli, Dierker, & Grillon, 1999). Adolescent high-risk children also have increased startle (Grillon, Dierker, & Merikangas, 1998). Females showed increased startle during baseline and during fear provoking conditions, whereas high-risk males demonstrated increased startle during the threat condition.

This series of studies of the fear-potentiated SR is interesting because it links human anxiety with both human clinical studies (Lang, 1995) and animal models for anxiety (Davis, 1986). This will allow us to identify some of the brain systems involved in the state and trait of anxiety.

PSYCHOPHARMACOLOGY

Theories
Gray's (1982, 1987) theory of the trait anxiety dimension of personality identified a primary brain locus in the dorsal ascending noradrenergic system (DANB) originating in the locus coeruleus (LC) and ascending to the cerebellum, thalamus, limbic system and virtually the entire neocortex (see Figure 2-16). The model is based on laboratory experiments, primarily with rats as subjects, showing that destruction of the system impairs passive-avoidance learning, and conditioned inhibition. In humans most of the drugs that reduce anxiety and neurotic inhibition act on the noradrenergic system. Drugs that increase anxiety increase the activation of the system as estimated by increases in the norepinephrine (NE) metabolite MHPG. The latter effect is more pronounced in panic disorders as will be discussed in Chapter 7.

Redmond (1985, 1987) proposed that the DANB and LC consititute an "alarm system" at lower levels and panic at the higher levels of activation. The alarm system idea is similar to Gray's function for the system as serving "sensitivity" to stimuli associated with punishment or novel stimuli.

Redmond's evidence was based on research on primates, primarily monkeys, but also humans. His findings included:

1. Antianxiety drugs, such as benzodiazepines and opiates, reduce LC activity and NE release.
2. Alpha-2 receptor antagonists, which increase LC activity and NE release, induce anxiety in monkeys and humans as reflected in facial expression in the former and verbal reports in the latter.
3. Electrical stimulation of the LC in monkeys produces facial expressions and reactions that are ordinarily seen in response to threats in the environment. The restrained monkey looks around as if trying to identify the source of his anxiety.
4. Drugs that decrease LC function attenuate reactions to a threatening stimulus.
5. Threatening stimuli, such as slides of monkeys with threatening facial expressions, produce increased LC activity and LC lesions abolish these responses to threat.
6. Symptoms produced by opiate withdrawal result in increases in LC activity in rats, MHPG in monkey brain, and CSF MHPG in humans.

Thus, there is ample evidence that the LC response is biased toward either aversive or ambiguous stimuli with potential threat. The LC is the only source for NE in the forebrain and the major source to other regions (Valentino & Aston-Jones, 1995). Stress increases NE activity in brain regions that receive their sole input from the LC. The DANB is involved in activation of the entire neocortex and therefore serves an alerting reaction to significant stimuli, primarily those of a threatening nature. The LC also responds to unconditioned aversive stimuli, that is, pain.

Gray (1987) also sees an involvement of the serotonergic system in anxiety, but it is a smaller one than that for NE. Serotonin is involved in that part of the output of the Behavioral Inhibition System, which inhibits motor behavior in the immediate response to threat. NE is involved in the sensitivity to stimuli associated with threat and the experience of anxiety. Indeed, the major function of the serotonergic system is in the inhibition of behavior (Soubrié, 1986), suggesting a primary role of the system in other personality traits involving restraint (high conscientiousness, low impulsivity).

Cloninger (1987) defines harm avoidance in the same way as Gray does: sensitivity to conditioned signals for punishment, novelty, or frustrative nonreward and behavioral expression in passive-avoidance, and resistance to extinction of fear-conditioned responses. Unlike Gray, however, he regards serotonin as the principal monoamine involved in this trait. NE is regarded as the principal neuromodulator for the trait he calls "reward dependence." Serotonergic activity is said to be positively related to harm avoidance. Gray (1986) and Zuckerman (1995) have criticized the idea that one neurotransmitter is responsible for one personality trait. Apart from this, however, is the disagreement on the role of serotonin in trait anxiety or neuroticism. Perhaps the research on human psychopharmacology and personality can provide some answers.

Studies of Monoamines and Neuroticism

The first studies of monoamines used metabolites from CSF, plasma, or urine correlated with various personality traits. Ballenger et al. (1983) studied monoamine metabolites in a group of normal subjects. CSF MHPG correlated only with state anxiety, assessed just before the spinal tap. Plasma MHPG, however, correlated substantially with N and anxiety scales from the MMPI. Contrary to the hypothesis, the correlations were negative. In other words, those high on N showed low levels of the NE metabolite. The serotonin metabolite in CSF did not correlate with N but correlated with two indices of N in the MMPI, but in opposite directions.

Redmond et al. (1986) found no significant correlations in normals between CSF MHPG or 5-HIAA and measures of anxiety from self-ratings, or ratings by interviewers or observers of videotapes of the interviews. In depressed patients, there were some low but significant positive correlations between CSF MHPG and ratings of anxiety, a distressed appearance, somatization, and sleep disturbance. The serotonin metabolite did not correlate significantly with any measures of anxiety in either normals or patients.

Anxiety disorders, particularly panic disorder, show decreased alpha-2 receptors. Alpha-2 receptors (see Figure 2-14) regulate the levels of NE and therefore are inversely related to reactivity of NE, at least in patients (Cameron et al., 1996). The question is: Is this a state or trait phenomenon in the patients? Based on the finding that binding of the receptors are normal in the well-relatives of patients and increase in response to treatment, it would seem to be a state phenomenon. Receptor binding was negatively related to symptoms in patients but not in nonpatients. Cameron et al. conclude that the binding abnormality tends to be a state rather than a trait. However, they did find that the NE levels, taken in the standing position, were increased in both panic patients and their well-relatives, suggesting evidence of trait for NE reactivity itself.

Many of the following studies used small patient samples in which state and trait anxiety may be difficult to distinguish. Manuck et al. (1998) used a large sample of 119 normals. Rather than just measuring resting levels of metabolites, they used a challenge method, using a serotonergic stimulant, fenfluramine, measuring prolactin response (PRL) as an index of serotonergic responsivity. Among men, PRL response correlated negatively with NEO measured neuroticism, but only with the Angry-Hostility subscore. Negative correlations with life history of aggression and self-report measures of assault and impulsivity suggest that low scores on serotonergic activity are more indicative of impulsive aggression than neuroticism or general anxiety. Indeed, clinical studies show low serotonin found in those who are violent against themselves or others (Åsberg, 1994; Mann, 1995).

A smaller study of only 22 normals, all males, used a fenfluramine challenge for serotonin, a clonidine challege for NE, and a bromocriptine challenge for dopamine (Gerra et al., 2000). Harm-avoidance scores correlated positively with both prolactin and cortisol indices of serotonergic response but not with responses to the NE challange. In a study by Ruegg et al. (1997) harm-avoidance was related positively with cortisol but not significantly with prolactin measures of serotonergic response. Peirson et al. (1999) found a positive relationship between all of the harm-avoidance subscales and 5HT2 receptor sensitivity.

Tryptophan is the first step in the production of serotonin (see Figure 2-15). A depletion of tryptophan results in a loss of serotonin. Rapid tryptophan depletion has been reported to increase depression with a temporary relapse in recovered depressed patients (Delgado et al., 1990) and in nonpatients with a family history of depression, but not in normal men without such a history (Benkelfat, Ellenbogen, Dean, Palmour, & Young, 1994). Stewart, Deary, and Ebmeier (2002) did the tryptophan depletion experiment on normals selected from high and low ranges of the EPQ N scale to see if N was a vulnerability factor for reaction to the depletion of serotonin. Overall, there was no change in mood scores produced by the procedure and no interaction with N in the change in mood scores, but N did affect scores on a verbal fluency test on the day of depletion, with high N subjects performing worse than low N subjects.

Drugs that increase the availability of serotonin, notably selective serotonin reuptake inhibitors (SSRIs), are effective in the treatment of depression (Montgomery, 1995) and panic disorders (Shader & Greenblatt, 1995). A study was made of the effectiveness of one SSRI (fluoxetine) on NEO measures of personality in persons with major depressive disorder (Du, Bakish, Ravindran, & Hrdina, 2002). Therapy produced significant decreases in N and increases in E in the total group of depressive patients, but these changes were mostly observed in the responders to treatment. It is possible that the SSRI was directly responsible for the personality changes, but the absence of a placebo control group or measures of the changes in serotonin produced by the drug preclude this conclusion.

Two studies of depressed patients show a positive relationship between indices of serotonin activity and neuroticism or harm avoidance. Roy (1999), using a simple CSF assessment, found a very high correlation between CSF 5-HIAA and EPQ N, and Hansenne et al. (1997) found a moderate correlation between the prolactin response to a serotonin challenge and harm avoidance scores.

Patients with posttraumatic stress disorder (PTSD) showed significantly higher levels of plasma NE and lower serotonin levels than controls, and the serotonin levels correlated negatively with a scale for anxiety (Spivak et al., 1999). In a group of abstinent alcoholics, self-rated depression and scores on an anxiety scale were positively correlated with CSF MHPG (Heinz et al., 1999). Self-rated depression also correlated positively with 5-HIAA.

The serotonin (5HT) receptor 5HT-1A receptor has a role in anxiety. Mice in whom the gene controlling this receptor has been "knocked out" show greater anxiety expressed in inhibition and fear of aversive environments (Ramboz et al., 1998). Drugs that are receptor agonists show some antianxiety effects (Coplan, Wolk, & Klein, 1995). Tauscher et al. (2001) correlated the NEO scales with PET imaging studies of regional 5HT-1A receptor binding. None of the five major factors of the NEO correlated with receptor binding, but the anxiety facet of the N scale correlated negatively and significantly with binding in the dorsolateral prefrontal, parietal, and occipital cortices and the anterior cingulate. The vulnerability facet of N correlated with receptor binding in the anterior cingulate and the occipital cortex. The finding is remarkable for the specificity of the personality trait (anxiety) and its generality to some of the major brain sites associated with anxiety and anxiety disorders, particularly prefrontal cortex and anterior cingulate.

Separation Stress

Social separation is a powerful stressor in both human and monkey infants. Abrupt separation from peers in peer-reared and from mothers in mother-reared rhesus monkey infants produced increases in the norepinephrine metabolite MHPG in all separations (Higley, Suomi, & Linnoila, 1992). MHPG was consistently increased by the stress of separation over a series of separations, whereas the serotonin metabolite 5-HIAA increased during the first separation but habituated, returning to baseline, during a series of separations. Rearing conditions affected MHPG across the years and conditions (separations) but did not affect 5-HIAA or the dopamine metabolite HVA. Peer-reared monkeys had consistently higher levels of MHPG than mother-reared monkeys. These results suggest that nore-pinephrine is the monoamine most closely related to both trait and state anxiety and, by inference, neuroticism in humans.

If any of the monoamines are an influence in the development of stable individual differences they should show reliability, if not stability, across time. In the Higley et al. study, levels of MHPG were stable across years and conditions, but HVA and 5-HIAA declined during development (year 1 to 2). However, interindividual differences were moderately reliable both within and between years for all three monoamine baselines (rs = MHPG. 58; HVA .69; 5-HIAA, 64).

GABA

The amino acid GABA which functions as an inhibitory neurotransmitter is described in Chapter 2. GABA is estimated to be the primary neurotrans-mitter in 30–40% of all CNS neurons throughout the CNS (Paul, 1995). Ben-zodiazepine antianxiety drugs, barbiturates, and alcohol all bind to GABA-A receptors; therefore, GABA could be relevant to trait anxiety or neuroticism. The benzodiazepine receptors are linked to GABA receptors and potenti-ate the effects of these receptors. Benzodiazepine receptor agonists reduce anxiety and inverse agonists increase anxiety. GABA could be a crucial factor in state or trait anxiety, particularly in its modulation of parts of the brain mediating anxiety arousal, such as the locus coeruleus (Gray, 1982). How-ever, the widespread distribution of GABA receptors throughout the brain suggests that fear modulation is only one of its functions.

GABA has been found to be lower in depressed patients than in controls in several studies (Muscettola, Casiello, Giannini, & Bosi, 1986). Flumazenil, a GABA antagonist, induced panic attacks in 80% of patients with panic disorder, but not in normal controls (Nutt, Glue, Lawson, & Wilson, 1990). GABA measures from plasma taken after traumatic road accidents predicted which survivors had developed acute posttraumatic stress disorder (PTSD) at 6 weeks posttrauma (Valva et al., 2004). Low levels of GABA were found in those who developed PTSD. It is possible that the panic disorder patients were already low in GABA neuron density. Weizman et al. (1987) did find a 24% reduction in benzodiazepine binding sites in a group of patients with general anxiety disorder. Drug treatment increased the binding capacity of these sites to normal levels, suggesting a state anxiety interpretation.

Hormones
The HYPAC System. Hormones are produced in glands or in the hypothala-mus and travel through the blood stream to target loci in the brain and

elsewhere. The hypothalamus initiates reactions in the pituitary gland, which in turn sends tropic hormones to stimulate glands to secrete their hormones. Several of these systems are shown in Figure 2-19. Cortisol is one of the products of the hypothalamic-pituitary adrenocortical (HYPAC) system. This system is activated by stress and associated with major depressive disorder. In depressed patients there is a correlation between cortisol and the MHPG metabolite of NE, suggesting the joint activation of the HYPAC and noradrenergic arousal systems by stress (Schatzberg & Schildkraut, 1995). Drugs that activate the noradrenergic system, producing panic in patients with panic disorder, also produce increased levels of cortisol (Charney & Heninger, 1986).

The dexamethasone (DEX) suppression test has been used as a measure of activity in the HYPAC system. DEX suppresses ACTH and cortisol release for more than 24 hours in most normal subjects as well as in persons with anxiety disorders, but fails to suppress cortisol release in most patients with major depression particularly those of the more severe melancholic type (Arana & Baldessarini, 1987). Neuroticism is a predisposing factor for major depression, so it is possible that overactive cortisol activity also may be characteristic of high N persons not currently suffering from clinical depression. High N is, however, also a predisposing factor for anxiety disorders in which there is only a slightly higher rate of nonsuppression.

Kagan (1994), in his longitudinal study of inhibited children, reported that these children had significantly higher saliva cortisol levels at 5, but not at 7 years of age. However, those who had consistently high levels of cortisol at both 5 and 7 years of age were more likely to be inhibited than uninhibited.

Corticotropin-Releasing Hormone (CRH) that stimulates ACTH release from the pituitary gland has been used as a further challenge to the HYPAC system after DEX suppression. Elevated circulating cortisol levels can suppress the ACTH response to a CRH challenge (Holsboer, 1995). Depressive patients still show a greater response to the combined DEX-CRH test than normals indicating a dysregulated HYPAC system.

McCleery and Goodwin (2001) gave the DEX-CRH challenge to *currently* nondepressed subjects, selected from the extreme high and low ends of the distribution of scores on the EPQ. Currently nondepressed, about half of the high N subjects, had experienced a major depressive disorder in the past. High and low N subjects did not differ on basal cortisol levels, but low N subjects had a greater cortisol response to the the DEX-CRH challenge! The authors attempted to explain the unexpected results in terms of a "down-regulated" HPA axis following exposure to trauma in the high N subjects. Studies of patients with posttraumatic stress disorder, in contrast to depressives, had an enhanced negative feedback control of the HYPAC. This explanation is somewhat weakened by the fact of the absence of such trauma reported by high N subjects, although most reported poor parenting and more family breakdown in their past.

The role of the HYPAC system in clinical anxiety disorders and those simply high on N remains a mystery. Cortisol reaction to stress may be a state rather than a trait indicator of HYPAC vulnerability to anxiety and depression disorders. Of course, the HYPAC system is stimulated by nore-pinephrine and the hypothalamic response, and cortisol may represent a secondary reaction to prolonged stress. On the other side, CRH activates the NE system and increases defensive withdrawal in reaction to novel situations. CRH applied to neurons produces excitatory effects in amygdala, locus coeruleus, cortex, and hypothalamus (Feldman, Meyer, & Quenzer, 1997). Ventricular infusion of CRH produces EEG arousal. Stress involves mutual positive feedback systems, and it is hard to say which is cause and which is effect in the chain of reactions.

Experimental studies of rhesus monkeys showed clearer evidence for cortisol as a state and a trait indicator for anxiety. Baseline levels of cortisol were moderately reliable ($r = .42$) across two years (Higley et al., 1992). Plasma cortisol was significantly elevated by separation from peers or mothers in young monkeys. Cortisol levels were higher in peer-reared monkeys, a reflection of the chronic stress produced by this kind of mother-absent rearing.

Corticotropin Releasing Hormone (CRH), the first step in the HYPAC stress response system, is associated with a greater right prefrontal cortex activity, a pattern correlated with fearful behavior in rhesus monkeys (Kalin, Shelten, & Davidson, 2000).

Testosterone. The sex hormone testosterone is also affected by stress, but in this case it is lowered by stress from defeat in competitive activities and increased by success or victory in such activities (Dabbs, 2000). Daitzman and Zuckerman (1980) and Dabbs, Hopper, and Jurkovic (1990) found negative correlations between testosterone and N and other scales assessing anxiety, but Dabbs et al. could not replicate their findings in a subsequent larger study. Like cortisol, testosterone seems to be a stress-related hormone, and one exhibiting trait qualities only in cases in which stress is chronic, as in major or chronic depression. In persons suffering from such long-term stress, sexual desire may be influenced by lowered testosterone levels. This is true for women as well as men, as androgens such as testosterone seem to influence sexual desire in both sexes.

The preceding sections have implicated various areas of the brain, peripheral autonomic, and HYPAC hormonal systems in the trait of neuroticism-anxiety. This is, however, like identifying all the parts of an automobile without describing how they function together. The next section on neuropsychology attempts to do this, drawing on clinical studies of humans with brain damage and those with anxiety disorders, experimental studies of animals, and most recently the brain-imaging studies of humans. There has been a great deal of progress since the first edition of this book (Zuckerman, 1991) in mapping the neurological mechanisms of fear and anxiety. Anxiety is the core trait of neuroticism, but a description of the mechanisms of anxiety response as a state do not fully account for the type of persistent trait anxiety that makes high N persons vulnerable to full-blown anxiety and depressive disorders.

NEUROPSYCHOLOGY
The attempt to define the source of emotional feelings in physiology goes back to the beginning of psychological science. William James's (1884) theory of emotional feelings attributed them to the perception of peripheral bodily responses. An emotional stimulus is received in the sensory areas of the brain, which triggers responses from the periphery of the body. According to James, it is the perception of these responses that leads to the feelings characteristic of emotions. According to this view we are afraid because our heart races and we run, rather than we feel fear causing our heart to race and our running. There is some evidence of this sequence in the responses of persons with panic disorders who respond to internal cues like increases in heart rate with a feeling of panic even though these responses may have no conscious external source.

Four decades later, James's theory was challenged by Cannon (1929) and Bard (1929). Like others before him, Bard found that ablations of large areas of the cerebral cortex did not affect the capacity for emotional reactions in cats. Organized emotional expression was disrupted only when he removed the hypothalamus. Because the hypothalamus was known to control the autonomic nervous system, it made sense to regard it as the place where emotions originated. Emotional feelings were the reaction in the cortex to events in the hypothalamus rather than the peripheral autonomic responses controlled by this brain center. James and Cannon and Bard were in agreement on one point: conscious feelings in the higher cortical centers did not produce bodily effects but were a function of activity in lower

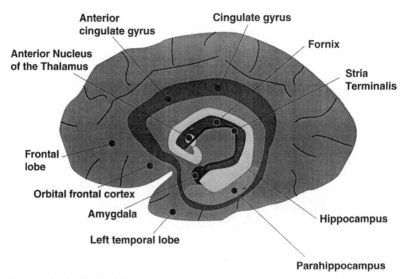

Figure 4-1. Cortical and limbic structures implicated in anxiety. Note that limbic brain structures, for example, the hippocampus (stippled) lie under and inside the lobes of the cerebrum. From M. Zuckerman, 1999, *Vulnerability to psychopathology: A biosocial model*, p. 106, Washington, DC: American Psychological Association. Copyright 1999 by American Psychological Association. Reprinted by permission.

brain centers (Cannon-Bard) or bodily responses (James), which were not initially conscious. Cannon and Bard took the psychology of emotion out of the armchair and into the operating laboratory and observation room. Their theory was based on the findings that although cortical excisions did not abolish emotional expression in cats, a transection of midbrain above the hypothalamus (and other midbrain structures) abolished intergrated emotional expression.

The focus of Cannon and Bard on the hypothalamus ignored the fact that it was part of a larger brain neighborhood called the *limbic system*. Papez (1937) was a neuroanatomist who never did actual experiments on emotions. But, on the basis of reports on human patients with brain damage and animal studies, he put the hypothalamus in the context of a larger system shown in schematic form in Figure 2-11. The reader may consult Figures 2-9 and 4-1 for anatomical views of the limbic system. Readers can refer back to these figures for the location of specific nuclei involved in the experience of anxiety and overactive in some of the anxiety disorders.

Papez suggested that emotional stimuli bifurcated at the thalamus with simultaneous transmission to the hypothalamus, where emotional responses originate, and the higher sensory cortex, where a more cognitive analysis is made. The cingulate cortex, which forms the roof of the limbic brain, is where emotion is experienced. The dorsal thalamus projects directly to the lateral cortex conveying the sensory and perceptual aspects of stimuli, whereas the ventral thalamus projects to the hypothalamus, anterior thalamus, cingulate gyrus, and hippocampus, which "elaborate the functions of emotional expression" (Papez, 1937). The cingulate conveys this experience to the neocortex and the hippocampus. The amygdala, absent in this early model, assumed a central importance in models, to be discussed shortly.

MacLean's (1982) concept of the "triune brain" was described in Chapter 2. Recall that he described the three brains of humans as they appeared in evolution: the "reptillian," "paleomammalian," and "neomamalian" brains. The paleomammalian brain corresponded to what already has been described as the limbic system, plus some additional structures. The paleommalian brain is also called the "visceral brain" at the core of which is the hippocampus. He regarded the hippocampus as the center mediating emotional experience, just as Papez regarded the cingulate gyrus as serving this function. Unlike Papez, however, MacLean regarded the hippocampal formation as inclusive of the dentate gyrus and amygdala. But the hippocampus was regarded as the center where stimuli were received and evaluated, the dentate gyrus as the output center for the sympathetic nervous system, and the amygdala as the output center for the parasympathetic nervous system. Actually, it is known today that the amygdala participates in both sympathetic and parasympathetic outputs (LeDoux, 1987).

Eysenck (1967) regarded the visceral (limbic) brain as a basis for the trait of neuroticism, speaking of "differential thresholds of arousal" in visceral brain in those low or high on N. Eysenck did not define any pathways in the system or describe the different roles of the various structures within the system. His student Jeffrey Gray (1982) delved much further into the neuropsychology of of anxiety.

Gray's "bottom-up" approach to personality is described in Chapter 1. He worked entirely with rats as subjects and extrapolated to humans by analogy. But, in recent years, in collaboration with Pickering, he has been testing his behavioral model on humans (Pickering et al., 1997). The biological model, however, is a comparative one still based on an extensive survey of research, performed on rats, including his own studies. The model for neuroticism is described in two editions of his book on "The Psychology of Fear and Stress" (Gray, 1971, 1987) as well as his book *The Neuropsychology of Anxiety: An Enquiry into the Functions of the Septo-Hippocampal System* (Gray 1982a).

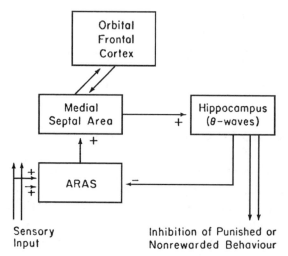

Figure 4-2. Schematized septohippocampal system: Inputs from orbital frontal cortex and arousal produced by sensory input into the ARAS stimulate the medial septal area, which produces theta waves in the hippocampus. Output of the hippocampus inhibits punished or nonrewarded behavior. From "Causal theories of personality and how to test them," by J. A. Gray, 1973, in *Multivariate analysis and psychological theory*, p. 424, J. R. Royce, Ed. New York: Academic Press. Copyright 1973 by Academic Press. Reprinted by permission.

Gray conceives of a behavioral inhibition system (BIS) underlying the trait of anxiety. The BIS is sensitive to four kinds of stimuli: signals of punishment, nonreward (frustration), innate fear stimuli, and novel stimuli. The output of the system results in behavioral inhibition, increased arousal, and increased attention to the eliciting stimulus. As Gray puts it, the anxiety stimulus causes the animal to "stop, look, and listen." The BIS can be inhibited by (or inhibit) the two other systems: the reward system and the fight/flight system. The latter will be discussed in subsequent chapters in connection with other major personality traits.

At the heart of the system involved in fear is the septo-hippocampal system schematized in Figure 4-2. Input from the sensory cortex is organized in the orbital frontal cortex, transmitted through the medial septal area and hippocampus to the ascending reticular activating system (ARAS) which elicits arousal in the prefrontal cortex. The hippocampus produces inhibition of punished or nonrewarded behavior in mechanisms described more fully in the extended schematic (Figure 4-3).

Figure 4-3 shows the extended plan for the BIS in connection with the Papez circuit. There is a great deal of specific structures or substructures within the schematic accounting for the various inputs and outputs of the BIS. Information from the prefrontal cortex (PFC) and the neocortical association areas, where incoming signals are analyzed for form, enters the hippocampal formation (HF) from the entorhinal cortex (EC). The subicular area (SUB) of the HF acts as a comparator, comparing the current signals from the EC with past signals that may have been associated with punishment. The hippocampus selects stimuli with strong biological significance, that is, connected with primary reinforcement. Arousal output is mediated via the locus coeruleus (LC), the source of the noradrenergic system, and the hypothalamus (HYP) stimulating the HYPAC hormonal system. Behavioral inhibition is triggered in the pathway from the SUB comparator to the cingulate gyrus (CING).

Gray's neuropsychological model is notable for the absence of the amygdala. Actually Gray regarded the amygdala as the basis for another system, the fight/flight system. In contrast, Le Doux (1987, 1998) makes the amygdala the core of the anxiety system, serving the role of comparator receiving both the thalamic and cortical inputs and organizing the pattern of emotional response to fear-provoking stimuli.

Aggleton and Mishkin (1986) described the amygdala as the "sensory gateway to the emotions." The central role of the amygdala in emotion is also supported by Davidson (1992, 2002), Davis (1986), and Le Doux (1987, 1998). Davis (1986) suggested that the amygdala is the major locus for fear and anxiety based on his studies of the fear potentiated startle reflex (FPSR). The FPSR is a conditioned acoustic startle response elicted by a cue previously associated with shock or some other aversive stimulus. The CS precedes the loud startle UCS and the degree to which it augments the response to the UCS is the FPSR. His evidence is much of the same kind that Gray produced for his assertion that the septo-hippocampal system is the core of the fear circuit. Drugs that increase anxiety in humans increase the FPSR and drugs that reduce anxiety decrease the FPSR. Brain stimulation and lesioning studies in rats point to the role of the central nucleus (CN) of the amygdala in the fear response. The various outputs of the CN are shown in Figure 2-12. These include the criteria for Gray's BIS, such as behavioral inhibition, autonomic sympathetic system arousal (increase in heart and breathing rates), increased vigilance, and activation of the ascending norepinephrine arousal system originating in the locus coeruleus, and others such as cardiovascular conditioning, startle increase, and facial expressions of fear.

Inputs from somatosensory, visual, and auditory cortex converge on the amygdala at various stages of analysis and integration as shown in Figure 4-4, from Le Doux (1987). A unimodal stimulus might be the roar of a lion (auditory); a polymodal stimulus would be the roar plus the

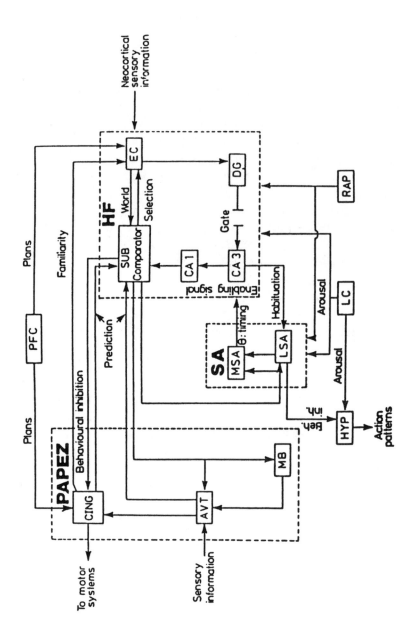

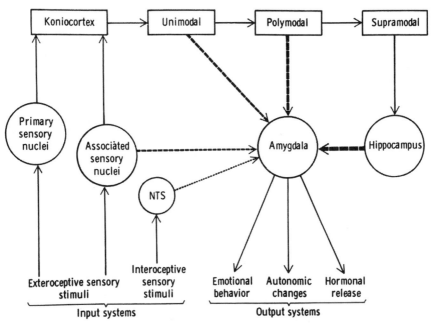

Figure 4-4. Sensory projections to amygdala and emotional evaluation. Amygdala receives inputs from various exteroceptive and interoceptive sensory modalities (dashed lines). Density of *dashed input lines* to amygdala signifies extent to which sensory signal is processed before reaching the amygdala. Inputs arriving from various cortical association fields have been transformed more than inputs arriving directly from thalamus or nucleus tractus solitarii (NTS). Different inputs may mediate unique aspects of emotional processing, each capable of initiating changes in emotional behavior and autonomic and humoral (hormonal) activity. From "Emotion" by J. E. LeDoux, 1987, in *Handbook of physiology: The nervous system, Vol. V*, p. 437, F. Plum, Ed. Bethesda, MD: American Physiological Society. Copyright 1987 by American Physiological Society. Reprinted by permission.

←———

Figure 4-3. The neurology of the behavioral inhibition system. The three major building blocks are shown in heavy print and outlined by dashed boxes: the hippocampal formation (HF) made up of the entorhinal cortex (EC), the dentate gyrus (DG), areas CA 3 and CA 1 of the hippocampus proper; the subicular area (SUB); the septal area (SA), containing the medial septal area (MSA), and the lateral septal area (LSA); and the Papex circuit, which receives projections from and returns them to the subicular area via the mammillary bodies (MB), anteroventral thalamus (AVT), and the cingulate cortex (CING). Other structures shown are the hypothalamus (HYP), the locus coeruleus (LC), the raphe nuclei (RAP), and the prefrontal cortex (PFC). Arrows show direction of projection; the projection from the SUB to MSA lacks anatomical confirmation. Words in lower case show postulated functions; beh. inh. is behavioral inhibition. From "The neuropsychology of emotion and personality," by J. A. Gray, 1987, in *Cognitive Neurochemistry*, p. 177, S. M. Stahl, S. D. Iverson, and E. C. Goodman, Eds. Oxford: Oxford University Press. Copyright 1987 by Oxford University Press. Reprinted by permission.

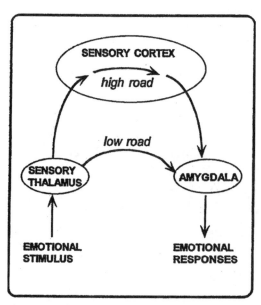

Figure 4-5. The low and high roads to the amygdala. Information about external stimuli may reach the amygdala by way of direct pathways from the thalamus (low road) as well as pathways from the thalamus to the cortex and then to the amygdala (high road). The low road direct from thalamus to amygdala is faster but involves no cortical processing and less awareness of the stimulus or even any awareness of what is making us anxious. From J. LeDoux, 1998, *The emotional brain*, Fig. 6-13, p. 164. London: Weidenfeld & Nicholson. Copyright 1998 by Joseph LeDoux. Reprinted by permission.

sight (visual), plus the smell (olfactory) of a lion; a supramodal would be the integration of all of these retrieving a memory of previously experienced lion attacks in the hippocampus. The result would be the responses described in Figure 4-4: emotional behavior, autonomic changes, and hormonal release (the HYPAC stress response).

External stimuli may trigger the amygdala-initiated responses before they are fully processed by cortical centers. Le Doux (1998) describes the "high road" and the "low road" to the amygdala as shown in Figure 4-5. An emotional stimulus reaching the sensory thalamus may be transmitted directly to the amygdala without appraisal in higher cortical centers. This "low-road" mechanism would be the basis of the type of anxiety in which the sufferer cannot identify the stimulus or thought that is making them anxious. These responses are quicker than those involving the thalamo-cortical-amygdal circuit (the high road), which may modify or even inhibit the emotional responses from the amygdala. LeDoux (1998) suggests that the amygdala system is involved in implicit emotional memory, whereas

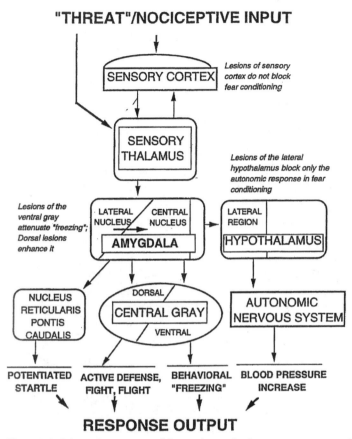

Figure 4-6. Schematic summary of fear pathways in the nervous system and their behavioral and physiological response outputs. Fear stimuli ("threat") are received in the sensory thalamus and sent to the sensory cortex for additional processing. The sensory thalamus transmits to the lateral nucleus and then to the central nucleus of the amygdala. The central nucleus projects to the lateral hypothalamus that mediates the autonomic components of the fear response. Projections to the central gray results in defensive immobility ("freezing") and escape behavior. A direct projection to the nucleus reticularis pontis caudalis modulates the startle reflex. From "Emotion: Behavior, feeling and physiology" by M. Bradley & P. J. Lang, 2000, in E. Richard & D. Lane, Eds., *Cognitive neuroscience of emotion*, p. 250. London: Oxford University Press. Reprinted by permission.

the hippocampal system in explicit or conscious memory. Both mechanisms blend in immediately conscious working memory. Figure 4-6 summarizes the inputs, their sources, and primary contributions to the fear experience.

Davidson (2002) proposes a role for the prefrontal cortex (PFC) (3), particularly the medial and orbital PFC, in modulating the time course of emotional responding. In the absence of this inhibitory influence, the amygdala does not extinguish the emotional response, despite repeated exposures to the emotional stimulus. The persistence of anxiety in spite of opportunities for extinction in clinical anxiety disorders could be a function of a weak PFC. Davidson also suggests a distinction in the role of right and left PFC. The left PFC seems to be involved in the inhibition of anxiety through extinction, whereas the right PFC appears to potentiate the fear reaction. According to Davidson this lateralization difference extends down to the amygdala itself, with right amygdaloid reactions predicting dispositions to experience, negative emotions, and negative memory bias. He also maintains that the right amygdala is involved in unconscious processing of emotions, whereas the left amygdala serves more conscious emotional learning.

Of what relevance is the description of the role of the amygdala relevant to individual differences in neuroticism? Davidson believes that the amygdala is involved in the learning of fear responses but is not the crucial factor in what he calls "affective style." Individual differences, he believes, are more a function of the prefrontal regulation of emotion rather than the amygdala. But it is difficult to see why a structure that is central to the ease of acquisition of fear would not also be relevant to the trait of "fearfulness."

The emphasis of these investigators has been on the role of the amygdala in fear and anxiety. Davidson claims that neuroimaging studies using induced emotions find that the amygdala activation is primarily related to negative rather than positive emotions. However, this could be a function of the greater intensity of negative emotions than most positive emotions. A study using intracranial stimulation of the amygdala in cats found that higher voltages (intensities) produced fear or anger responses at the same sites that produced mere orienting (interest) at lower intensities (Ursin & Kaada, 1960). However, fear and anger appear at different sites in the amygdala. Gray describes a "fight-flight" system in the amygdala, but fear and flight appear as a sequence in response to stimulation, and neither is linked to anger.

Lesioning of the amygdala in monkeys reduces fear, but it also reduces normal affiliative behavior and dominance. Kling and Stelkis (1976) suggest that the amygdala and its inputs from the orbital and temporal cortex may be a neural substrate for sociability in primates. This could be a secondary effect of the loss of emotional response, but it does suggest that the amygdala also may play a role in positive emotionality of the type linked to social relations.

LeDoux (1998) describes an interaction between the amygdala and hippocampus in their effects on the HYPAC stress system as shown

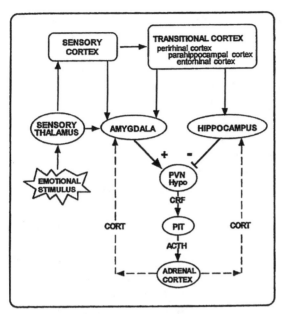

Figure 4-7. Stress pathways in the brain and their activation or inhibition of the Hypothalamic-Pituitary-Adrenocortical (HYPAC) system. Stimuli associated with danger activate the amygdala. By way of pathways from the amygdala to the paraventricular (PVN) nucleus of the hypothalamus (Hypo), corticotrophin-releasing factor (CRF) is sent to the pituitary gland, which, in turn, releases adrenocorticotropic hormone (ACTH) into the bloodstream. ACTH then acts on the adrenal cortex, causing it to release corticosteroids (CORT) into the blood stream. CORT travels from the blood into the brain where it binds to specialized receptors on neurons in the regions of the hippocampus and amygdala as well as other regions. However, as long as the emotional stimulus is present, the amygdala will attempt to cause PVN to release CRF. The balance between the excitatory inputs (+) from the amygdala and the inhibitory inputs (−) from the hippocampus to PVN determine how much CRF, ACTH, and ultimately CORT will be released. From J. Le Doux, 1998, *The emotional brain*, p. 241. London: Weidenfeld & Nicholson. Copyright 1998 by Joseph Ledoux. Reprinted by permission.

in Figure 4-7. Fear stimulus inputs processed in the thalamus and/or sensory cortex pass to the transitional cortex and then to the amygdala and/or hippocampus. The amygdala has a stimulatory effect on the paraventricular nucleus of the hypothalamus (PVN Hypo), whereas the hippocampus has an inhibitory effect on this nucleus. If the excitatory effect predominates the PVN Hypo releases CRF causing the pituitary to release ACTH, resulting in secretion of cortisol from the adrenal cortex. Cortisol travels through the blood to the amygdala and hippocampus where it binds to receptors on the neurons of these structures. The effect on the hippocampus is a negative feedback inhibiting further activation of the HYPAC system, but the amygdala continues to stimulate the HYPAC as long as the stimulus is present.

Prolonged stress can result in the failure of the hippocampus to dampen the stress response and in actual damage to the hippocampal neurons. The hippocampus is diminished in mice after prolonged social stress (Blanchard et al., 1995) and in Vietnam veterans with posttraumatic stress disorder (Bremner et al., 1995). Schizophrenics show loss of neuronal tissue in amygdala and hippocampus (Breier et al., 1992; Torrey et al., 1994). Damage to the hippocampus produced by prolonged stress can affect memory function, and this is a demonstrable loss of function in these disorders.

The entire brain volume relative to the remainder of the intracranial volume was found to be negatively related to NEO measured neuroticism with age and gender control (Knutson, Momenan, Rawlings, Fong, & Hommer, 2001). None of the other four NEO personality factors were related to brain volume. Within the N factor, only anxiety and self-consciousness facets were related to brain volume. The measure of brain volume that was related to N was related to changes occurring after the brain reached its maximal growth rather than during brain development. The results indicate that stress in adolescent through adult life was the factor involved in reduction of brain volume. This would be consistent with the reductions in specific areas found in posttraumatic stress disorder.

SUMMARY

Neuroticism is the only basic personality factor directly linked with clinical disorders. This is because the core of the factor is negative emotions, particularly anxiety and depression. The ancient Greeks called it the "melancholic" disposition. The definitions of the trait in personality tests varies among test constructors, with some including subfactors such as impulsiveness and aggression/hostility, whereas others regard these as separate and distinctive factors on their own. But all agree on anxiety and depression as components and despite the differences in content the various measures of neuroticism are highly intercorrelated.

Twin studies of heritability yield heritabilities of .4 to .5, although there is variation among the studies depending on the methods used to assess personality and their reliabilities. But it must always be remembered that heritability is a population based statistic. Nontwin adoption studies are inconclusive because most correlations, with either adoptive or biological parents or between adoptive and biological siblings, are low with inconsistent findings on which are significant or higher. Heritabilities for measures of temperament in children are about the same or even a little lower than those for personality in adults.

In the molecular genetics studies, a major candidate for a gene involved in neuroticism has emerged: the serotonin transporter gene. The shorter form of the genetic marker is associated with behavioral abnormalities in humans and monkeys, including anxiety, angry-hostility and impulsiveness. These kinds of reactions also are associated with serotonin deficits in humans and other primates. The short form of the gene marker also is associated with greater activation of the amygdala in humans during exposure to images of angry or fearful faces. Studies of monkeys, however, suggest an interaction between the genotype and early rearing conditions. Monkeys reared by their mothers are less susceptible to the deleterious effects of the differences in genetic form.

Neuroticism tends to be associated with high activation of brain as assessed by EEG, particularly at right-frontal sites. Differences in infant temperament also have been related to right-sided cortical activation, suggesting that negative emotions tend to activate the right brain hemisphere. fMRI studies show that activation of the right prefrontal cortex tends to modulate activation in the amygdala during stimulation with fear provoking stimuli. Findings on cortical evoked potentials are not entirely consistent, but investigators usually find large EPs, particularly later component ones, associated with neuroticism.

Simple measures of autonomic sympathetic system activation, such as heart rate or skin conductance, taken in baseline or stressful conditions, have not shown any correlation with neuroticism as a trait. However, acceleration of heart rate as an immediate response to an intense stimulus did correlate with both neuroticism and introversion, as predicted from the theories of Eysenck and Gray. Neuroticism and Harm Avoidance are related to the magnitude of the fear-potentiated auditory startle reflex, particularly during the presentation of fearful visual stimuli. These correlations in normals are consistent with studies of children of parents with anxiety disorders.

Simple correlational studies of monoamine metabolites in normal humans have not revealed any consistent correlations of these metabolites with neuroticism or anxiety trait. However, studies of brain stimulation in monkeys, and the effects of antianxiety and panic-provoking drugs in humans with panic disorder, suggest that the activation of the noradrenergic system originating in the locus coeruleus is a major factor in anxiety. Some theories have proposed that serotonin reactivity is also a factor in anxiety. Although there is some evidence for serotonin reactivity in the initial stages of anxiety provocation this reaction tends to habituate. It may be related to the tendency for inhibition of all ongoing behavior during periods of intense fear. However, some drugs used to treat anxiety disorders

(SSRIs) potentiate serotonin by preventing its uptake. Low levels of serotonin are found in depression and anxious, depressed, and hostile persons who commit or attempt violent acts of aggression toward themselves (suicide) or others. Patients with posttraumatic stress disorder, and chronic anxiety, show higher levels of norepinephrine and lower levels of serotonin than controls. The evidence from clinical studies is fairly consistent in suggesting that high norepinephrine and *low* serotonin levels are characteristic in those with extreme chronic anxiety. The evidence is less clear in normals, perhaps because of a restriction of range of anxiety and neurotransmitter activity.

The connection between the action of the benzodiazepine anti-anxiety drugs and the GABA-A receptors suggests that GABA could be associated with human neuroticism. GABA is lower in depressed patients and a GABA antagonist induces panic attacks in most patients with panic disorders. But as with norepinephrine the association between neurotransmitter and degree of neuroticism has not been reported in normals.

Stress activates the HYPAC hormonal system in humans and other species, and cortisol, an end-product of the system, is elevated in stressful conditions. Studies of humans suggest that cortisol is more of a state indicator than a vulnerability trait related to neuroticism. In monkeys, however, prolonged stress induced by nonoptimal rearing conditions (mother absent), and immediate stress induced by sudden maternal separation, resulted in elevated cortisol levels. Prolonged stress can probably change cortisol levels more permanently. In a similar manner, testosterone is lowered by stress and chronic stress may produce semipermanent changes affecting sexual behavior.

James's 19th-century theory of emotions gave the brain a secondary role in emotional feeling, conceiving the feelings in the brain as a reaction to peripheral changes in autonomic and muscular activations. The Cannon-Bard theory suggested that the hypothalamus stimulated emotional responses in the higher cortical brain centers and responses in the peripheral nervous system and musculature simultaneously. Papez defined a broader emotional mechanism in the entire limbic system with experience a function of activity in the cingulate cortex. Gray's theory included much of the Papez circuit but with the central role of appraisal of emotional stimuli attributed to the septo-hippocampal circuit. In contrast to these older theories, Le Doux, Davis, and Aggleton and Mishkin identified the amygdala as the center of the limbic system controlling fear and anxiety. Fear conditioning and the fear-potentiated startle reflex, lesioning, and stimulation studies in animals, as well as the actions of drugs suppressing or initiating anxiety supplied the major evidence for this model. The amygdala receives inputs directly from the thalamus and from higher cortical centers and the outputs of the central nucleus include most of the classical behavioral and physiological signs of fear or anxiety. The right prefrontal cortex has been proposed by Davidson as the modulating factor in the immediate emotional effects in the amygdala, as well as the long-term effects through extinction. The amygdala may not necessarily be related only to fear or anxiety, but indications are that the central nucleus is primarily involved in negative emotionality and other amygdaloid nuclei are involved in anger. Animal studies also suggest that some sites may mediate positive affiliative behavior.

The hippocampus also may play a role in anxiety by processing more explicit emotional memories from the higher cortical centers and modulating the amygdala responses and the output of the HYPAC system originating in the hypothalamus. Prolonged stress can damage the hippocampus producing deficits in the memory processing function and ability to inhibit emotional reactions. Such damage has been found in mice and humans, veterans with postraumatic stress disorder and schizophrenics. Actually, the volume of the whole brain has been found to be negatively related to neuroticism. Prolonged emotional stress can be a killer of neurons and may alter the trait of neuroticism, sometimes irreversibly.

Freud (1922/1961) contrasted what he called "the crudest form of the 'shock' theory" of traumatic neurosis with his psychological theory. The shock theory [as in 'shell-shock'] "takes the essential nature of the shock as residing in the direct injury to the molecular structure, or even to the histological structure, of the nervous elements." In contrast, his own theory involves "the breaking through of the barrier with which the psychic organ [is provided against stimuli, and from the tasks with which this is thereby placed" (p. 25). The recent neurological findings show that there may have been more truth in the "crude" theory than Freud was willing to concede. However, Freud recognized the possibility that the psychological level of analysis might someday be rooted in a biological explanation.

Biology is truly a realm of limitless possibilities; we have the most surprising revelations to expect from it, and cannot conjecture what answers it will offer in some decades to the questions we have put to it. Perhaps they may be such as to overthrow the whole artificial structures of hypotheses. (Freud, 1922/1961, p. 56)

CHAPTER 5

Psychoticism (Psychopathy), Impulsivity, Sensation and/or Novelty Seeking, Conscientiousness

The diverse array of traits in the title for this chapter reflects the disagreements among personality classifiers as to the nature of "personality in the third dimension." The Eysencks proposed the label of "Psychoticism" for this higher order factor. Both Block (1977) and Zuckerman (1989) suggested that if a clinical term was appropriate for the scale called "Psychoticism" (P) (Eysenck & Eysenck, 1976), it should be "Psychopathy" (Antisocial Personality Disorder in the current psychiatric nomenclature). The subtraits of P described by Eysenck and Eysenck (1985) include: aggressive, cold, egocentric, impersonal, impulsive, *antisocial*, unempathic, creative, and tough-minded. With the possible exception of creativity, these are all traits of the psychopath rather than the psychotic, particularly if one includes the endogenous depressives among the psychotic. The highest scoring clinical groups among males and females are: prisoners, drug addicts, alcoholics, and personality disorders (Eysenck & Eysenck, 1976), all of which contain high proportions of antisocial personality disorders. Psychotics, among females at least, score low on the P scale relative to other clinical groups. The concept of a P dimension came from ratings of clinical groups that largely included psychotics and neurotics, but not psychopaths (S. B. G. Eysenck, 1956), and this may account for the conceptualization of the P dimension as psychoticism. Revisions of the P scale have tended to eliminate most of the psychotic sounding items except for a few with a mildly paranoid flavor. Psychopaths often voice the opinion that everyone is "against them."

Factor analyses of the P scale along with many other types of scales have shown it to be one of the best markers for the dimension called "Impulsive Unsocialized Sensation Seeking (ImpUSS), which includes impulsivity, sensation seeking, autonomy and aggression at one pole and socialization, responsibility, cognitive structure, and inhibition of aggression at the other

(Zuckerman et al., 1988, 1991, 1993). This is a factor dimension that could have been labeled socialization or psychopathy. In a four- and five-factor analysis, aggression and hostility split off from the broader P-ImpUSS factor to form a separate major factor (Zuckerman, 2002). In a three-factor analysis, the broad P factor would include both Conscientiousness and Agreeableness factors in the Big Five (Eysenck, 1992). Costa and McCrae (1992b), however, insist that "five factors are basic."

Tellegen's (1985) third dimension is called "Constraint" and includes scales for control, harm avoidance, and traditionalism. This would seem to be the ImpUSS factor reversed. Cloninger's Novelty Seeking factor includes impulsivity as well as "exploratory excitability" and thus resembles the ImpSS scale in the ZKPQ more than the form V SS Total scale. Although Costa and McCrae (1992a) place "excitement seeking" in their extraversion factor, sensation seeking, measured by the SSS, correlates more highly with and loads more highly on the conscientiousness factor than the extraversion one (Zuckerman, 2002; Zuckerman et al., 1993).

"Personality in the third dimension" is obviously complex, but as will be seen it has strong biological roots and is a vital factor in human social adjustment. Psychopathy, or antisocial personality disorder, represents the clinical extreme of asocialization and some of the psychobiological evidence from studies of that diagnosis will be used in this chapter. Aggression is usually part of the psychopathic trait profile. Although aggression is part of the broad ImpUSS trait in a three-factor model, it can be distinguished as an independent dimension in five-factor models and will be dealt with in the next chapter rather than this one.

GENETICS

Biometric Twin Studies

Many scales have been used to measure the third major dimension of personality. Most of these scales are moderately correlated among themselves, but each seems to have some unique variance so that the presentations of the results of biometric studies will be by individual scales.

Psychoticism. The Psychoticism scale developed by Eysenck and Eysenck (1975) has many psychometric problems including extreme skewness of distributions and relatively lower reliabilities than the other two major factors, extraversion and neuroticism (Loehlin & Martin, 2001). These problems might lower its potential in measurement of heritability.

Table 5-1. Twin correlations and heritabilities for the psychoticism scale

Study	MZ *rs*	DZ *rs*	h²
Eaves & Eysenck (1977)	.47	.28	.46
Eaves et al. (1989) 15 studies	.46	.23	.49
Loehlin & Martin (2001)			
Males young	.22	.12	Total: .28
middle	.37	.24	
old	.30	.17	
Females young	.40	.20	
middle	.35	.20	
old	.30	.18	

The studies using the P scale are shown in Table 5-1. Eaves and Eysenck (1977) first studied the trait using a large heterogeneous sample of English twins. Using a modeling ANOVA technique (Jinks & Fulker, 1970), they found that 46% of the total variance in P could be attributed to genetic factors. Correcting for the unreliability of the P measure, they calculated the corrected heritability at 81%. But this dramatic increase in heritability is a function of the low reliability of the measure, with sampling error accounting for 40% of the variance. Heritability measures are not usually corrected for reliability of measurement, although perhaps they should be.

Eaves et al. (1989), summarizing 15 studies that used the P scale, reported a heritability of .49 with no evidence of shared environment. They did report, however, that the heritability is almost as strongly due to nonadditive as to additive genetic mechanisms (21% and 28%, respectively). The more recent study by Loehlin and Martin (2001) was performed on a large Australian twin sample and was analyzed by gender and age. Their results show a smaller heritability for P, only .28 overall, perhaps because of their use of a short form of the EPQ with lower reliabilities than the long form. Age and gender did not markedly affect the heritabilities.

Impulsivity. The first studies of the heritability of impulsivity (Imp) were done using an Imp subscale of the EPI extraversion scale. The other component was sociability. A twin study showed that the heritability of Imp was .36 compared to .46 for sociability (Eaves and Eysenck, 1975). Later Eysenck and Eysenck (1977) developed special scales to measure impulsivity, and these were used in a genetic twin study (Eaves, Martin, & Eysenck, 1977; Eysenck, 1983). The four scales of impulsivity were: (1) impulsivity in the narrow sense (acting quickly without forethought); (2) nonplanning (not planning ahead for some task to be done); (3) risk-taking (engaging in risky

Table 5-2. Twin correlations and heritabilities for impulsivity type scales

Study	Nationality	Scale	Twin Type#	MZ r	DZ r	h^2
Pederson et al. (1988)	Swedish	KSP-Impulsivity	twins together	.45	.09	.45
			twins apart	.40	.15	
Saudino et al. (1999)	Russian	KSP-Impulsivity	twins together	.48	−.06	.49
Loehlin (1992)	American	TTS-Impulsivity	high school	.39	−.11	.39*
			WWII Vets	.52	.02	.52*
Bouchard (1993)	American	MPQ-Constraint	twins together	.59	.38	.42*
			twins apart	.61	−.04	.61*
Jang et al. (1998)	Canadian	NEO-Impulsivity	twins together	.38	.27	.37
	German			.36	.21	

Twin type refers to raising: together means raised together; apart means twins adopted away and raised in different families. If specified by sample, e.g. high school, it refers to twins raised together.
* These heritabilities (h^2) were calculated using the Falconer Index, but when MZ-DZ rs exceed the MZ, the MZ correlations is used as the index. The other heritabilites were calculated from models.
Note: KSP = Karolinska Scales of Personality; TTS = Thurstone Temperament Schedule; MPQ = Multidimensional Personality Questionnaire

activities for fun); (4) liveliness (high activity and exuberance). Total genetical effects for males for the four subscales varied between .15 and .40; for females they ranged from .17 to .37. Narrow impulsivity had the highest and liveliness had the lowest heritabilities for both men and women. The specific (to the subtrait) component of the broad heritability exceeded the common (across all subtraits) component for nearly all of the scales for both genders. There were small shared environmental effects for all scales, but the specific (nonshared) effects were stronger.

Loehlin (1992) analyzed the effects for various kinds of impulsivity-type scales from several studies as shown in Table 5-2. Most of the correlations for dizygotic twins are either negative or close to zero, perhaps because of the low sample sizes or reflection of an influence of nonadditive type genetic mechanisms. The heritabilities, defined simply by the size of the MZ twin correlations alone because of the low DZ, are .52 in the veterans and .39 in the high school age twins.

Two studies used the impulsivity scale from the KSP. Saudino et al. (1999) found a heritability of .49. Pederson et al. (1988) analyzed data from the Swedish adoption study. The correlation for identical twins raised together was almost the same as that for identical twins raised in separate

Table 5-3. Twin correlations and heritabilities for conscientiousness (cons.)

Study	Country	Scale	Twin Types	MZ r	DZ r	h^2
Jang et al. (1996)	Canada	NEO Cons.	from gen. pop.	.37	.27	.44
Riemann et al. (1997)	Germany	NEO Cons.	from gen.pop.	.54	.18	.53
		peer ratings		.41	.17	.71
Loehlin et al. (1998)	America	self-ratings	H.S. students	.42	.21	overall: .52
		CPI		.53	.34	
		ACL		.37	.14	
Bergeman et al. (1993)	Sweden	NEO Cons.	raised together	.47	.11	.29
			raised apart	.19	.10	
Cattell (1982)	America	HSPQ Cons.	from gen. pop.	.50	.17	.50

families indicating no effect of shared environment. An analysis of all four groups showed that 45% of the variance could be accounted for by genetics factors, but nearly all of this was due to a nonadditive type of genetic mechanism.

Bouchard (1993) reported results from the Minnesota twin adoption study using the Constraint factor of the MPQ. The correlations of twins raised together and raised apart were nearly identical and both were high, again indicating no effect of twins sharing a common environment. Looking over the range of heritabilities, we can see they range from .3 to .5. Heritabilities from the studies by Eysenck and his colleagues would fall in this same range. The general lack of correlation between dizygotic twins may indicate the presence of a nonadditive type of genetic mechanism operating on this trait.

Impulsivity in the NEO is classified as a subtrait of Neuroticism. Jang et al. (1998) analyzed the heritability of impulsivity along with the other subtraits in Canadian and German populations. The correlations for identical twins were somewhat lower and those for fraternal twins were higher than those in the other studies shown in this table. The heritability for the combined sample was .37, at the lower end of the range of heritability for other impulsivity scales shown in this table.

Conscientiousness. Conscientiousness is a trait that emerged from the ascendancy of the Big Five in personality. It is not a trait that one can identify in most other species but it may have evolved in humans living in social groups with explicit rules for approved behaviors. Table 5-3 shows genetic studies using scales actually called "conscientiousness," rather than those extrapolated from other scales.

The first study is one by Cattell using a scale for conscientiousness from the HSPQ. The study yielded a moderate heritability of .50. Following this are the studies by Jang et al. (1996) and Rieman et al. (1997) in Canada and Germany using the NEO Conscientiousness scale. Peer ratings on conscientiousness were used in addition to the questionnaire. The high heritability of .71 was a result of using a model which took out the error variance, thereby raising the genetic component. If we use the Falconer formula the heritability for peer ratings would be .48 close to those obtained for the self-report NEO, .53.

Loehlin et al. (1998) derived conscientiousness measures from three different methods: self-ratings on bipolar trait scales, the CPI questionnaire, and the Adjective Check List. The results were fairly similar using all three methods and the overall heritability was .52.

Bergeman et al. (1993) collected data from participants in the Swedish twin adoption study using a short form of the NEO conscientiousness scale. Unlike the results of Pederson et al. (1988) using the KSP Impulsivity scale in the same population or the Bouchard (1993) results in the Minnesota twin adoption study (see Table 5-2), there was a substantial difference between identical twins raised together and those raised in separate families. This reduced heritability to .29 and resulted in a significant shared environment effect of .11. Other than this atypical result, the other heritabilities for conscientiousness are in the range .4 to .5.

Sensation Seeking. The original Sensation Seeking Scale was based on the construct "optimal level of stimulation" with the idea of individual differences in optimal levels. Optimal levels of arousal also were considered basic to the trait (Zuckerman, Kolin, Price, & Zoob, 1964). Optimal levels refer to the levels of stimulation and arousal at which persons functioned and felt best. Level of stimulation was, however, not limited to intensity but included novelty, complexity, incongruity, and change (Zuckerman, 1979, 1994). Over time, four subfactors in the general trait were discovered using factor analyses. These were incorporated in forms IV (Zuckerman, 1971) and V (Zuckerman, Eysenck, & Eysenck, 1978). Form V substitutes a total score for the general scale in form IV. The existence of a general trait incorporating all four subtraits has been questioned, even though moderate correlations among scores on all four have been found. These were higher in form IV, but in form V a deliberate attempt was made to increase the discriminant validity of the subscales through item selection so that the

Table 5-4. Twin correlations and heritabilities for sensation seeking type scales

Study	Country	Scale	Twin types	MZ r	DZ r	h^2
Fulker et al. (1980)	England	SSS-Total	males	.63	.21	.58
			females	.56	.21	
Hur & Bouchard (1997)	America	SSS-Total	raised separate	.54	.32	.59
Saudino et al. (1999)	Russia	KSP-MA		.54	.14	.53
Pederson (1988)	Sweden	KSP-MA	raised together	.26	.16	.23
			raised separate	.20	.14	
Jang et al. (1998)	Canada	NEO-Excit. Seeking		.48	.10	.46
	Germany			.45	.31	
						combined sample

Note: SSS = Sensation Seeking Scale (form V); KSP-MA = Karolinska Scales of Personality-Monotony Avoidance Scale; NEO Excit. = NEO Excitement Seeking facet scale

correlations are somewhat lower but still significant. The subscales of the SSS V may be described in terms of content as follows:

Thrill and Adventure Seeking (TAS) items include a desire to engage in risky sports or activities involving speed, adventure, defiance of gravity, or other unusual sensations. The items ask about desires or intentions rather than actual experience.

Experience Seeking (ES) items refer to experience through the mind and senses, travel, art, music, food, dress, and living a nonconformist life with unusual friends.

Disinhibition (Dis) items reflect attitudes or experiences regarding seeking of social and sexual stimulation through partying and variety in sexual partners.

Boredom Susceptibility items concern intolerance for monotonous conditions or boring people, and restlessness when alone in familiar surrounding for any length of time.

There are many other similar scales, including monotony avoidance (MA) from the KSP and excitement seeking (ExcS) from the NEO, although most of these scales cover only a limited range of the content of the four subscales of the SSS V and are much shorter. Table 5-4 shows the genetic studies done with the SSS and the other two scales.

Table 5-5. Heritabilities of the SSS form V subscales

SSS Subscales	Eysenck (1983)		Koopmans et al. (1995)		Hur & Bouchard 1997	
	Males	Females	Males	Females	M & F	Med. all 5
Thrill & Adventure Seeking	.45	.44	.62	.63	.54	.54
Experience Seeking	.58	.57	.56	.58	.55	.57
Disinhibition	.51	.41	.62	.60	.46	.51
Boredom Susceptibility	.41	.34	.48	.54	.40	.41

The first study using the SSS was done with English twins residing in the London area (Fulker, Eysenck, & Zuckerman, 1980). Heritability was 58%, at the upper range of what is found for most personality traits. The second study using the SSS used twins from the Minnesota twin-adoption study, separated near birth and raised in different families (Hur & Boucharad, 1997). The heritability from the separated identical twins was .54 (the correlation) and that from the separated fraternal twins was .64 (double the correlation). Averaging these two would give a heritability of .59, almost exactly what was obtained from nonseparated twins in the Fulker et al. study. There was no evidence of a shared environmental effect in these studies.

Saudino et al. (1999) and Pederson et al. (1988) used the KSP MA scale. In the former study, the heritability was .53, close to the results from the studies using the SSS. The Pederson et al. study used twins from the Swedish Adoption Study and contrasted twins raised together with those raised apart. The correlations between both together and separated identical twins were lower than in the previous studies, and the heritability was only .23. Nearly all of the remainder was due to the nonshared environment and error of measurement.

Jang et al. (1998) analyzed the subscales of the NEO including excitement seeking, a sensation seeking type subscale, grouped under the major factor of extraversion. The results were similar in the Canadian and German samples, yielding a total heritability of .46 for the combined sample.

The SSS subscales were analyzed by Eysenck (1983) for the English twins, Hur and Bouchard (1997) for the separated twins from the Minnesota study, and Koopmans et al. (1995) for a Dutch sample of twins. The results are shown in Table 5-5. Eysenck found substantial heritabilities for all of the subscales but particularly for ES and Dis. The heritability for Dis was higher in men than in women. The genetic results were broken down into those due to a common or general factor in all of the subscales and factors specific to each of them. Nearly all of the genetic variance in ES was due to a general factor, whereas for the others about two thirds of their genetic variances were due to factors specific to the individual scales.

Koopmans used a Dutch version of the SSS IV, which contains the same subscales as in V but the items were put into a Likert-type format. Heritabilities were high for both men (.48–.62) and women (.54–.63). The highest heritabilities were for Dis and TAS, but those for ES were the same as in the English study. There was no evidence that different genes influenced sensation seeking in men and women. The genetic correlations among the scales were substantial but, instead of a general genetic factor, the data suggested one including ES and TAS and another composed of Dis and BS. Dis and BS are the scales most highly related to antisocial forms of sensation seeking whereas ES and TAS represent more neutral forms. In this study, TAS and ES had the highest heritabilites.

The Hur and Bouchard study also included a scale for self-control (the inverse of impulsivity). The control scale was negatively correlated with all of the SS subscales. The covariance between the SSS and the Control scale was determined largely by shared genetic influences. This supports the rationale for combining sensation seeking and impulsivity in the form of an Impulsive Sensation Seeking scale in the ZKPQ version of the trait. The genetic correlation between the two scales was highest for the Dis, ES, and BS scales but much lower with the TAS scale.

The median heritabilities across all groups are shown in the last column of the table. Heritabilites for Dis, TAS, and ES, are very close, only that for BS is below those of the first three. This, like other results using BS, may be due to the lower reliability of the BS scale.

As with most other personality traits, the genetic analyses of sensation seeking show little effect of a shared environment. However, shared environment encompasses a broad variety of factors, including parents, social class, schools, and so on. A focus on specific shared environmental factors could reveal some interactions of genetics and environment. A group of Dutch investigators looked at the role of religious upbringing on the disinhibition (Dis) subscale of the SSS (Boomsma, de Geus, van Baal, & Koopmans, 1999). Table 5-6 shows the twin correlations and heritabilites on Dis for two groups, those raised with a religious upbringing, and those raised in a nonreligious family setting.

For those twins raised in a nonreligious setting, the results were like the other studies of Dis with a substantial heritability for men and women and

Table 5-6. Twin correlations and proportions of variance on the disinhibition subscale of the SSS due to genetics (G), shared environment (SE), and nonshared environment (NSE) as a function of religious upbringing[*]

	Religious upbringing		Non-Religious upbringing	
	Males	Females	Males	Females
MZ twin *r*s	.62	.61	.62	.58
DZ twin *r*s	.62	.50	.35	.35
G	00	.37	.49	.61
SE	.62	.25	.11	00
NSE	.38	.38	.40	.39

Adapted from "A religious upbringing reduces the influence of genetic factors on disinhibition: Evidence for interaction between genotype and environment on personality" by D. I. Boomsa et al. (1999), *Twin Research*, *2*, Tables 5A and 5B, p. 122. Copyright, 1999 by Stockton Press. Reprinted by permission.

minimal or no effects of shared environment. But for those twins raised in a religious environment there was no genetic effect for men and a strong effect of shared environment. For women raised in religious families there was some genetic effect but the shared environment effect was nearly as strong. Apparently, a religious upbringing may increase the correspondence between the traits in fraternal twins overriding the genetic influences, but in a more permissive rearing environment the genetic effects are free to express themselves, modified only by specific peer influences outside of the home.

Part of the broad P-ImpUSS factor found in factor analyses of personality tests (Zuckerman et al., 1988; Zuckerman et al., 1991) is "unsocialized" ("U"). The other factors – psychoticism, impulsivity, and sensation seeking – are all related to psychopathy, an extreme form of the lack of socialization. Twin studies of adult psychopathy, or antisocial behavioral histories, and criminality show significant heritabilities (.43–.54) with no effects of shared environment (Cloninger & Gottesman, 1987; Lyons et al., 1995). However, twin studies of juvenile delinquency show minimal genetic effects but substantial effects of shared environments as well as specific environments. Lyons et al. said: "We hypothesize that there are psychological characteristics (for example, sensation-seeking and impulsivity) that mediate the relationships between genes and observable antisocial behavior" (p. 913).

The P and SS scales and a scale for socialization all correlated significantly with ratings of prisoners on the Hare and Cox (1978) Psychopathy Check List (PCL, Harpur, Hare, & Hakstian, 1989). The newer ImpSS scale and the P scale also correlated with PCL ratings in another study (Thornquist &

Table 5-7. Correlations and heritabilities of MMPI scales relevant to socialization in twins raised separately (DiLalla et al., 1996)

MMPI Scale	MZ twin *r*s	DZ twin *r*s	h^2
Psychopathic Deviate	.62	.14	.61
Hypomania	.56	.23	.55
Authority Conflict	.41	.19	.42
Family Conflict	.50	.32	.50

Zuckerman, 1995). The Psychopathic Deviate (Pd) and Hypomania (Ma) scales from the MMPI are two indicators of psychopathic personality when both are peak scores in the MMPI profile. The dual peaks are also indicative of antisocial behaviors, even in nonpsychopathic adolescents and adults. These two scales also correlated with ratings of antisocial behavior on the PCL (Harpur et al., 1989).

The MMPI scales were analyzed in the Minnesota twin-adoption study (DiLalla, Carey, Gottesman, & Bouchard, 1996). Table 5-7 shows the twin correlations for the two psychopathy-relevant clinical scales (Pd & Ma), and two relevant content scales, Authority Conflict (AuC) and Family Problems (Fam). The subjects were all separated twins raised in different families. The Pd scale had one of the two highest heritabilities among all of the MMPI scales (.61). The other scale with the same heritability was Schizophrenia. Ma also had a high heritability (.55). The two content scales, AuC and Fam, had moderate heritabilities (.42 and .50). Thus, both the personality trait components of P-ImpUSS and those for psychopathic behavior are at least moderately genetic in origin in adults. A study of the genetic covariance of these two categories of traits is needed to test the Lyons et al. (1995) hypothesis that the genetic component of antisocial behavior is mediated by personality traits such as impulsivity and sensation seeking.

Another twin study from the Minnesota adoption project used scales from the CPI (Bouchard, McGue, Hur, & Horn, 1998). Table 5-8 shows the results on the scales relevant to the ImpUSS dimension. Correlations for twins raised apart and those raised together were very close showing no effect for shared environment. Heritabilities were close to .5 for all four scales, but for responsibility and socialization the genetic mechanism was entirely additive, whereas for self-control and tough-mindedness it was nonadditive, indicating dominance or epistatic mechanisms.

The Psychopathic Personality Inventory (PPI) is a self-report index of the personality component of psychopathy including subscales such as

Table 5-8. Twin correlations and heritabilities of CPI scales relevant to socialization in twins raised apart (A) and together (T) (Bouchard et al., 1998)

CPI Scales	MZ-A	DZ-A	MZ-T	DZ-T	h^2
Responsibility	.54	.40	.41	.34	.49*
Socialization	.56	.28	.48	.21	.50*
Self-Control	.61	−.04	.47	.08	.50**
Tough-Minded	.45	.13	.42	.12	.45**

* Primarily Additive Genetic Variance
** Primarily Non-Additive Genetic Variance

egocentricity, carefree nonplanfulness, social potency, fearlessness, impulsive nonconformity, coldheartedness, and blame externalization. A study using the PPI was done with twins from the Minnesota Twin registry ((Bloningen, Carlson, Krueger, & Patrick, 2003). The genetic variance was .47, most of which was epistatic variance. The pattern of zero or negative dizygotic twin correlations suggested a nonadditive genetic mechanism for all of the subscales except social potency (an extraversion type scale).

Family Studies

Adoption studies have investigated the relative influences of the adoptive (social) relationships with those in biological relationships to the parents of rearing (social + biological), and in some cases with the original biological parents (genetic) of adopted-away children. Table 5-9 shows the results from the Texas Adoption Study when the children reached late adolescence

Table 5-9. Correlations between biological as contrasted with adoptive relations on CPI scales relevant to socialization and impulsivity (Loehlin, Willerman, & Horn, 1985)

	Biological		Adoptive		Sibling Relationships		
CPI Scale	Father-Child	Mother-Child	Father-Child	Mother-Child	Biologic Siblings	Adopt-Adopt	Adopt-Biologic
Responsibility	.12	.06	.06	.05	.61**	.00	.33*
Socialization	.16	.06	−.03	−.02	−.01	.03	.10
Self-Control	.00	.07	.08	.03	.34	−.06	.03
Impulsivity	.13	.05	.07	.01	.23	.27*	.10

* p ¡ .05
** p ¡ .01

(Loehlin, Willerman, & Horn, 1985, 1987). Hardly any of these correlations, whether with biological or adoptive relatives, are significant, although those with the biological relatives tend to be somewhat higher than those with the adoptive relatives. Most of the latter are close to zero or even negative in the case of siblings. The correlations of the biological relatives are in the same low range as those for fraternal twins in the studies of conscientiousness (Table 5-3). Loehlin et al. (1987), summarizing the results, estimate the heritability at only .25 with no effect of shared environment and a strong effect of nonshared environment. The heritability is about half of that estimated from the twin study using the CPI (Bouchard et al., 1998).

The biological mothers of the adopted-away children had been given the MMPI before they gave birth. The correlations of the children with both adoptive and same family biological fathers and mothers on the Pd scale were all small and nonsignificant (.01–.12). The correlation on Pd between the birth mother, who they never knew, and their children was .27 and highly significant. Additional evidence of a latent effect of the genetic factor was that the social and emotional adjustment of the adoptive childen, as rated by their parents, fell significantly at adolescence in contrast to the stability of adjustment in their biological children.

Adoption studies in several countries have contrasted the genetic influence of the biological parents, the social influence of the adopting parents, and their interaction in the prevalence of criminal behavior in children. Ishikawa and Raine (2002) reviewed 15 such studies in Denmark, Sweden, and the United States. Nearly all studies support a genetic influence of criminality in biological parents and criminality in their adopted-away offspring. Most show little independent influence of purely social factors in the influence of the adoptive parents alone. Several do support the idea of an interaction or additive effects of genetic and environmental influences.

The largest of these took place in Denmark involving over 14,000 adoptions and nearly 66,000 court records on parents and children (Mednick, Gabrielli, & Hutchings, 1984, 1987). Their results are shown in Table 5-10. Having a biological parent who had a criminal record significantly increased the chances of criminality in the adopted-away sons, even though they never had any contact with these parents. But having an adoptive parent who was criminal did not increase the criminality in adopted sons. Furthermore, the risk to adoptive sons increased linearly with the number of convictions of the biological parents. This increase was particularly dramatic among the sons of the most chronic criminals. Although these adoptees constituted only 1% of the adoptee population they accounted for 30% of

Table 5-10. Cross-Fostering analysis: percentages of adoptive sons convicted of criminal law offenses as a function of criminality in biological and adoptive parents*

		Are biological parents criminal?	
		Yes	No
Are adoptive parents criminal?	Yes	24.5%	14.7%
	No	20.0%	13.5%

* From Chapter 3 by S. A. Mednick et al. (1996), in *Development of antisocial and prosocial behavior: Research, theories and issues*. D. Olweus, J. Block, & M. Radke-Yarrow, Eds., p. 40. Copyright 1986 by Academic Press. Reprinted by permission.

the convictions among male adoptees! Biological siblings raised in different homes had an increased concordance (20%) for criminality, a rate that was twice as high as that for nonrelated adoptees raised in the same family (8.5%).

There are some caveats to these analyses. Criminality in the adoptive parents is much less common than in the biological parents and is generally less severe and chronic. Furthermore, in the Scandinavian countries an extensive welfare system reduces the extremes of socioeconomic environment found in the United States. Even so, interactions between genetic and environmental influences have been found in Sweden (Cloninger & Gottesman, 1987; Cloninger, Sigvardsson, Bohman, & von Knorring, 1982) and the United States (Cadoret, O'Gorman, Troughton, & Haywood, 1985).

The Swedish study used more than criminal convictions to classify congenital and postnatal factors. Postnatal factors included the occupational status of the adoptive parent and multiple temporary placements prior to adoption. The results of this broader classification are shown in Table 5-11.

Table 5-11. Cross-Fostering: analysis of predisposition to petty crime in adoptees classified by congenital and postnatal risk factors (Cloninger & Gottesman, 1987)

		Male adoptees congenital		Female adoptees congenital	
		Low	High	Low	High
Postnatal Factors	Low	2.9%	12.1%	0.5%	2.9%
	High	6.7%	40.0%	2.9%	11.1%

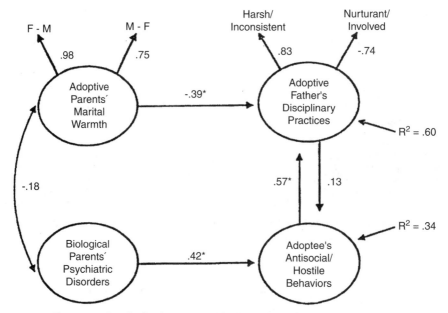

Figure 5-1. Standardized maximum likelihood estimates of a a model of mutual influences between adoptive fathers' (F's) parenting and adoptive children's antisocial/hostile behaviors (*p < .05). M = mothers. Goodness of fit = .91.
From "The developmental interface between nature and nuture: A mutual influence model of child antisocial behavior and parent behaviors," by X. Ge et al., 1996, *Developmental Psychology, 32*, Fig. 3, p. 585. Copyright 1996 by American Psychological Association, Reprinted by permission.

The Swedish study showed a strong nonadditive interaction effect. The group having both congenital and prenatal dispositions had a three times greater risk (males) and a four times greater risk (females) than the adoptees in the group having only a congenital disposition.

The Iowa adoption study took this research further by analyzing the role of parenting practices within the adoptive family in the interaction with the influences of antisocial and substance abuse diagnoses in the biological parents (Ge et al., 1996). Studies of family environments as perceived by children have shown a genetic influence (Hur & Bouchard, 1995; Plomin, Reiss, Hetherington, & Howe, 1994). This could be produced by evocative influences of children on parents. A child with a genetically influenced antisocial temperament can evoke more punitive reactions from parents than a more docile child. Their results as shown in the models pictured in Figures 5-1 and 5-2 indicate such interactions.

The biological parents' psychiatric disorders (antisocial personality and/or substance abuse) independently influenced the presence of

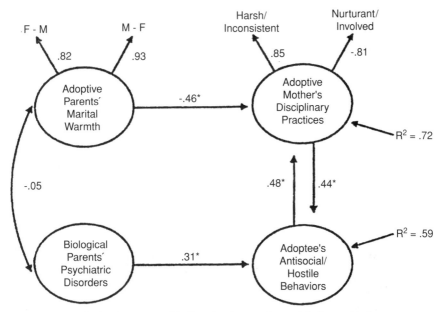

Figure 5-2. Standardized maximum likelihood estimates of a model of mutual influence between adoptive mothers' (Ms') parenting and adopted children's antisocial/hostile behaviors (*p < .05). F = father. Goodness of fit = .94.

From "the developmental interface between nature and nurture: A mutual influence model of child antisocial behavior and parent behaviors," by X. Ge et al., 1996, *Developmental Psychology, 32*, Fig. 4, p. 585. Copyright 1996 by American Psychological Association. Reprinted by permission.

adoptees' antisocial and hostile behaviors. The warmth of the marital relationship in the adoptive parents influenced the adoptive parents disciplinary practices. A lack of warmth was related to harsh and inconsistent practices and negatively related to nuturant practices. Adoptive fathers' disciplinary practices were more a reaction to adoptees antisocial behaviors than a cause of such behaviors. The relation between mothers' disciplinary practices and the adoptees' antisocial behaviors, however, was a reciprocal one. This could lead to an escalating cycle of rebelliousness and hostility in the child eliciting harsh reactions or rejection from the mother, in turn aggravating the antisocial reaction in the child. These factors would emerge as specific rather than shared environmental influences in the family, because different children would be treated differently as a function of their own genetically influenced behaviors.

The results of this study have implications for the twin studies of personality traits, which usually conclude that there is no effect of shared environment. This is based on the idea that parental influences are the same for all the children in the family. But parental reactions to children with different personalities may be different. Parents are human and consistency is an ideal but not always a practical way to deal with children who have different responses to discipline and unconditional love.

Molecular Genetics

Ebstein et al. (1996) reported the first association between the dopamine D4 (D4DR) receptor exon III polymorphism and the personality trait of novelty seeking. Novelty seeking was based on a scale developed by Cloninger, which closely resembles sensation seeking scales, particularly the recent ImpSS that is part of the Alternative Five. A correlation of .68 was found between the two scales. If this were corrected for attenuation the two scales would correlate between .8 and 1.00 depending on their reliabilities.

The D4DR has two primary allele forms in Israeli and Western cultures, one with four repeats and the other with seven repeats of the base sequence. The longer form is associated with high novelty (sensation) seeking (NS) and the shorter form with moderate or low NS. In the same year, Benjamin et al. (1996) showed an association between NS as extrapolated from combinations of NEO-PI-R scales and the long forms of the D4DR. Prolo and Licino (2002) reviewed 21 studies between 1996 and 1999. Techniques of assessment varied, some using tests and some clinical interviews, and varied populations, some normal and some abnormal, were used. Excluding infant studies, 11 found significant relationships between NS (however assessed) and the longer forms of the D4DR. Meta-analyses by Schinkin, Letsch, and Crawford (2002) found no relationship in comparisons between the seven-repeat form and others, but when the analyses compared long and short forms of the gene, a small positive effect was found. A somewhat larger effect was found in the few studies of the D4DR-521 C/T promotor polymorphism.

The weakness of the D4DR effect is not surprising, as the D4DR polymorphism only accounts for 10% of the genetic variance and 4% of the total variance of the trait. Many other genes may be involved, and if the genetic variance is additive or interactive the power to detect the influence of any one gene is limited.

The importance of the gene is also indicated by its association with forms of psychopathology related to impulsive sensation seeking: substance abuse (heroin and nicotine) (Ebstein & Kotler (2002), attention-deficit hyperactivity disorder, and pathological gambling disorder (Castro et al., 1997).

Studies of infants extend the phenomenal associations of the gene to an age preceding any significant social influence (Ebstein & Auerbach, 2002). At 2 weeks of age, infants with the longer form of the gene showed stronger orientation and motor organization and a greater range and regulation of states (Ebstein et al., 1998). The effect on orientation was in interaction with the serotonin transporter gene. At 2 months of age, infants with the long D4DR had lower scores on negative emotionality, including distress in reaction to novel or suddenly presented stimuli, daily routines, and limitations, than those with the short forms. These differences continue to 1 year of age and those with the long form also show less social distress in reactions to strangers.

The infants with the short form are closer to what Kagan described as the inhibited type of infant. Adult sensation seekers (Disinhibition scale) also show strong orientation reactions to novel stimuli, as measured by heart rate deceleration, but low sensation seekers show accelerations of heart rate, particularly at high intensities of stimulation (Orlebeke & Feij, 1979; Ridgeway & Hare, 1981; Zuckerman, Simons, & Como, 1988). These adult patterns could reflect early infant differences in reaction to novelty and intensity of stimulation.

The serotonin transporter genotype (5-HTTLPR) in the short form has been associated with anxiety, depression, and angry hostility, as described in the previous chapter. However, in both infants and adults, the short alleles of the 5-HTTLPR and long alleles of the dopamine receptor 4 (DRD4) have opposite effects on orientation or interest in infants and novelty seeking trait in adults (Ebstein & Kotler, 2002). The short allele of the serotonin transporter increase avoidance behaviors, whereas the long form of the dopamine receptor 4 increases approach behavior. This kind of genetic interaction in influencing behavioral and personality traits is probably the rule rather than the exception. Comings, Saucier, and MacMurray (2002) investigated the role of all five of the dopamine receptor genes in several personality traits. Four dopamine receptor genes, DRD1, DRD2, DRD4, DAT1) contributed to the 5.25% of the variance in novelty seeking. DRD1 actually contributed the most. They also found that all of the personality traits have genes in common.

Because the DRD4 is associated with personality traits which are in turn associated with substance use and abuse it might be expected that the long form of this gene would be associated with these behavioral expressions of sensation seeking. In fact, this allele is associated with heroin and alcohol dependence and smoking in several studies (Ebstein & Kotler, 2002). Duaux et al. (1998) failed to find a significant differences between opiate addicts and controls on the frequency of a polymorphism for the DRD3 receptor gene, but within the opiate dependent population those with high sensation seeking scores had more frequent homozygous forms of the allele associated with the reinforcing properties of cocaine in monkeys and rats. The high sensation seekers among the drug addicts had a particular predilection for the stimulants amphetamine and cocaine in addition to opiates. The dopamine D3 receptor is specifically expressed in the mesolimbic-mesocortical dopamine pathways hypothesized to be a primary locus for the traits of sensation seeking (Zuckerman, 1995) and impulsivity (Gray, 1987).

A number of studies have found associations between substance abuse and the TAQ A1 RFLP located near the dopamine D2 receptor gene (DRD2) (Uhl, Persico, & Smith, 1992). Uhl et al. found that 44% of substance abusers in seven studies showed the presence of this A1 RFLP contrasted with 27% of controls. The presence was higher in the more severe than in the less severe substance abusers. Similar findings were reported by Smith et al. (1992), who also found a difference between substance abusers and controls on the B1 RFLP (DRD2). O'Hara et al. (1993) found differences in the frequencies of the A1 and B1 RFLP's between substance users in the white general population but not in the black population. The A1 allele was present in 51% of a cocaine dependent sample contrasted with 31% of nonsubstance abusing controls (Noble et al., 1993). The B1 allele also was found more frequently in cocaine dependent persons. The A1 allele was associated with indicators of severity of cocaine abuse, such as use of "crack" and early risk factors, alcoholism in parents, and deviant behaviors prior to cocaine abuse. The association between these DRD2 variants and substance use, abuse, and dependence, as well as an association with predrug risk factors, and pathological gambling disorder (Comings et al., 1996), suggests that these alleles may be associated with antisocial personality and/or impulsive unsocialized sensation seeking.

A recent meta-analysis of 15 studies comparing about 1,000 alcoholics and 900 controls found that alcoholics had a higher prevalence and frequency of the A1 allele of the DRD2 gene than controls (Noble, 1998). Furthermore, the allele was more prevalent in the more severe than in the less severe alcoholics. The prevalence of the A1 allele in severe alcoholics (48%) was three times its prevalence in controls, screened to eliminate alcoholics and drug abusers (16%).

Homozygosity of the DRD3 gene also has been associated with opiate dependence but only in those with high sensation seeking scores (Duaux et al., 1998). Sensation seeking was much higher in the opiate dependent group than in controls and those with high sensation seeking scores in the opiate group also were more frequently cocaine and amphetamine addicts.

Biometric genetic studies of criminality and psychopathy have shown some evidence of interaction between genetic influences from the biological parents and environmental ones from the adoptive family. A recent study has shown an interaction between the gene for monoamine oxidase-type A (MAO-A) and a childhood history of maltreatment (Caspi et al., 2002). In this longitudinal study of male children from 3 to 26 years of age, it was found that conduct disorder during childhood and antisocial personality disorder by age 26 were associated with childhood maltreatment, but only in those men who had the polymorphism producing low MAO-A activity. Those with the other allele associated with high MAO-A activity showed no significant relationship between childhood maltreatment and antisocial diagnoses (see Figure 5-3). Childhood maltreatment seems to affect only the children with a genetic vulnerability in the MAO-A gene. More about the differental psychopharmacology of MAO-A and MAO-B types will be presented in the section on psychopharmacology.

Whether looking at personality or psychopathology, it is increasingly apparent that the idea of a specific gene for any one trait or disorder is unlikely. At least several genes may be associated with a trait and the same genes may be associated with several or many traits. Whether the combinations of genes are additive or epistatic (interactive) it is easy to see why gene-trait associations are so difficult to establish, particularly when only one gene and one trait are analyzed in a given study. This is not to say that genetic research should be atheoretical. The particular candidate genes to be studied can be selected according to what is known about the biochemical or neurological correlates of behavior in animals or humans. The findings indicate a connection between genes involved in dopaminergic systems and antisocial personality and the personality traits involved in this disorder.

PSYCHOPHYSIOLOGY

Autonomic Arousal

Lower basal levels of skin conductance level (SCL) have been found in high compared to low sensation seekers in some studies, but these have been found in females not males (Zahn, Schooler, & Murphy, 1986), and young females as opposed to older ones (Plouffe & Stelmack, 1986). But several other studies found no differences at all between high and low sensation seekers in baseline SCL. Similar inconsistent results with baseline SCL have

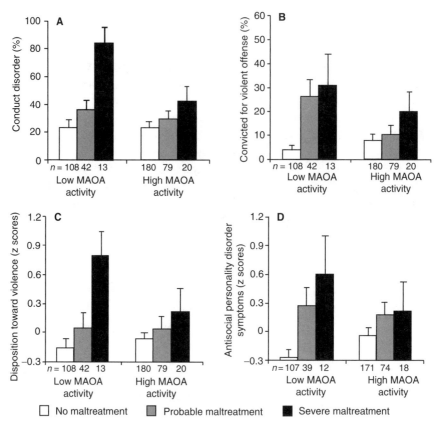

Figure 5-3. The association between childhood maltreatment and subsequent antisocial behavior as a function of MAO activity (expressed in polymorphisms for the gene for MAO type A). Figure A: Percentage of males (and standard error) meeting diagnostic criteria for Conduct Disorder between ages 10 and 18. Figure B: Percentage of males convicted of a violent crime by age 26. Figure C: Mean z scores on the Disposition Toward Violence at age 26. Figure D: The antisocial Personality Disorder symptom scale at age 26. In all of these the effect of maltreatment was significant in the low MAO-A allele group but not in the high MAO-A allele group. From "Role of genotype in the cycle of violence in maltreated children," by A. Caspi et al., 2002, *Science, 297,* Fig. 2, p. 852. Copyright 2002 by *Science* magazine. Reprinted by permission.

been found for psychopathy (Hare, 1978; Raine, 1996). However, in reaction to a socially stressful situation, giving a videotaped talk about their personal faults, persons with antisocial personality disorder showed lower SCR than control and drug-dependent groups (Raine, Lencz, Bihrle, LaCasse, & Colletti, 2000).

Neary and Zuckerman (1976) found no differences between high and low sensation seekers in baseline SCL but they found a difference in strength of the orienting reflex (OR) in response to a simple visual stimulus. On the first presentation of the stimulus the ampitude of the SC OR was greater in the high than in the low sensation seekers, but on the second and subsequent presentations there was no difference. On presentation of a new visual stimulus, the difference reappeared only to disappear on the subsequent presentations. The authors speculated that the OR to a novel stimulus reflected the greater interest of high sensation seekers in novel sensations. A few subsequent studies were able to replicate this finding (Feij, Orlebeke, Gazendam, & van Zuilen, 1985; Robinson & Zahn, 1983; Smith, Perlstein, Davidson, & Michael, 1986), but five others could not.

Smith et al. demonstrated the OR difference for auditory as well as visual stimuli, but they also found an influence of word content on the OR. High sensation seekers had stronger responses to "loaded" words selected for their potential interest to sensation seekers even after the first presentation of the words. In a subsequent study, they also showed that high sensation seekers had stronger SC ORs to high intensity sexual and aggressive words (Smith, Davidson, Smith, Goldstein, & Perlstein, 1989). These are strong areas of interest for sensation seekers and those with antisocial personalities.

No differences are found between antisocial individuals and controls on the SC OR except for a subgroup of schizoid or schizotypal psychopaths who show reduced SC ORs, perhaps an indication of their lack of interest in the environment or attention deficits (Ishikawa & Raine, 2002). In fact, strong SC ORs may indicate a protective factor against criminality in those who have some genetic disposition inherited from their fathers. Potentially antisocial males who manage to avoid criminal convictions have higher SC ORs than those who grow up to be convicted (Ishikawa, Raine, Lencz, Bihrle, & Lacasse, 2001).

As with basal SC levels, mixed results have been found for basal heart rate (HR) measures. Some investigators found lower HR in high sensation seekers (Ridgeway & Hare, 1981; Robinson & Zahn, 1983) but others have not (Cox, 1977; Stern, Cox, & Shanan, 1981; Zuckerman, Simons, & Como, 1988). Higher blood pressures have been found in low sensation seekers during physical exams but these tend to disappear on subsequent readings suggesting they are response to stress rather than a true basal difference in arousal (Carrol, Zuckerman, & Vogel, 1982; von Knorring, Oreland, & Winblad, 1984).

Basal HR has been found to be consistently lower in antisocial children and adolescents compared to controls (Raine, 1996, 2002). The average effect size from a meta-analysis is a moderate .56. Other psychiatric disorders are associated with high heart rates, so this effect is diagnostically specific. Longitudinal studies show that low resting HR is found before antisocial behavior develops, even in children as young as 3 years old. Low HR interacts with various psychosocial risk factors in increasing risk for becoming adult offenders (Farrington, 1997). Individuals with antisocial personality disorder show a weaker HR response to a stressful social situation than controls or substance dependent persons (Raine et al., 2000).

The HR orienting reflex (OR) is characterized by a deceleration of HR following a novel, nonaversive stimulus, such as a low to moderate intensity tone, and lasting from 2 to 4 seconds before returning to baseline. Evidence of a stronger HR OR in high than in low scorers on the Disinhibition subscale of the SSS have been found by several investigators (Cox, 1977, Orlebeke & Feij, 1979; Ridgeway & Hare, 1981; Zuckerman et al., 1988). The difference usually disappears on the second or third presentation of the stimulus, perhaps reflecting the interest in novel aspects of the environment in high sensation seekers that quickly dissipates with repetition.

There is no evidence that men with antisocial personality differ in HR OR reactions. But psychopaths tend to show increased anticipatory HR but decreased SCR responses when confronted with unavoidable punishment (Ishikawa & Raine, 2002). The increase in HR has been interpreted as a coping mechanism to tune out cues of punishment and the low SCR indicates it is successful.

Sensation seeking and impulsivity are not characterized by underarousal, as suggested by earlier theories, but show a strong response to intense stimuli in contrast to more controlled, low sensation seeking individuals. The latter tend to show inhibition of arousal at higher intensities of stimulation. Sensation seekers are also more responsive to novel stimuli or stimuli with interesting and sensational content. There is more evidence for the underarousal hypothesis for antisocial personality disorder, particularly as indicated by EEG and HR studies under monotonous recording conditions.

Cortical Arousal

In Chapter 3, I discussed the evidence bearing on Eysenck's theory that extraversion was a function of cortical underarousal and as a consequence extraverts were less conditionable than introverts. However, at the time most of these studies were done, extraversion actually contained two factors: sociability and impulsivity. Studies that analyzed these components separately found that conditionability was a function of impulsivity rather than sociability (Barratt, 1971; Eysenck & Levey, 1972). Later, Eysenck and

Eysenck (1985) realigned the subtraits in their three factor model, assigning impulsivity to the P rather than the E dimension. Cortical arousal, as measured by the EEG also showed that low arousal was related to impulsivity rather than to sociability (Goldring & Richards, 1985; O'Gorman & Lloyd, 1987). A PET study found negative relationships between P and glucose use in cortical, thalamic, and cingulate areas (Haier et al., 1987). Low cortical arousal is also found in studies of psychopathic personality, consistent with the association of this trait with P as a personality dimension (Ishikawa & Raine, 2002).

In contrast to impulsivity, sensation seeking has not been found to be related to low levels of *tonic* cortical arousal. However, sensation seeking, particularly of the disinhibitory type, has been related with some consistency to a particular measure of cortical *arousability* called *augmenting-reducing* (A-R), (Buchsbaum, 1971). It is unfortunate that Buchsbaum used this term to describe the cortical paradigm that he developed, because it gets confused with the same label applied by Petrie, Collins, and Solomon (1958) to a procedure involving the Kinesthetic After Effect (KAE). The KAE is a psychophysical, not a psychophysiological measure, in which inferences about brain reactivity are made on the basis of estimates of the width of a block of wood after stimulation by rubbing another block. I have argued that the KAE lacks retest reliability and that the inferences made about brain processes from it are questionable (Zuckerman, 1984, 1986). Vando (1974) developed a questionnaire based on the Petrie concept, but the scale correlates only minimally or not all with the KAE.

The A-R, based on actual cortical EP measurements, represents the relationship between amplitude of the cortical EP and stimulus intensity. The EP component is an early one representing the first impact of stimulus intensity on the cortex. A strong positive relationship is called "augmenting" and a weak positive or negative relationship is called "reducing," although the measures such as slopes are continuous. The measure is like Pavlov's (1922/1960) construct "Strength of the Nervous System," based on the nervous system's capacity to respond to high intensities of stimulation without showing "transmarginal inhibition."

The first study relating sensation seeking to A-R showed a substantial relationship between the slope of the visual EP amplitude and the Disinhibition subscale of the SSS as pictured in Figure 5-4 (Zuckerman, Murtaugh, & Siegel, 1974). High scorers on the Dis scale showed an augmenting pattern and low scorers showed a reducing pattern with little increase in amplitude through the first four levels of intensity and a significant decrease at the highest intensity. The same relationship has been found for the auditory

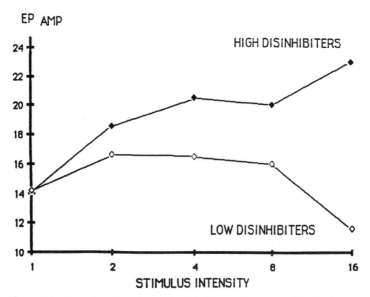

Figure 5-4. Mean visually evoked potential (EP) amplitudes (P1-N1) of high and low scorers on the Disinhibition subscale of the Sensation Seeking Scale as a function of stimulus intensity. From "Sensation seeking and cortical augmenting-reducing," by M. Zuckerman et al., 1974, *Psychophysiology, 11,* p. 539, Copyright 1974 by the Society for Psychophysiological Research. Reprinted by permission.

evoked potential as shown in Figure 5-5 from a study by Zuckerman, Simons, and Como, 1988). A majority of replications have been successful, particularly for the auditory EP, despite variations in EP methods, subject populations, and the use of translated scales (Zuckerman, 1990). Replications continue to appear (Brocke, Beauducel, John, Debener, & Heileman, 2000; Stenberg, Rosen, & Risberg, 1990). A-R also has been related to impulsivity, (Barratt, Pritchard, Faulk, & Brandt, 1987; Carrilo-de-la-Pena, & Barratt, 1993). High augmenting scores have been found in delinquents and drug users, groups who typically score high on disinhibition (Zuckerman et al., 1980). Adult, nonpsychopathic criminals cortically augment visual stimuli in comparison with controls (Raine & Venables, 1990).

The P1-N1 component of the EP that is related to disinhibition in humans can be identified in cats and rats and therefore offers the possibility for comparative studies (Siegel & Driscoll, 1996). Furthermore, the complex shapes of the EP are very stable in cats as well as humans and show high similarity in human identical twins, suggesting genetic determination (Buchsbaum, 1974; Rust, 1975). Hall, Rappaport, Hopkins, Griffin, and Silverman (1970) classified cats as EP augmenters or reducers and compared their behavioral

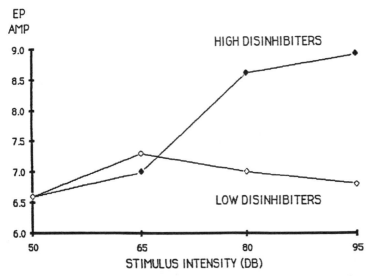

Figure 5-5. Mean auditory evoked potential (EP) amplitudes at four levels of sound intensity (50–95 dB) for high and low scorers on the Disinhibition subscale of the Sensation Seeking Scale. From "Sensation seeking and stimulus intensity as modulators of cortical, cardiovascular, and electrodermal response: A cross-modality study," by M. Zuckerman, R. F. Simons, and P. G. Como, 1988, *Personality and individual differences, 9,* p. 368. Elmsford, NY: Pergamon Press. Copyright 1988 by Pergamon Press. Reprinted by permission.

reactions to novel and/or frightening stimuli. EP augmenting was related to exploration, activity, and aggressiveness but not to fear, rage, or excitability. Lukas and Siegel (1977) also found more activity and exploration in the responses of augmenter cats to a frightening stimulus. Saxton, Siegel, and Lukas (1987) replicated these results and found that reducer cats were more emotional and tense and reacted to novel threatening stimuli by withdrawal rather than exploration or aggression. The behavioral reactions of augmenter cats fit the definition of sensation seeking, and its suggested animal model of exploration (Zuckerman, 1984).

Impulsivity, as a trait in cats, was investigated in two experimental paradigms (Saxton et al., 1987). A fixed internal (FI) bar pressing task for food reward assessed the strength of reward motivation, and a differential reinforcement for a low rate of response (DRL) bar pressing measured the capacity to inhibit or slow responses in order to get reward. Augmenting cats learned the FI task more quickly than reducers but the reducer cats were superior in the DRL task because they were able to inhibit their rate of response. In other words the augmenter cats were more impulsive and unable to restrain or delay response in pursuit of reward.

Table 5-12. Behavioral and physiological differences between roman high avoidance (RHA) and roman low avoidance (RLA) rat strains*

Variable	Difference
EP Augmenting vs. Reducing	RHAs augmenters, RLAs reducers.
Exploration (open-field test)	RHAs more active, less fearful.
Shock-induced Aggression	RHAs more and RLAs less aggressive.
Alcohol Drinking	RHAs drink alcohol in solution, RLAs abstain.
Barbiturates	RHAs high tolerance, RLAs low tolerance.
Maternal Behavior	RHA females less time in nest with young, RLAs more time in nest.
Hypothalamic Self-stimulation	RHAs less sensitive to high intensity of stimulation, more responsive to high intensities; RLAs escape from high intensities.
STRESS EFFECTS (Monoamines and Hormones)	
Prefrontal Cortex	RHAs increased dopamine, RLAs no change.
Hypothalamus	RLAs increased serotonin, RHAs less change. RLAs increased corticotropin releasing factor. RHAs less change in CRF.
Pituitary Gland	RLAs increased adrenocorticotropic hormone (ACTH). RHAs less change in ACTH.

* From M. Zuckerman, Personality and Psychopathy, Chap. 2 in J. Glicksohn (Ed.), *The neurobiology of criminal behavior*, Table 3, p. 41. Boston, MA: Kluwer Academic Publishers. Copyright 2002 by Kluwer Academic Publishers. Reprinted with permission.

Siegel, Sisson, and Driscoll (1993) extended the A-R paradigm to rats, using two strains selectively bred for their reactions to shock in a shuttle box. One strain was selected from those who were actively aggressive or avoidant and the other was frozen and passive in reaction to the aversive stimuli. Tested on the A-R model using a visual EP, nearly all of the Roman High Avoidance (RHA) rats were augmenters and nearly all of the Roman Low Avoidance (RLA) rats were reducers. The significance of this finding can be assessed by examining the behavioral and biological differences between the two strains, as shown in Table 5-12.

The RHA (augmenter) strain is more exploratory and less emotional in the open-field test, more aggressive when shocked, more likely to drink alcohol, and a high tolerance for barbiturates. The females show poor maternal behavior with little contact with their young. The RLA (reducer) strain are just the opposite on these behavioral traits. Brain self-stimulation in the lateral hypothalamus is highly reinforcing, but the reaction to the stimulation reward depends on its intensity. The RHA rats are sensitive and more responsive to high intensities of brain stimulation. In contrast, the RLA rats are more sensitive to the low intensities, and tend to escape from stimulation at high intensities. This seems to be an expression of the A-R paradigm at the motivational level.

The differences between the two strains on biological stress effects offers a model for the biochemistry of impulsive unsocialized sensation seeking. During stress the RHA rats show increased dopamine in the prefrontal cortex. Increased dopamine may be what enables the RHA rats to become active in response to stress since dopamine is involved in initiation of motor activity.

The RLAs show no change in dopamine but do show increased serotonin in the hypothalamus. Serotonin is associated with inhibition of behavior and thus may account for the freezing and passivity bred into this strain.

The two strains show differences in the HYPAC system in response to stress. The RLAs show increased secretion of the corticotropin releasing factor (CRF), and increased release of adrenocorticotropic hormone (ACTH). The RHAs show little arousal in this hormonal pathway for stress.

If this is a good model for the biology of human impulsive unsocialized sensation seeking, we would predict that high ImpUSS persons would have a reactive dopamine system and unreactive serotonergic and HYPAC systems, the latter expressed in low levels of cortisol. Antisocial personalities should also show some of the same characteristics.

There is another animal model based on comparisons of two groups of rats selected for their novelty seeking behaviors in several kinds of experimental situations (Dellu, Piazza, Mayo, Le Moal, & Simon, 1996). The high responders (HRs) show novelty seeking behaviors in these situations, whereas the low reactives (LRs) prefer the more familiar environments. The HRs show more self-administration of amphetamine than the LRs and there is a high correlation ($r = .62$) between reactivity to novelty and drug intake. The HRs also show a higher rate of food ingestion after food deprivation even though there is no difference in consumption under normal conditions. As with the RHA-RLA comparisons, the differences on biochemical reactions between HRs and LRs are interesting in that they suggest hypotheses for human personality correlation with such reactions.

The basal dopaminergic activity measured by the ratio of the dopamine metabolite DOPAC to dopamine was measured in autopsy. The HRs had a higher ratio in the nucleus accumbens (NA), a primary site for self-stimulation reward and the effects of stimulant drugs, and the response to novelty correlated with the DOPAC content in the NA ($r = .54$). Opposite results were obtained for DOPAC in the prefrontal cortex where LRs were higher and DOPAC correlated negatively with responses to novelty.

The differences were attributed to evidence that dopamine release in the prefrontal cortex inhibits its release in the nucleus accumbens. Pain stress increases dopamine release in the NA more in HRs than in LRs. The findings of Dellu et al. are consistent with those of Bardo et al. (1996), who found that exposure to novelty in rats stimulates release of dopamine in the NA and injection of a dopamine antagonist reduces or eliminates novelty seeking activity.

If these results can be extrapolated to humans, we would expect higher basal levels of dopaminergic activity and more release of dopamine in reaction to stress or novelty in high sensation or novelty seekers and stimulant drug users. However, the contrasting results in prefrontal cortex and the NA make predictions of general dopamine reactivity problematic.

The comparisons of RHA and RLA rats on reactions to stress suggested that there was more reactivity of the HYPAC stress system in the RLA strain. This should result in lower levels of cortisol as an end product hormone of the system. Stress and extreme anxiety as well as depression are related to cortisol as described in the last chapter. However, administration of corticosterone to rats increases extracellular dopamine content in the NA and corticosterone has positively reinforcing effects in humans and rats. HR rats, in particular, are susceptible to the reinforcing properties of the hormone as shown by self-administration experiments. The investigators found that although the corticosterone response to novel situations was equivalent in HRs and LRs, the HRs showed a continued response for two hours post exposure, whereas the LR's levels of the hormone dropped. These results may suggest results in the relation of novelty seeking to HYPAC activity in high and low sensation seekers opposite to those found in the RHA/RLA studies. Comparions of comparative studies of other species with human correlational studies poses many problems, particularly if different models lead to different predictions.

Human Studies of Biochemical and Genetic Correlates of Augmenting-Reducing

Platelet MAO-B levels are negatively correlated with augmenting of visual EP's in patient groups, consistent with the low levels of MAO-B in high sensation seekers and those exhibiting antisocial or high drug and alcohol use (Buchsbaum, Landau, Murphy, & Goodwin, 1973; Haier, Buchsbaum, Murphy, Gottesman, & Coursey, 1980). Visual EP augmenters in patient groups had lower levels of 5-HIAA (the serotonin metabolite), HVA (the dopamine metabolite) in CSF and lower levels of endorphins than reducers (von Knorring & Perris, 1981). Zimeldine (a selective inhibitor of serotonin uptake) reduced the EP amplitude-stimulus intensity slope, consistent with the negative relationship between serotonin and augmenting-reducing (von Knorring & Johansson, 1980). Persons consuming the drug "Ecstasy," which damages serotonergic systems in the brain, exhibit more EP augmenting than controls (Croft, Klugman, Baldeweg, & Gruzelier, 2001; Tuchtenhagen et al., 2000). These studies are all consistent with the hypothesis of a role of serotonergic activity in the reducing of the cortical reaction to intense stimuli.

Strohel et al. (2003) investigated the role of the serotonin transporter gene (5-HTTLPR) and the D4 receptor gene (DRD4, exon III) in augmenting-reducing of the auditory EP. The DRD4 has been related to novelty seeking as discussed previously. Individuals homozygous for the long form of the serotonin transporter gene tended to be EP augmenters compared to those heterozygous for the allele (but not to those homozygous for the short form). Those with the long form of the D4 receptor also tended to be augmenters, but this was primarily found among those homozygous on the long form of the serotonin transporter. The interaction of the two polymorphisms approached significance ($p = .09$). This is an important study that should be replicated with large ns because it is one of the few actually showing an interaction between genes in affecting a physiological-personality trait marker.

BIOCHEMISTRY

Hormones

The differences between RHA and RLA rats in reactions to stress (Table 5-12) suggest that cortisol would be lower in those high in impulsive sensation seeking or antisocial tendencies than in those low in this dimension. In a simple correlational study of normals, cortisol in CSF correlated negatively with the EPQ P scale, the SSS Disinhibition scale, and the MMPI Ego Strength scale, suggesting low levels of the hormone in antisocial, disinhibited types (Ballenger et al., 1983). Low cortisol is also associated with novelty seeking in veterans with posttraumatic stress disorder (Wang, Mason, Charney, & Yehuda, 1997). Low levels of urinary cortisol are found in prisoners who are psychopathic and/or violent (Virkunen, 1985). Because high levels of cortisol are found in major depression and in reaction to stress in anxiety disorders, the low levels of cortisol in more externalizing types may show the lack of anxiety and stress reactivity in psychopathic personality.

Epinephrine (Epi), or adrenaline, is a hormone produced largely by the adrenal medulla although some small amounts are present in brain. The hormone is under control of the sympathetic branch of the autonomic nervous system and when released stimulates all organs innervated by this branch to increase general arousal. Low levels of Epi in basal states in boys aged 13 predicted criminal activity when they reached adult ages (Magnusson, 1987, 1996; Olweus, 1987).

Testosterone has been associated in public stereotypes with aggressive and antisocial traits, but studies of normals suggest that it is also associated with healthy traits such as sociability, activity, and assertiveness (Daitzman & Zuckerman, 1980). Of course it is also related to traits such as low self-control, sensation seeking and impulsivity, which may cause problems in those with antisocial tendencies (Aluja & Torrubia, in press; Daitzman & Zuckerman, 1980). Testosterone is related to the behavioral expressions of these latter traits in subjects in terms of their number of sexual partners in their history (Bogaert & Fisher, 1995; Dabbs, 2000; Daitzman & Zuckerman, 1980), and antisocial behavior beginning in childhood (Dabbs, 2000). Very low levels of testosterone are associated with low sensation seeking and sexual dysfunctions in men (O'Carroll, 1984). But looking at the normal range of sensation seeking, high sensation seekers tend to have very high levels of testosterone whereas low sensation seekers have normal levels (Daitzman & Zuckerman, 1980).

Neurotransmitters and their Enzymes

Monoamine oxidase (MAO) is an enzyme that catabolizes the oxidative deamination of a number of biogenic amines in the brain, including the monoamines. MAO comes in two forms: the A and B types. MAO-A preferentially oxidizes serotonin and norepinephrine, whereas in human and primate brain (but not in rat brain) dopamine is primarily oxidized by MAO-B (Berry, Juorio, & Patterson, 1994; Murphy, Aulakh, Garrick, & Sunderland, 1987; Shih, Chen, & Ridd, 1999).

2-phenylethylamine (PEA) is the most selective endogenous substrate for MAO-B. It is metabolized mostly by MAO-B. PEA potentiates neuronal responses to dopaminergic and noradrenergic agonists. Inhibition of MAO-B potentiates dopaminergic responses by elevating endogenous PEA levels (Berry et al., 1994).

MAO-B increases gradually with age in both brain, blood platelets and plasma (Robinson, Davis, Nies, Revarics, & Sylvester, 1971). Increased oxidation of dopamine by MAO-B may be responsible for the loss of dopaminergic neurons in Parkinson's Disease. MAO-B has a lower affinity for serotonin than MAO-A (Asmitia & Whitaker-Azmita (1995), but Swedish investigators have suggested that there is a positive relationship between MAO-B and serotonin turnover based on a common genetic determination and a similar distribution in brain areas (Adolfsson, Gottfries, Oreland, Ross, & Winblad, 1978; Oreland, Wiberg, & Fowler, 1981).

MAO A and B are based on different genes on the X chromosone and are nearly totally genetically determined, although they may be affected by chronic alcoholism or smoking. Studies of mice in which either or both of the genes for MAO-A and MAO-B have been "knocked out" (KO) show different effects. Eliminating the MAO-A gene results in increases of serotonin and norepinephrine in cerebellum, frontal cortex, and hippocampus (Shih & Chen, 1999). These mice show increased aggressiveness and decreased freezing or defensive postures when paired with other mice. MAO-B KO mice showed a large increase in PEA, which potentiates the actions of both dopamine and norepinephrine. Mice deficient in MAO-B did not show increases in aggression. Mice with both types of MAO KO showed increased reactivity to stress, perhaps as a function of increased catecholamines in both.

A study of newborns using MAO-B obtained from the umbilical cord at birth showed behavioral differences in the first 3 days of life between infants with high or low MAO levels (Sostek, Sostek, Murphy, Martin, & Born, 1981). Low MAO infants were more aroused, active and reactive, cried more, and were "less cuddly," but showed more optimal motor behavior and motor developmental maturity. Adult levels of MAO-B are very reliable and stable with only a gradual increase with age (Murphy et al., 1976).

The association between MAO-B obtained from blood platelets and the trait of sensation seeking has been extensively studied. A survey of results through 1990 showed low but significant negative correlations between the SSS in 9 of 13 groups, and in 11 of the 13 groups the correlations were negative in sign (high sensation seekers tend to have low levels of MAO) (Zuckerman, 1994). Low MAO is found in a number of personality and clinical disorders characterized by high sensation seeking and impulsivity, as shown in Table 5-13. The exception might be the paranoid schizophrenics. Although schizophrenics as a group score low on sensation seeking, it is the more apathetic and inactive schizophrenics who are the lowest on the trait (Kish, 1970). Younger paranoid schizophrenics are not generally apathetic.

Low MAO-B is found in relatives of alcoholics and bipolar disorders who are not necessarily suffering from the disorder themselves. This finding suggests that MAO is a genetic marker for the disorder, perhaps increasing the risk through its association with personality traits like impulsivity and sensation seeking. Among alcoholics, low MAO and sensation seeking

Table 5-13. Personality and clinical disorders characterized by low levels of MAO-B

Low MAO-B is found in:	Reference
High Sensation Seekers (normal populations)	see Zuckerman, 1994, for refs
Attention Deficit Hyperactivity Disorder	Shekim et al., 1986
Antisocial Personality Disorder	Lidberg et al., 1985
Chronic Criminality	Alm et al., 1994
Borderline Personality Disorder	Reist et al., 1990
Alcoholism	Major & Murphy, 1978
Relatives of Alcoholics	Schukit, 1994; Sher, 1993
Drug Abuse	Von Knorring et al., 1987
Bipolar Mood Disorder	Murphy & Weiss, 1972
Relatives of Patients with Bipolar Disorder	Leckman et al., 1977
Paranoid Schizophrenics	Zureik & Meltzer, 1988

are associated with the type II alcoholism, characterized by a younger on-set, more antisocial behavior when intoxicated, and a family history of alcoholism.

Apart from personality and clinical disorders, low MAO-B levels are found among those in the general population who smoke, drink heavily, and use drugs (Arque, Unzeta & Torrubia, 1988; Coursey, Buchsbaum, & Murphy, 1979; Hallman, von Knorring, von Knorring, & Oreland, 1990; Kuperman, Kramer, & Loney, 1988). Low MAO in the general population, even among college students, is associated with convictions for offenses other than mere traffic violations (Coursey et al., 1979). Over a third of male college students with low MAO reported such convictions compared with only 6% in a high MAO group.

MAO-B is lower in men than women at all ages, and increases in human brain, platelets, and plasma with age (Murphy et al., 1976; Robinson, Davis et al., 1971). These data are consistent with the finding that sensation seeking (Zuckerman, 1994) and psychoticism (Eysenck & Eysenck, 1976) are higher in men than in women and decrease with age after peaking in the late adolescent group. Agreeableness and conscientiousness increased with age in four different cultures (Costa et al., 2000). Women are higher in agreeableness and men are higher on excitement seeking in U.S. adults and college age samples (Costa, Terracciano, & McCrae, 2001). The results on personality traits are also consistent with the finding that the behavioral factor in the psychopathy check list declines with age (Harpur & Hare, 1994), and the 1-year prevalence of antisocial personality disorder is much higher in men than women and declines with age in both sexes (Robins & Regier, 1991). Of course, this parallelism of gender and age differences is not limited to MAO but also could fit the demographic characteristics of the hormone testosterone. Biochemical factors may underlie gender and age changes in personality and its expressions. The increased wisdom, constraint, conservatism, and benevolence of age may be due as much to changes in our biochemistry as to experience alone.

A comparative study of MAO-B in monkeys living in a natural colony found that low MAO monkeys were more active, social, aggressive, dominant, and more playful and sexually active than high MAO monkeys of both sexes (Redmond, Murphy, & Baulu, 1979). Sexual activity would be a factor in the evolutionary selection of low MAO, the monoamine functions it serves, and sensation seeking.

MAO type A has been related to aggression in mice and these associations will be discussed in the next chapter. Because MAO-A is not found in blood but is found in the brain, studies of humans have used the MAO-A gene polymorphism to classify individuals as low or high MAO activity types. A rare mutation in a Dutch family produced a null allele resulting in the absence of MAO-A enzyme (Brunner, Nelsen, Breakefield, Ropers, & Van Oost, 1993). The members of the family with this mutation were characterized by antisocial and aggressive behavior. A polymorphism in the promoter region of the MAO-A gene associated with low MAO-A activity had an increased frequency in alcoholics with antisocial personality (Samochowiec et al., 1999). Nonpsychopathic alcoholics did not differ from controls in the frequency of this polymorphism.

In the previous section on genetics, I discussed the study by Caspi et al. (2002) in which those with an allele producing low MAO-A activity *and* who also were exposed to severe maltreatment as children tended to develop conduct disorder in childhood and adolescence and antisocial personality disorder as adults. Apparently, the absence or low amount of MAO-A in the brain in interaction with childhood maltreatment produces unsocialized personalities. High levels of MAO-A, regardless of childhood maltreatment, seem to innoculate children against chronic unsocialized behavior typical of antisocial personality. The changes produced by inhibition of both types of MAO in mice increase the disinhibitory effects of either type A or B inhibition alone (Mejia, Ervin, Baker, & Palmour, 2002). One of the tests used was the differential reinforcement for a low rate of reinforcement, the same test on which cats who were "reducers" on EP augmenting-reducing were superior to "augmenters" because they were more capable of restraint (Saxton et al., 1987). Prenatal treatment with MAO-B inhibition in mice reduced the ratio of success out of total attempts to get rewards, but the

MAO-A inhibition by itself did not affect this measure of constraint versus impulsivity.

The general association of the monoamine enzymes with personality and behavior in the P-ImpUSS dimension suggests the importance of the monoamine neurotransmitters regulated by these enzymes in the brain: the catecholamines, dopamine (DA) and norepinephrine (NE), and the indoleamine, serotonin (SE). The comparative literature, using experimental methods, has uncovered some broad functions of the monoamines in behavioral reactions relevant to personality differences in humans. In general, DA circuits in the brain are involved in appetitive approach and exploration (Cloninger, 1987; Dellu et al., 1993; Depue & Iacono, 1989; Gray, 1987; Panksepp, 1982; Zuckerman, 1984, 1991), SE in behavioral control and inhibition of approach in response to signals of danger (Soubrié, 1986), and NE to arousal, alarm, and fear (Gray, 1982; Redmond, 1987). More specific monoamine pathways will be outlined in the last section on neuropsychology.

Studies of the monamines in humans are less direct and experimental since their activity in the brain is less accessible. One can study metabolite products of activity in the CSF, blood, and urine, but these may be in part related to neurotransmitter or hormone activity in the peripheral systems. One can also assess the hormonal and behavioral responses to agonists and antagonists of the systems. This has been the more popular methodology in current research.

In the exploratory study by Ballenger et al. (1983), NE in the CSF and plasma dopamine-beta-hydroxylase (DBH) both correlated negatively with the SSS Total scale, but not significantly with the P scale. The metabolites of DA and NE were not correlated with either P or the SSS. The DBH correlation with sensation seeking was inconsistently replicated. Noone has attempted to replicate the one with CSF NE but another approach, to be discussed later, does support the relationship. Limson et al. (1991) found no significant relationships between NE or any other monoamine metabolites in CSF and any of the novelty seeking, harm-avoidance, or reward-dependence scales of Cloninger's (1987) TPQ. Low levels of CSF NE have been more consistently associated with antisocial behavior. A meta-analysis of this association found a significant negative effect size of .41 (Raine, 1993).

Another approach is to test the effects of neurotransmitter agonists or antagonists on subjects, measuring subjective, behavioral, or hormone responses of neurotransmitter activity. Amphetamine and nicotine are stimulant drugs favored by high sensation seekers. Both are dopamine agonists and in the case of amphetamine the release of dopamine in the mesolimbic reward system probably accounts for its euphoric effects, called "highs" in the vernacular. Hutchison, Wood, and Swift (1999) gave d-amphetamine or a placebo to normal subjects on different occasions. The drug itself significantly increased self-reported elation, vigor, and positive affect in all subjects, but this stimulation effect interacted with the personality scales for Disinhibiton (SSS) and Novelty Seeking (TPQ). Those scoring high on both scales reported more arousal from amphetamine, but those high on Disinhibiton (Dis) also reported more elation and positive affect in response to the drug. One problem is that amphetamine stimulates the release of NE as well as DA. NE could mediate the subjective report of arousal, but DA mediates the reward effects in rats and may very well account for reports of elation and positive affect in the high disinhibiters.

A similar interaction between drug effects and nicotine (adminstered by nasal spray) was found in nonsmokers (Perkins, Gerlack, Broge, Grobe, & Wilson, 2000). High scorers on the Dis and Experience Seeking (ES) subscales of the SSS reported a stronger head "rush," vigor, and arousal even at lower doses of nicotine. The fact that this relationship was found in nonsmokers suggests that it was their intial reaction to the drug not influenced by extended experience with nicotine through smoking. The two studies might suggest a greater dopaminergic reactivity, perhaps accounting for the greater use of drugs and smoking among high sensation seekers.

This sensitivity to DA stimulants could be based on several factors including low levels of DA synthesis and a resultant supersensitivity or multiplicity of receptors or simply a low level of receptor density due to genetic factors. Cloninger's (Cloninger et al., 1993) model suggests the first possibility. But, the extreme case of low dopamine levels in humans is found in Parkinson's disease (PD). Persons with PD are lower on Cloninger's Novelty Seeking scale than controls suffering from rheumatoid and other orthopedically impairing disorders (Menza, Golbe, Cody, & Forman, 1993). In PD, there are major decreases of the ventral-tegmental as well as the nigrostriatal dopamine systems. PD patients suffer from depression and a loss of interest in their environment but this did not account for their low NS scores in the study. PD is an abnormal degree of DA loss and the relationship between tonic DA activity and novelty or sensation seeking may hold within a more normal range of activity.

In a PET study of personality, the Dis and ES subscales of the SSS correlated positively with glucose uptake in the caudate and putamen parts of the striatal dopaminergic system (Haier et al., 1987). However, this was found in a group of patients with Generalized Anxiety Disorder, and the results were not found in a very small control group.

Gray, Pickering, and Gray (1994) used Single Photon Emission Tomography to locate DA D2 receptor binding and had EPQ personality measures from a small group of normals. There was a very high negative correlation ($r = -.82$) between the P scale and DA D2 binding in left and right basal ganglia. A low number of DA receptors, as found in the highest P subjects, indicates a high supply of DA. This would be consistent with the results of the Haier et al. study, in patients. However, studies of normals (Hansenne et al., 2002) and alcoholic subjects (Wiesbeck, Mauerer, Thome, Jacob, & Boening, 1995) using the DA D2 receptor agonist, apomorphine, found positive relationships between growth hormone (an index of DA response) and novelty seeking. This would indicate a higher sensitivity of D2 receptors and presumably low basal DA supplies. Gera et al. (2000) also found a positive relationship between novelty seeking and response to a DA agonist (bromocriptine).

Depue (1995), using a DA agonist and measuring prolactin (PRL) response, found a relationship between the EPQ P scale and a blunted PRL indicating DA receptor insensitivity and therefore a high supply of DA. Although he did not find a relationship between PRL response and disinhibition and boredom susceptiblity scales of the SSS, he did find one with Eysenck's SS type scales, venturesomeness and risk taking, indicating increased sensitivity of DA receptors in high sensation seekers and perhaps decreased DA levels. As previously mentioned, increased receptor sensitivity also could be a compensation for a low density of DA receptors.

Netter and her colleagues in Germany have been studying the relationships between personality and the monoamine systems using agonist and antagonist drugs and measuring their effects on hormonal indicators of monoamine reactivity. Most of these were done in the context of studying nicotine addiction. Because prolactin (PRL) is inhibited by DA, PRL response (a decrease in PRL) is increased by DA agonists and decreased or blunted by DA antagonists. The PRL response (increase or decrease) would in both cases indicate receptor sensitivity. No relation between PRL responses to DA agonists and antagonists and sensation seeking was found in the study by Netter, Hennig, and Roed (1996). However, the craving for nicotine was increased by a dopamine agonist in high experience seekers.

This group investigated the responses to dopamine agonists and antagonists compared with placebo responses in the same group of subjects (Reuter, Netter, Toll, & Hennig, 2002). Most of the subjects could be classified as either agonist responders or antagonist responders both indicating sensitive DA receptors and low DA levels. High scores on SSS Thrill and

Adventure Seeking (TAS) and ES subscales were found in the "pure" agonist responders and low scores were found in the "pure" antagonist responders together with high scores on extraversion. The former group developed more nicotine craving when given an agonist, suggesting that dopamine has an incentive motivating effect in high sensation seekers. The group responding with increased nicotine craving to a DA antagonist, consisting of extraverted low sensation seekers, respond to nicotine to remedy a DA deficit caused by a temporary reduction in levels.

Depue (1995), using a dopamine agonist and measuring PRL response, found no relationship with Dis and Boredom Susceptibility (BS) SS scales, but he did find a negative relationship with the EPQ P scale indicating increased dopamine receptor sensitivity in high P scorers. He also found positive relationships with Eysenck's Venturesomeness and Risk Taking scales indicating decreased sensitivity and perhaps increased DA levels.

Netter (personal communication, 2003) has data showing greater responsivity or sensitivity of the dopamine system to a DA agonist in those high on novelty seeking, extraversion, impulsivity, Dis, and BS (the entire spectrum of approach related traits).

Most studies suggest that those high in approach behavior tendencies, as represented in sensation or novelty seeking, have an increased sensitivity to chemical stimulation of the dopaminergic systems. This could explain their special attraction to drugs, not because of a deficit but from their enhanced incentive motivation ("a bigger bang"). The level of basal activity in the system is more problematic. It certainly is not pathologically low as in Parkinson's disease (PD) in which there is markedly reduced interest in sensation seeking. It is interesting that the DA agonists used in therapy for PD may cause an increase in drive and well-being in additon to their beneficial effect on motor disturbances.

The relationship between serotonin (SE) and the traits involved in the P-ImpUSS dimension of personality is quite clear and consistent. Low levels of serotonergic activity or response are related to a lack of inhibitory capacity expressed in impulsivity, sensation seeking, and antisocial behavior.

Netter et al. (1996) used a SE agonist and measured cortisol and PRL responses. There were no differences between participants high and low on the SSS ES scale in reaction to a placebo, but reacting to the agonist the expected increase in cortisol was found in the low ES participants. The high ES individuals actually showed a decrease in cortisol back to baseline merely reflecting the diurnal slope of cortisol. With the PRL measure of response there was no difference on ES, but the high Dis showed a weaker response than low Dis subjects. Hennig et al. (1998) gave a SE antagonist and found that high Dis and impulsive subjects showed low responsivity to the antagonist, whereas the low disinhibitors showed the expected decrease in PRL.

Depue (1995) found that PRL response to a serotonergic agonist was negatively related to scales representing the entire range of the P-ImpUSS dimension: EPQ-P, SSS Dis and BS, and Barratt's impulsivity scale. Siever and Trestman (1993) found weaker PRL responses to a serotonergic agonist in patients with borderline personality disorder and response was more blunted in those with higher impulsivity. Netter, Toll, Reuter, and Hennig (2003) used cortisol responses to an SE reuptake inhibiter. They found that low responders had significantly lower heart rate, and higher EPQ P, and SSS ES scores than high responders, but these differences were not significant when corrected for the higher weight of the low responders.

These authors also used cortisol responses to a noradrenergic agonist. Low responders to the agonist showed higher motor impulsivity on Barratt's scales, higher Dis on the SSS, higher exploratory excitability (a subscale of NS on the TPQ) and lower scores on physical anhedonia and traditionalism on the MPQ. These findings support an earlier finding of a negative relationship between CSF levels of norepinephrine and sensation seeking (Ballenger et al., 1983).

The lack of reactivity in the SE system in impulsive, unsocialized, high sensation seekers is consistent with the clinical literature, which reports low serotonin activity in personality disorders characterized by impulsivity and aggression (Coccaro & Siever, 1995; Mann, 1995; Zalsman & Apter, 2002). Studies relating low SE to aggression will be discussed in the next chapter. Low SE is related to suicide as well as homicide. What the two kinds of aggression (toward self and others) have in common is their impulsivity. Long-planned and passionless murders or suicides are not related to low SE. The comparative literature also shows that serotonin is vital in behavioral control and restraint (Soubrié, 1986).

Interactive effects between the monoamines are rarely considered in research projects. DA and NE often respond together in arousing or stressful situations and the two catecholamines are inhibited by SE activation. To use a loose automotive analogy, NE is the accelerator, DA the steering (toward reward or away from punishment), and SE provides the brakes. A faulty mechanism in any of these can lead to the accidents of psychopathology. The ancient Greeks believed that a proper balance of bodily "humors" was the essence of health, both physical and mental (Zuckerman, 1995). They were probably right in terms of the neurotransmitters, enzymes, and hormones that regulate behavior.

There is still much uncertainty about the molecular mechanisms in neurotransmission that may account for differences in reactivity. There are many kinds of receptors in each system and they serve different functions.

Differences in reactivities may be due to differences in transmitter production, which in turn depends on enzymes. Differences may be due to sensitivities and densities of postsynaptic and presynaptic receptors. They may be due to transporter and uptake mechanisms or to regulating enzymes like MAO. Genetic regulation of the systems is not a fixed constraint but an ongoing process. Advances in molecular methods and connections of results to personality differences are hopes for the future.

NEUROPSYCHOLOGY

The frontal lobes have been described as serving the "executive function" in behavior, such as decision making and moderation of impulsive tendencies to react without planning or forethought. Cognitive functions such as attention, flexibility to adjust to changing contingencies, working memory, self-regulation, and abstract thinking involve the frontal cortex. Even since the classical case study of Phineas Gage, the railworker whose prefrontal cortices were largely destroyed in an accident in 1848 (Damasio, et al., 1994), neuropsychological studies of brain damage and the after effects of lobotomy operations have suggested that frontal lobe reduction reduces anxiety and increases impulsive, disinhibited behavior and the expression of angry aggressive feelings (Zuckerman, 1991).

Brain injuries, prenatal, perinatal (during birth), or postnatal, are much more frequent in criminal offenders, particularly violent ones (Miller, 2002; Raine, 2002). Persons with damage to the ventromedial frontal cortex tend to be autonomically unreactive to normally disturbing stimuli and tend to ignore possibilities of punishment in reward seeking tasks (Blair, 2002).

An MRI study of antisocial personality disorder (APD) showed an 11–14% reduction in prefrontal gray matter compared with a normal control group and a group of substance dependent individuals (Raine et al., 2000). Within the APD group those with less gray matter showed less autonomic response (SCR & HR) to a social stressful situation than those with more gray matter. It is interesting that the substance dependent group had a psychopathy rating and record of arrests that was intermediate between the normal control and the APD group. They were not intermediate, however, in amount of frontal gray matter deficit and autonomic reactivity, suggesting that the brain deficit may be one qualitatively rather than quantitatively related to APD. This could mean that the personality traits comprising the P-ImpUSS dimension may not be linearly related to amount of frontal brain matter. Studies of personality and brain imaging are needed in normals to resolve this issue.

Antisocial persons tend to have decreased right hemisphere functioning, as shown by functional MRI, CT brain imaging, neuropsychological tests, spatial IQ measures, EEG, and cortical EPs (Raine, 2002). The right hemisphere is dominant in control of HR and other autonomic responses, therefore the decreased right hemispheric activity could influence the decreased HR found in those with antisocial personality. Differences in size between right and left hippocampus (R > L) were found comparing successful (not yet caught) and unsuccessful psychopaths (Raine et al., 2004). The unsuccessful psychopaths showed a greater relative right size anterior hippocampus. Successful psychopaths (from the community) did not differ from controls on this structural lateralization. This kind of abnormality has been found in schizophrenics and children exposed to physical trauma or abuse although these possibilities were ruled out in this study. The authors suggest, instead, that the R > L may be associated with disruption to normal brain development.

If any traits are related to frontal lobe and hippocampal deficits it is likely to be impulsivity and socialization. Persons with these deficits have difficulty in learning to restrain or delay responding for reward in the presence of signals of possible punishment. Poor socialization may be a function of these emotional deficits.

The lack of emotional reaction, particularly anxiety, in the primary psychopathic personality, suggests more than frontal brain involvement. Circuits from the frontal to temporal lobe and thence to the amygdala also may be impaired in APD. The ascending serotonergic system originating in the raphe nuclei and innervating the amygdala, hippocampus, hypothalamus and the orbital cortex may be involved in the impulsivity aspect of APD (see Figure 2-18). Serotonin tends to inhibit emotional and behavioral responses and, as discussed in the previous section, and seems to be less reactive in impulsive sensation seekers and those with APD.

The specific lack of capacity for anxiety arousal in the primary psychopath may reflect deficits of norepinephrine in the dorsal ascending noradrenergic system which begins in the locus coeruleus, connects with most limbic structures and the entire neocortex (see Figure 2-16). This is a diffuse arousal system, which has been theorized to underlie sensitivity to signals of punishment (Gray, 1982). A weakness of the system would account for the notorious lack of attention to signals of punishment in the psychopathic personality. Raine (2002) suggests that the weak autonomic and NE responses are related to personality traits characteristic in psychopathy, particularly "stimulation seeking and fearlessness."

Impulsive sensation seeking is motivated by a strong attraction to sensory rewards, particularly intense and novel sensations. This is one reason why the mesolimbic dopamine system (MDS) is a prime candidate for involvement in this motive. The MDS begins in the ventrotegmental (VT) area and projects to the nucleus accumbens (NA) via the medial forebrain bundle (MFB) through the lateral hypothalamus and terminating in the lateral and medial prefrontal cortex (see Figure 2-17). It is in this pathway that we find the highest rates of electrical brain self-stimulation in rats (Stellar & Stellar, 1985). Athough self-stimulation also can be obtained through electrodes planted in another dopamine system, the nigrostriatal, beginning in the substantia nigra and extending to the caudate nucleus, the highest rates are found in the MFB and the lateral hypothalamus. Stimulant drugs have their major effect when infused into the NA and opiate rewards occur more in the VT (Bozarth, 1987). We have speculated that the attraction of drugs for the impulsive sensation seeker is based on a stronger dopaminergic response in this intrinsic reward system. Whether this is based on sensitivity of receptors, low levels of basal activity, or simply stronger mechanisms of reactivity is an open question.

SUMMARY

The third major dimension of personality includes socialization, conscientiousness, cautiousness, and self-control at one pole and sensation seeking, impulsivity, and antisocial personality at the other. The antisocial personality disorder is the obvious clinical extreme, although it typically includes another trait – aggression – to be discussed in the next chapter.

The traits included in this dimension, as well as antisocial personality disorder, are about 50% genetic. Heritabilities for impulsivity range from .3 to .5 depending on how the trait is defined. Conscientiousness heritabilities are generally around .5. Sensation seeking or novelty seeking heritabilities are .5 to .6, closer to .6. Self-control (vs. Impulsivity) and sensation seeking share a substantial degree of common genetic variance. Some but not all studies of impulsivity show nonadditive types of genetic variance. Studies of sensation seeking in the general population show no evidence of shared environment but a study that divided the population into those with and without a religious upbringing showed strong shared environmental and weak genetic influences on disinhibition in the former, and no shared environmental and strong genetic influence in the latter.

Adoption studies of criminality show interactions between genetic influences from the biological parents and environmental ones from the adoptive parents. Environmental influences alone are not sufficient to produce a lifelong pattern of antisocial behavior, but in interaction with a genetic predisposition they increase the risk of later criminal behavior to a significant degree. There also is evidence of a correlational genetic-environment factor. Genetically influenced antisocial behavior in adoptees can elicit harsh parenting in the adopting parents, which may in turn reinforce aggressive, antisocial behavior in the adoptees.

Dopamine receptor genes have been associated with novelty seeking in a number of studies, although an equal number of studies could not replicate the association. The alleles of the dopamine-4 receptor gene also have been associated with infant behavior and substance abuse. A region near the D-2 receptor also has been associated with substance abuse. The MAO-A gene has been associated with antisocial personality disorder.

Measures of basal skin conductance (SC) and heart rate (HR) have shown little association with personality traits in this dimension, but basal HR is consistently lower in antisocial children and adolescents and low basal HR in children is predictive of adult criminal behavior. The SC and HR orienting reflexes (ORs) to novel stimuli tend to be stronger in high sensation seekers, particularly if the stimulus content is relevant to their interests. However, the stronger response rarely persists beyond the inital stimulus presentations, suggesting a rapid boredom reaction overwhelming the interest in the novel stimulus.

Low levels of cortical arousal have been found in those high on psychoticism and in those with antisocial personalities but not in high sensation seekers. However, sensation seekers, particularly disinhibiter types, show a cortical augmenting pattern in the relationship between visual and auditory evoked potential (EP) amplitudes and intensities of stimulation, whereas low sensation seekers tend to show a reducing pattern, suggestive of cortical inhibition. Impulsivity also is related to cortical augmenting-reducing. Comparisons of EP augmenters and reducers among cats and rats show behavioral characteristics similar to those differentiating high and low human sensation seekers, such as explorativeness and fearlessness in reaction to novel stimuli. They also show an inability to restrain response in reaction to stimuli associated with reward, that is, impulsiveness. Two strains of rats characterized by augmenting or reducing show different physiological reactions to stress. The augmenting strain shows a strong dopaminergic reaction and weak serotonergic one. The reducing strain shows a strong serotonergic one in the hypothalamus and increased hypothalamic-pituitary-adrenocorticotropic response.

Hormonal studies in humans show low cortisol levels in those with antisocial and disinhibition traits. Low epinephrine levels in early adolescence predicts criminal behavior at adult ages. High testosterone levels are found in sensation seekers, particularly those of the disinhibiter type, as well as in those with impulsivity and antisocial traits.

Monoamine oxidase (MAO) type B is associated with high sensation seeking and with various disorders characterized by impulsivity and antisocial sensation seeking. It is also found in the near-relatives of some of those with the disorders suggesting that MAO mediates a genetic connection. The MAO-A gene is associated with a more aggressive type of impulsivity and antisocial behavior. Studies of MAO-B in normal human populations and in monkeys living in natural colonies show behavioral correlations consistent with impulsivity and disinhibition as personality traits. The MAO-B type is preferentially associated with catabolism of the dopaminergic systems in the brain in contrast to the MAO-A type, which is preferentially associated with serotonergic and noradrenergic systems, although both have some influence in the other systems. Low levels of MAO-B inhibition may elevate dopamine reactivity through the lowered inhibition of PEA, an enzyme that potentiates dopamine response.

Correlational studies of monoamine metabolites in CSF, blood, or urine during the basal state have not shown much relationship with personality traits. However, stimulating the monoamine systems with agonists, antagonists, or reuptake inhibitors and measuring reactivity with self-reports, behavior, or hormones has revealed some relationships with personality in the ImpUSS dimension. High sensation seekers show a self-reported high reactivity to dopamine stimulants such as amphetamine and nicotine. They also show evidence of increased sensitivity to dopamine receptors, possibly an indicator of low dopamine availability in neurons. This sensitivity may explain their particular attraction to drugs, which stimulate dopamine reward systems in the mesolimbic dopaminergic system. However, extremely low dopamine availability, as in Parkinson's disease, is associated with low sensation seeking motivation, even controlling for the movement problems endemic to the disease.

In the case of serotonin, low levels of the transmitter are characteristic of impulsive clinical types and a blunted reactivity to serotonergic releasers is shown by those high on sensation seeking, impulsivity, and psychopathy traits. The findings on human subjects are consistent with the comparative research, showing a behavioral inhibition factor associated with serotonin in other species.

Low levels of norepinephrine were found in the CSF of high sensation seekers and high disinhibition sensation seeking and motor impulsivity were related to low reactivity to a noradrenergic agonist.

Both comparative studies of nonhuman species and studies of humans show that the frontal lobes are important in modulation of behavior and the cognitive processes that are necessary for such regulation. Frontal lobe damage increases impulsivity and reduces anxiety and its inhibiting effects. Reduced prefrontal gray matter has been found in persons with antisocial personality disorder and these reductions are related to the unreactive autonomic responses characteristic of this group. But the deficit in emotional responses also may involve the amygdala and temporal lobes. Sensation seeking may have a biological substrate in the mesolimbic dopaminergic system running from the ventrotegmental area to the nucleus accumbens (a major site supporting drug reinforcement effects), and to the lateral hypothalamus (another positive reinforcement site) and lateral and medial prefrontal cortex.

The ascending serotonergic system originating in the raphe nuclei and innervating the amygdala, hippocampus, hypothalamus, and frontal orbital cortex may be the system connected with self-control and capacity for delay. A weakness or nonresponsivity of this system could lead to impulsive behavior.

The dorsal ascending noradrenergic system beginning in the locus coeruleus and ascending to the entire limbic system and cortex is connected with arousal, particularly fear arousal. The lack of fear in the impulsive sensation seeker and the primary antisocial personality type may be related to a weakness or lack of responsivity in this system.

At each level from the genetic to the behavioral there are bound to be interactions between systems: for example, sensitivity to signals of punishment versus sensitivity to signals of reward, approach versus inhibition, dopaminergic versus serotonergic activation. The relative weights of opposing systems must determine behavioral outcomes in any given situation. It is the relative balance between systems that is related to personality or psychopathology. The higher order personality trait of ImpUSS consists of a strong approach incentive to appetitive or novel stimuli, a weak inhibitory system, and a weak emotional arousal system. The antisocial personality shows all three mechanisms plus a lack of empathy and increased aggressiveness. The next chapter concerns the latter factor.

CHAPTER 6

Aggression-Hostility/Agreeableness

Aggressiveness is a major individual difference, or "personality," factor in most species of animals (Gosling, 2001), including monkeys (Chamove, Eysenck, & Harlow, 1972) and dogs (Svartberg & Forkman, 2002). Strains of mice and rats differ markedly in aggressiveness. In nonhuman animals, aggression is classified by the provoking conditions including: pain, fear, maternal protection of the young, an intruder in the animal's territory, mating competition, and prey to a predator. The last of these, called "predatory aggression," differs from intraspecies or "defensive aggression" in that it does not require anger or even strong emotion. If anything, the excitement of a predator is more like the positive excitement during sensation seeking in humans. Even well-fed cats seem to enjoy hunting and when there is no real prey they play at stalking and pouncing. Human predators, however, are different in that they stalk their own species, but some of the sensation seeking motivation may be the same as in other species. Sexual sadists are generally unemotional and detached but get pleasurable excitement from the suffering of their victims (Cosyns, 1998). Humans who hunt other species are most like predator animals. Like cats, they hunt for the challenge and pleasure of the kill even when they are not at all hungry.

Human aggression is classified by the form it takes. Human aggressiveness involves three types of expression: the behavioral, as in physical or verbal aggression; the emotional, as in anger; and the attitudinal, as in hostility. Buss and Perry (1992) did a factor analysis of items in their hostility inventory and found four intercorrelated subfactors: physical aggression, verbal aggression, anger, and hostility.

Verbal aggression is more frequently expressed than physical aggression. Even in those who are occasionally physically aggressive, like child or spouse abusers, the aggression is not as frequently expressed as is verbal aggression. Many adults have not engaged in real physical aggression since they were children. Even in a population of prison inmates in which physical assault is common, most inmates exhibit assaults less than once a month (Sheard, Marini, Bridges, & Wapner, 1976).

Anger may or may not accompany aggression, but trait emotionality and state anger make aggression more probable in a provoking situation (Verona, Patrick, & Lang, 2002). Hostility is a more persistent trait, a mixture of attitude and anger. It may be directed primarily at a single target or generalized to many others, or abstract stereotyped groups, as in prejudice.

Homicide is an extreme form of aggression but can come in many forms. Impulsive murders are committed in the "heat" (anger) of the situation and immediately on some provocation such as an argument or perceived threat. Premeditated murder is less immediately reactive, less intensely emotional, and more instrumental in nature (Stanford, Houston, Villemarette-Pittman, & Greve, 2003). Impulsive aggression seems to have more biological substrates than premeditated aggression. Psychopaths are a more violent group than criminals without a psychopathic personality. Degree of psychopathy is related to likelihood of violence, both in prison and after release from prison (Hart, Hare, & Forth, 1994). Woodworth and Porter (2002) contrasted murderers who were classified as psychopathic with those who were not. Most of the homicides committed by psychopaths were primarily instrumental in nature, whereas nonpsychopaths committed more reactive and fewer instrumental murders than those with psychopathic personalities.

Aggression in the form of fighting can be entertainment for some persons. The traditional Saturday night fight or gang battles in some subcultures seem to be positively reinforcing for the participants despite the risks involved. Joireman, Anderson, and Strathman (2003) showed relationships between sensation seeking (boredom susceptibility and disinhibition), impulsivity, and "consideration of future consequences," a cognitive trait, and physical and verbal aggression. The connections between these traits and aggression was mediated by hostile cognitions and negative trait affect (anger). Boredom susceptibility showed a stronger correlation with verbal aggression, whereas disinhibition was more strongly related to physical aggression.

Alcohol and other drugs, including opiates, cocaine, amphetamine, phencyclidine and anabolic steroids (but *not* marijuana) are associated with violent behavior for various reasons (Volavka & Citrone, 1998). Suppressant drugs such as alcohol and opiates have a disinhibitory effect, reducing whatever control there is in violently predisposed persons. Drug withdrawal may induce irritable states. Drugs like amphetamine and cocaine can cause paranoid type psychoses and delusion-induced violence.

The illegal drug trade can lead to territorial fights among dealers or violent crimes among drug-dependent users desperate to obtain the drugs. Amphetamine and cocaine intoxication seem to have some direct effects on anger and aggression thresholds, perhaps because of their agonistic effects on brain catecholamines. In most cases, drugs act in interaction with predispositions toward antisocial behavior in general and violence in particular. But in some cases the drugs seem to cause a change in personality or a "Jekyll and Hyde" effect. Perhaps they release unconscious or latent tendencies by reduction of inhibition. More likely they simply lower the threshold for aggression existent as a potential in all humans with the exception of a few saints.

The influences of socialization or psychopathy, impulsivity, and sensation seeking in aggression suggest that they may all be involved in one factor. Indeed, in a three-factor analysis this is true (Zuckerman et al., 1988, 1991). When four or five factors are analyzed, however, aggression-hostility (Agg-Host) emerges from the P-ImpUSS factor to form a separate dimension (see Chapter 1). This dimension is most highly related to trait anger, although it also is correlated with trait depression and anxiety (Zuckerman et al., 1999).

In the standard Big-Five model of Costa and McCrea (1992), the Agreeableness (A) factor is most closely related to Agg-Host in the Zuckerman-Kuhlman model (Zuckerman et al., 1993). However, A is not conceptually the opposite of Agg-Host. One may be disagreeable without being aggressive or even hostile. The facets of agreeableness in the NEO are: trust, straightforwardness, altruism, compliance, modesty, and tender-mindedness. One may be low on all of these without manifesting aggression in any direct way. Altruism, for example, has no relationship to antisocial expressions, including aggression (Krueger, Hicks, & McGue, 2001). In fact, altruism, in this study, was shown to come from environmental factors (shared and nonshared), whereas antisocial behavior was a function of genetics and unshared environment only. Curiously, Costa and McCrea place the subtrait of angry-hostility in their neuroticism major factor. Eysenck and Eysenck's (1985) three-factor model puts anger in the neuroticism dimension and aggression and hostility in the psychoticism factor. Indeed, a closer look at the results in our own factor analyses show that the aggression, hostility, and anger tend to fall in the quadrant between Neuroticism and P-Impulsive Unsocialized Sensation Seeking in a three-dimensional analysis (Zuckerman et al., 1988). However, aggression loads relatively more highly on the P-ImpUSS dimension and anger and hostility relatively more highly on the N dimension. Thus, the cognitive and emotional aspects of the trait without the physical or verbal expression of it are neurotic. But when the expression of anger and hostility are not inhibited by anxiety and aggression is overt, the combination falls into the P-ImpUSS pattern.

GENETICS

Biometric Studies

In their review of genetic influences on aggression and impulsivity, Bergeman and Seroczynski (1998) note the wide variation in heritabilities among different studies. They attribute this to the effects of nonadditive genetic variance, changes in the balance between genetic and environment over age, gender differences, measurement issues, and differences between the different expressions of aggression. If there is nonadditive genetic variance, twin studies will overestimate, and family studies will underestimate, heritability. Heritability for aggression is higher for older and lower for younger twins, whereas shared environment is higher for younger twins (Miles & Carey, 1997). Heritability of aggression is somewhat higher for men than for women. Shared environment was a factor in observational but not in parent or self-reported indices of aggression. Different dimensions of aggression may yield different results, as will be described later.

The review of "the environmental architecture" of human aggression by Miles and Carey (1997) concluded from a meta-analysis of 24 studies that an overall genetic effect may account for up to 50% of the variance in aggression. However, they included many scales, like socialization and psychopathic deviate which are not specific to the trait of aggression. I will confine this discussion to specific aggression scales except for agreeableness measures from the Big Five, widely used in large-scale twin studies of adults. Twin studies of this trait in adolescents and adults are shown in Table 6-1.

The studies by Jang et al. (1996) in Canada and Rieman et al. in Germany (1997) both suggest that between 40 and 50% of the trait of agreeableness is determined by genetic factors and the rest is almost entirely due to nonshared environment and error. Loehlin et al.'s (1998) study of American high school students reached a similar conclusion, using three different assessment techniques for measuring agreeableness. However, the study of twins raised together and separated twins in Sweden reached different conclusions (Bergeman et al., 1993). These investigators used a very short version of the A scale with only eight items. The twins raised together showed a pattern seen in most other studies. But the adopted twins raised apart showed little correlation in either MZ or DZ twins suggesting a primary effect of nonshared, specific environments. Taken together, the two discrepant sets

Table 6-1. Twin correlations and heritabilities of agreeableness

Study	Country	Test	MZ *r*	DZ *r*	h^2
Bergeman	Sweden	NEO-S			
et al. (1993)		Twins together	.41	.23	.35 (both
		Twins apart	.15	−.03	types twins)
Jang et al. (1996)	Canada	NEO-R	.41	.26	.41
Loehlin et al. (1998)	US H.S	Self-Rating	.32	.06	
	students	CPI	.46	.34	all .51
		ACL	.29	.18	
Rieman et al. (1997)	Germany	NEO	.42	.24	.42
		Peer Rating	.32	.21	.57
		Self & Peer			.66

Note: CPI = California Psychological Inventory; ACL = Adjective Check List

of data yield a primarily nonadditive type of heredity accounting for 35% of the variance in the trait and a relatively large shared environment effect of 46%.

Jang et al. (2001) analyzed the facet scales in the NEO, including the angry-hostility subscale of Neuroticism in samples from three countries, as shown in Table 6-2. The results are similar to those for the Agreeableness factor, with about half of the variance in Canada and Germany and 40% in Japan attributable to heredity. The ratio of MZ to DZ correlations also suggests a primarily additive type of genetic mechanism.

The Minnesota separated twin study compared twin correlations on the aggression subscale of the MPQ as shown in Table 6-3 (Tellegen et al., 1988, data updated 1990). The correlations for twins raised together are consistent with other studies showing close to 50% heritability. But the correlations

Table 6-2. Twin correlations and heritabilities for the angry-hostility subscale of the NEO in three countries (Jang et al., 2001)

Country	MZ *r*	DZ *r*	h^{2*}
Canada	.50	.24	.52
Germany	.44	.18	.52
Japan	.33	.13	.40

* These are computed using the Falconer formula. If the rule that heritabilities should not exceed the correlations for MZ twins is applied, then these heritabilities would be slightly lower: .50, .44, .40 for Canadian, German, and Japanese samples respectively.

Table 6-3. Twin correlations and heritabilities from the minnesota twin study (Tellegen et al., 1988, updated) & Di Lalla et al., 1996)

Study	Scale/Twin type	MZ *r*	DZ *r*	h²
Tellegen et al. (1988)	MPQ-Aggression/ Twins Together	.41	.18	.46
	Twins Apart	.32	.09	.25
Di Lalla et al. (1996)	MMPI-Host/ Twins Apart	.42	.05	.37

Note: MPQ = Multidimensional Personality Questionnaire; MMPI-Host = Minnesota Multiphasic Personality Inventory-Hostility (content scale)

for twins raised apart indicate a lower heritability of only 25%. This table also shows the data from the adopted twins in the Minnesota study on a hostility scale from the MMPI (DiLalla et al., 1996). Heritability for hostility was .37.

Table 6-4 shows additional twin studies of aggression-type ratings and test scales obtained from studies listed in the Miles and Carey (1997) review. Two studies used peer ratings of children on aggression in the first, and "bullying" in the second (Ghodsian-Carpey & Baker, 1987; O'Connor, Foch, Sherry, & Plomin, 1980). The results from both of these suggest a high heritability for aggression. However, the study of children using observer ratings of aggression showed no effect of heritability and a moderate effect of shared environment, because the moderate correlations were nearly the same for identical and fraternal twins (Plomin, Foch, & Rowe, 1981). Similarly, some studies of self ratings for hostility and aggression in adult

Table 6-4. Twin correlations and heritabilities for aggression scales and ratings in children and adults

Study	Method	Age range	MZ *r*	DZ *r*	h²
Ghodsian-Carpey (1987)	Agg rating parents	4–7	.78	.31.	.78
O'Connor et al. (1980)	Bullying, peer reports	5–11	.72	.42	.60
Plomin et al. (1981)	Agg-observer ratings	5–11	.39	.42	.00
Cantor (1973)	Hostility-self report	16–55	.14	.30	.00
Partanen et al. (1966)	Agg items-self report	28–37	.25	.16	.18
Rushton et al. (1986)	Agg items-self report	19–60	.40	.04	.39

Table 6-5. Twin correlations and heritabilities from genetic studies of Buss-Durkee hostility inventory (BDHI)

	BDHI Subscale	MZ r	DZ r	h^{2*}
Cates et al. (1993) Females	Direct Assault	.07	.41	.00
	Indirect Assault	.40	.01	.40
	Verbal Hostility	.41	.01	.40
	Irritability	.28	−.21	.28
Coccaro et al. (1997) Males	Direct Assault	.50	.19	.50
	Indirect Assault	.42	.02	.42
	Verbal Hostility	.28	.07	.28
	Irritability	.39	−.06	.39

* The Falconer formula was used but, because the heritability cannot exceed the correlation between identical (MZ) twins, every time it does when calculated by the formula (2x MZ r – DZ r) the correlation between identical twins is used as the heritability. This was the case for every variable except the Direct Assault for the females in the Cates et al. study, in which the DZ correlation actually exceeded the MZ correlation.

twins (Canter, 1973; Partanen, Bruun, & Markkanen, 1966) also indicate low heritabilities. However, a study of adults aged 19 to 60 using 23 aggression items from the Interpersonal Behavior Survey (IBS) showed a moderate heritability of about 40% for both men and women with some indication of nonadditive genetic variance (Rushton, Fulker, Neale, Nias, & Eysenck, 1986).

The older form of the Buss-Durkee (1957) Hostility Inventory (BDHI) was one of the most commonly used measures of self-report aggression inventories until recently. It had the advantage of assessing different types of aggression: direct assault, indirect assault, verbal assault, and irritability. These scales were developed rationally rather than through factor analysis, which is why Buss and Perry (1992) have revised the inventory. Two genetic studies, one for men and one for women, have been reported for the subscales (Cates, Houston, Vavak, & Crawford, 1993; Cocarro, Bergeman, Kavoussi, & Seroczynski, 1997). Their results are shown in Table 6-5.

Both studies found moderate heritabilities for indirect and verbal assault and irritability subscales (.28 to .47), but the study of females (Cates et al., 1993) found no heritability for direct assault, whereas the one of males (Coccaro et al., 1997) found their highest heritability for that scale. Perhaps this is a function of the lower expression of physical aggression in women, restricting the genetic variance in the trait. There is no effect of shared environment indicated for any of the scales in either study, but both show indications of a nonadditive genetic mechanism in the near-zero correlations for dizygotic twins.

There are remarkably few nontwin adoption studies in which aggression
or hostility were measured by specific scales for those traits. Miles and Carey
(1997) report a study of 4- to 6-year-old siblings by Parker (1989) based on
a paper presented at a conference in 1987, but apparently never published.
The correlations for an aggression scale were .47 for adoptive siblings and
.44 for biological siblings, indicating a strong effect of shared environment
but none for genetics. The correlations are suspiciously high for nontwin
relations and may reflect the biases of the peer raters to see similarity in
all siblings. The child-parent correlation between biologically related parents and children was only .19 and biologically related siblings were not
significantly correlated on the ACL aggression scale (Ahern et al., 1982).

Loehlin (1992) summarized family and adoption studies of agreeableness, using scales such as tender-mindedness, femininity, and empathy.
The correlations for biologically related parents and children and siblings
were quite varied (.02 to .57) with a median value of .13. Those for adoptive relations varied from −.03 to .16 with a median of .06, suggesting little
influence of family environment alone.

The inference of the absence of shared environmental factors, such as
home environment, from twin studies of a general population, is problematic without actual assessments of the environment. An adoption study in
which adoptive parents were interviewed and assessed showed an interaction effect as well as independent effects of genetics and an adverse home
environment in the adoptive families (Cadoret, Yates, Troughton, Woodworth, & Stewart, 1995). The genetic factor was having a biologic parent
with antisocial personality disorder, and adverse family environment was
judged from drug abuse and family disturbances such as separations, di-
vorce, and psychiatric problems in the adoptive family. Both of these factors and their additive interaction influenced childhood and adolescent
aggressivity and conduct disorder in the adopted children. In other words,
children with a genetic disposition were more likely to react to an adverse
environment with aggression than children without that disposition. But in
the absence of a genetic background for antisocial personality, an adverse
home environment alone did not increase aggressiveness in the adoptees.

Molecular Genetics

In the previous chapter, the relationships of MAO-A and -B genes and their
enzyme products to impulsivity, sensation seeking, and antisocial behavior
were discussed. Aggression is one type of that antisocial behavior. Studies of mice in which either or both genes were deleted showed that both
are involved in impulsivity, but the MAO-A deletion produced increased

aggressiveness, whereas the MAO-B deletion did not (Shih & Chen, 1999). The MAO-A knockout mice had increased levels of serotonin and norepinephrine in the cerebellum, frontal cortex, and hippocampus. Placed in a cage with other mice, they spent more time exploring and behaving aggressively and less time in stationary or defensive postures than wild, untreated mice. They bit and attacked other mice without provocation.

Both MAO-A and -B deficit mice show increased behavioral reactivity to stress. A mutation in a Dutch family produced a complete absence of MAO-A and the male members of this family were characterized by impulsive aggressive behavior against members of their own family as well as others. They also were mildly or borderline mentally retarded (Brunner et al., 1993).

Caspi et al. (2002) found an interaction between treatment in childhood and polymorphisms of the MAO-A gene which produce either low or high MAO-A activity. For both convictions for violent crimes and general disposition toward violence at age 26, the effects of childhood maltreatment were significant in those with the allele producing low MAO-A activity but not significant in those with the allele associated with high MAO-A activity. Those with maltreatment *and* a genetic disposition to low MAO-A activity had the stronger disposition toward violence.

Low levels of serotonin have been associated with impulsive aggression in animals and humans (New et al., 2002). In humans, the aggression may be directed toward self (suicide) or others (aggression and homicide). In humans, the serotonin transporter gene (5-HTTLPR) modulates transcriptional activity of the serotonin gene (5HT). A short form of 5-HTTLPR is associated with lower 5-HTT gene expression and function. Those homozygous for the long form have more 5-HTT activity. An association was found between the short form and scales of the NEO; those with the short form, in either homozygous or heterozygous form, scored higher on Angry Hostility and lower on Agreeableness than those with the long form (Lesch et al., 2002). The short form also was associated with neuroticism and anxiety, as was discussed in Chapter 4. A study of monkeys showed an association between the short form of the 5-HTTLPR and aggressive behavior in competitive situations.

Comings et al. (2002) examined the contributions of four dopamine receptor genes to a variety of personality traits. Typically, each gene only accounted for a small percentage of the variance of any trait (usually less than 2%). In the previous chapter, I discussed the role of dopamine receptor genes, particularly DRD4, in novelty seeking. The B-D Hostility scale was included in the study. The DRD4 was associated with subscales for negativism, and verbal hostility and the DRD5 with scales for assault, guilt, resentment, and suspicion. Most of these associations accounted for only 1–2% of the variance and none by itself reached the conventional level of significance (.05).

Catechol-O-Methyltransferase (COMT) is involved in the catabolic in-activation of the cathecholamine neurotransmitters, including dopamine and norepinephrine. A functional COMT (V158M) polymorphism has been related to violent suicide attempts and to direction of anger expression (Rujescu, Giegling, Gietl, Hartmann, & Möller, 2003). The allele form as-sociated with low COMT activity was more frequent in violent (but not nonviolent) suicide attempters. In a combined clinical and control group, those homozygous for the low activity allele scored higher on a measure of "anger-[directed] out," whereas those homozygous for the high activity allele were higher on "anger-in." COMT knock-out mice show increased ag-gressive behavior and increased prefrontal dopaminergic activity. A similar mechanism could explain the gene-anger-out and violent expressions in humans.

A study of genetic-personality relationships was done with 4-year-old children (Schmidt, Fox, Rubin, Hu, & Hamer, 2002). Their behavior was as-sessed through maternal ratings and observations in peer play groups. The alleles of the DRD4, the serotonin transporter (5-HTTLPR) and a serotonin receptor gene (5HT2C) were analyzed. Children with the long allele of the DRD4 were rated by their mothers as having more problems with aggression than the children with the short allele. No differences were observed on the classification based on observational ratings. The two serotonin genes were not associated with either measure of aggression.

Summarizing, there does appear to be wide variation in heritabilties of agreeableness/aggression across studies. Some of this is due to method vari-ance, and reliability differences in methods employed. Short forms usually yield lower heritabilities than long forms of questionnaire scales because of lower reliabilities. But both the Swedish and Minnesota separated twin studies showed lower heritabilites in the separated twins than in the twins raised together suggesting some shared environment effects, particularly in the Swedish twins. However, shared environment effects are not seen in higher DZ correlations in the twins together studies. Adoption studies also show weak to null effects of shared environments, but studies in which envi-ronments are actually assessed suggest an interaction of genetic and family environment effects. Bad home environments only influence aggressivity in children with a genetic vulnerability.

Impulsive aggressivity and impulsive, antisocial sensation seeking may share some of the same genetic makeup. Dopamine receptor and serotonin transporter genes may have a role in both. There is some preliminary, as yet nonreplicated, evidence for this supposition. However, there is some evidence of specificity in that the MAO-A gene may be more associated with violent expressions of antisocial, sensation seeking behaviors than the MAO-B gene.

There is also evidence for an interaction between MAO-A and childhood environments similar to that found in adoption studies. In the presence of the genetic disposition, those children experiencing childhood maltreatment are most likely to become violent adults. The strength of the environmental contribution to the interaction may be attenuated in adoption studies because of the restricted range of bad environments in adoptive families, as a result of screening of these families by social workers.

PSYCHOPHYSIOLOGY

Many of the studies of antisocial aggression deal with impulsive rather than premeditated aggression. Because many of the subjects, such as murderers and rapists, are drawn from prison populations, a high proportion could be classified as psychopathic or antisocial personality types. We would, therefore, expect some overlap between the physiological correlates of aggression and those for impulsive sensation seeking and antisocial personality as described in the last chapter. The question is, are there unique features to the psychophysiology of aggression that are different from or quantitatively different from those found in less aggressive antisocial types?

Autonomic Arousal

Low heart rate (HR) is the best replicated and cross-cultural correlate of antisocial behavior in child and adolescent samples (Raine, 2002). Low resting heart rate at 3 years of age has been shown to predict aggression at 11 years of age (Raine, Venables, & Mednick, 1997). Aggressive children at age 11 had lower HRs at age 3 than nonaggressive children, but children who scored high on nonaggressive antisocial behavior did not differ in age 3 HR from those low in this type of behavior. Of low HR children, 65.5% were classified as aggressive compared to 34.5% of high HR children. Other variables such as physical development, motor activity, temperament, family discord, and so on were related to aggressivity but did not abolish the relation between aggression and HR when statistically controlled.

Raine et al. (1997) suggest two explanations for the relationship between HR and aggressive behavior. One is that autonomic underarousal is related to fearlessness and a lack of fear makes antisocial violent behavior more likely, whereas fear of being hurt inhibits aggression. The other theory is that aggressive behavior may be a form of stimulation or sensation seeking as a reaction to aversive low-arousal states associated with boredom. Behavioral ratings of stimulation-seeking and fearfulness/fearlessness at age 3 predicted aggression at age 11 but were not related to nonaggressive antisociality at 11 (Raine, Reynolds, Venables, Mednick, & Farrington, 1998). Covariance analyses showed that the stimulation-seeking aggression relationship was independent of body size and fearlessness factors, but the fearlessness-aggression relationship was abolished when controlled for either body size or stimulation-seeking.

The studies describe above were conducted in the tropical island of Mauritius on children of African and Asiatic ethnicities. A study done in England showed that autonomic arousal and electrodermal orienting responses at age 15 predicted criminal behavior at age 29 (Raine, Venables, & Williams, 1995). The group of antisocial children were subdivided into those who subsequently, by age 29, had become criminals and those who had no criminal record (desistors). A third group had no antisocial problems at either age. Desistors had higher resting HRs than criminals, and normal controls fell between these two groups. Desistors also showed more electrodermal arousal (NS-GSRs) than criminals and tended to have higher arousal than normals as well. Both desistors and normals had greater electrodermal orienting responses (ORs) to tones than criminals but did not differ from each other. The weaker ORs of the criminals may be an indication of attention deficits. Children with attention deficits, particularly those with hyperactivity as well, are at risk for later antisocial behavior (Halperin & Newcorn, 1998). This study was not specifically addressed at antisocial aggression, but it is likely that the same psychophysiological factors that protect against criminality in general would prevent a child from becoming an antisocial aggressive personality. But some psychopaths are successful, in that they never get arrested, whereas others are repeatedly arrested and imprisoned. A study compared successful and unsuccessful psychopaths using official arrests as the criterion (Ishikawa, Raine, Lencz, Bihrle, & Lacasse, 2001). The unsuccessful psychopaths had a higher incidence of both self-reported theft and violent crimes than the successful ones. Heart rate (HR) was recorded before and during a stressful situation, consisting of preparing and giving a videotaped speech concerning one's faults and weaknesses. The two psychopathic groups and a nonpsychopathic control group did not differ in heart rate (HR) at baseline, but during the stressful periods the successful psychopaths and the controls showed strong increases in HR while the unsuccessful psychopaths showed little change at all. The low arousability of the unsuccessful psychopath may be what accounts for his impulsivity and insensitivity to cues for punishment.

In contrast to the studies described earlier showing a lowered autonomic arousal among aggressive antisocial persons, many studies show that persons who score high on hostility scales, usually among normal populations, show great anger and increases in blood pressure in response to stress or provocation. For instance, a study found that subjects who scored high on hostility and were harassed in an experiment showed enhanced and prolonged rises in blood pressure, forearm blood flow and vascular resistance, as well as increased norepinephrine, testosterone, and cortisol compared to low hostile subjects (Suarez, Kuhn, Schanberg, Williams, & Zimmerman, 1998). This kind of provocation can occur in everyday situations such as marital interactions (Smith & Gallo, 1999) and can result in cardiovascular disease, including hypertension. In a large prospective study of nearly 3,000 men in their 50s and 60s, suppressed anger was the most predictive factor of the incidence of isochemic heart disease even when other risk factors were controlled (Gallagher, Yarnell, Sweetnam, Elwood, & Stansfield, 1999).

Although hostility and anger often precede and accompany aggression, the emotional factors may not be fully expressed, and thus the cardiovascular conditions that are a normal state reaction to stress become chronic trait reactions.

Cortical and Subcortical Brain Arousal

Earlier studies of violent criminals using the EEG reported a high incidence of abnormal records in violent criminals including: diffused or focal slowing, spiking, or sharp waves in some areas (Volavka, 1995). The incidence of such abnormal records in prisoners convicted of homicide or habitual violence was 50 to 65% compared to 5 to 10% in nonviolent prisoners or normal controls. Quantitative analyses showed slowing of alpha activity and an increase of slow wave theta activity in violent prisoners. A limitation of most of these studies is that they used prisoners referred for neuropsychiatric evaluation.

However, one study used subjects selected from the general population of prisoners who had been rated for violent behavior (Wong, Lumsden, Fenton, & Fenwick, 1994). The low and middle groups in rated violence had 26% and 24% of abnormal EEGs, but there was 43% of abnormal EEGs within the most violent group. The most frequent site of the focalized abnormalities was the temporal lobe; 20% of the most violent had abnormalities in this lobe compared to only 2 to 3% of the other two less violent groups.

The cortical EP, particularly the P300 component, has also been used to study aggression. A study of detoxified alcoholics with a history of aggression showed a weaker P300 response than alcoholics without such a history (Branchey, Buydens-Branchey, & Lieber, 1988). Impulsive aggressive subjects screened from a college population showed lower P300 amplitudes at frontal sites (Gerstle, Mathias, & Stanford, 1998).

However, another study of prisoners rated as impulsive-aggressive or nonimpulsive-aggressive and noninmate controls, found that both inmate groups had significantly lower P300 amplitudes at all sites including the frontal, but the two inmate groups did not differ from each other at the frontal sites (Barratt, Stanford, Kent, & Felthous, 1997). There were differences on electrodes posterior to the frontal areas. Impulsiveness and anger measured by self-report trait tests were inversely related to P300 amplitudes. However, the groups rated as impulsive-aggressive and nonimpulsive-aggressive, on the basis of their behaviors in prison, did not differ on these two trait scales bringing the classification into question. Perhaps aggressive behavior in prison is not necessarily trait related but a function of factors specific to prison life.

Brain imaging PET studies have become more widely used in studies of violence. A summary of PET studies between 1982 and 1994 suggested reduced metabolism in the prefrontal cortex, particularly the orbital, is associated with impulsive-aggressive behavior (New, Novotny, Buchsbaum, & Siever, 1998).

A small PET study of psychiatric patients with a history of repetitive violent behavior leading to legal arrest showed that the violent patients had lower metabolism for bilateral prefrontal and temporal medial areas than normal controls (Volkow et al., 1995). The largest study of murderers using PET found that murderers had significantly lower glucose metabolism in both lateral and medial prefrontal cortical areas, including the right orbitofrontal cortex (Raine, Buchsbaum, & Lacasse, 1997). Similar differences were found in the parietal and occipital lobes, but no differences between murderers and controls were found in the temporal lobe.

Raine et al. (1997) also looked at activation in subcortical regions. Murderers had significantly lower metabolism in the corpus callosum. For the amygdala and medial temporal lobe, including the hippocampus, there were significant interactions involving differences by laterality. Murderers had significantly reduced left amydala and temporal/hippocampal activity and increased right activity relative to controls. A similar interaction was found for the thalamus, except that there were no differences at all for the left thalamus and the murderers were higher on right thalamic activity.

The differences in the corpus callosum are relevant to theories (Flor-Henry, 1976; Hare & McPherson, 1984; Raine et al., 1997) suggesting that persons with psychopathic personalities have less integration of verbal and emotional functions than others, that is, a kind of "semantic dementia"

(Cleckley, 1976), in which they use words without personal meaning to themselves or connection with real feelings. Because the corpus callosum connects the two hemispheres, a weakness in its functioning could be the basis for this cognitive dysfunction.

The sources of lateral differences among subcortical structures are less clear. They could have something to do with the connections between the cerebral hemispheres and these structures affecting aggression. The weaker left amygdala in the murderers may have to do with inhibition functions and the stronger right side may be related to the negative affect (anxiety and anger) said to be predominate in the right hemisphere.

EEGs were done on a subset of the murderers in the previous study by Raine et al. (Gatzke-Kopp, Raine, Buchsbaum, & LaCasse, 2001). In contrast to the PET findings of reduced prefrontal but not temporal glucose metabolism, the EEG study showed increases in slow-wave activity in the temporal but not the frontal activity. The differences in loci of the findings may be because the PET study was done during an active task that activates frontal lobes in particular, whereas the EEG was done during a resting state.

An interesting interaction between home backgrounds and prefrontal functioning was shown in a PET study by Raine, Stoddard, Bihrle, and Buchsbaum (1998). Bad home background in murderers was defined by psychosocial deprivation (early physical and sexual abuse, neglect, extreme poverty, foster home placement, a criminal parent, severe family conflict, and a broken home). One might think that such a background would increase the possibility of brain defects through bad prenatal care, head injuries, and bad diet. But actually it was the murderers with a good home background who had the reduced prefrontal metabolism, whereas the murderers from bad home environments showed relatively good prefrontal functioning! The findings suggest that the prefrontal deficit may be due to a genetic factor appearing most clearly in those without obvious environmental explanations.

The PET studies in particular suggest a pattern of hypoarousability in the prefrontal cortex and some studies suggest an involvement of the temporal cortex and subcortical structures such as the amygdala, thalamus, and hippocampus. Hypofrontality and low EEG arousal are also found in psychopathic personalities or criminals, in general, but the studies that use less aggressive prisoners as controls suggest that the pattern is more extreme in more violent criminals. The weakness of the prefrontal cortex may represent the impulsivity of most murderers and a lack of control during angry states. Hypofrontality is also found in schizophrenia and some of the studies (Raine et al., 1997; Volkow et al., 1995) included schizophrenics in their violence-prone groups. Only one of the studies used subjects from a general population of prisoners (Wong et al., 1994). In this study, abnormal EEGs appeared in only the most aggressive third of the sample and there was no difference between the low and middle range groups. Could this mean that extreme violent tendencies are due to qualitative genetic or postnatal sources of damage? I will look more closely at differences in brain structure and their possible interactions with environment in the later section on neuropsychology.

BIOCHEMISTRY

Hormones

Territorial aggression is a good illustration of the adaptive value of aggression in evolution. If a male rat is housed with a female and an intruding male rat is introduced into the cage the usual response is an attack on the intruder. In other species, including some of the primates, males control a harem of females for reproduction and attack any males approaching their mates. These dominant-aggressive males contribute a much larger proportion of the their genes to the offspring of the population than less aggressive males. The words of the song "As Time Goes By" put it more euphemistically: "It's still the same old story, a fight for love and glory." Not much "love" is involved in the systematic rape of the women in defeated populations in past and recent ethnic wars.

Testosterone plays an obvious role in both reproduction and aggression. Castrated males show a reduction in aggressiveness and sexual drive. However, the testosterone-aggression relationship is two way, raising the old "chicken and egg" problem of causation. A once dominant male who is defeated in a physical contest shows a drop in testosterone levels. Among humans testosterone is affected by the outcome of competition. In tennis and chess, the victors show increased, and the losers decreased testosterone (Dabbs, 2000). Even vicarious winning or losing can affect testosterone. Dabbs reports a study of reactions to their team's victory for Brazilians and their team's defeat by Italians. Nearly all of the Brazilians had increased testosterone and all of the Italians showed decreased testosterone after the game. Testosterone is both a trait and state variable. If one takes testosterone levels at the same time of day on several occasions the reliability of the trait is good. Levels of testosterone are moderately heritable. But, as the above studies show, levels of the hormone can be affected by day-to-day experiences and moods. Depression, for instance, can depress testosterone levels and sexual drive.

Correlational studies of the relationship between testosterone and hostility or aggression show a moderate effect size in the meta-analysis by Archer, Birring, & Wu, 1998). But the results are mixed with some positive results (e.g., Harris, Rushton, Hampson, & Jackson, 1996) and some negative results (e.g., Campbell, Muncer, & Odber, 1997). The results with questionnaire trait measures are less positive than those with behavioral assessments (Archer, 1991). The reasons may be the social undesirability of admitting hostility and aggression as traits or the partial dependence of the testosterone measure on the current state or mood of the subjects.

Behavioral records and observations of aggression in prison inmates tend to show significant relationships between testosterone and aggression. A large study of about 700 prison inmates found that a history of violent crimes (homicide, rape, child molestation) and violations of prison rules involving assault were positively related to levels of salivary testosterone (Dabbs, Carr, Frady, & Riad, 1995). A group of alcoholics with a history of violence had higher levels of serum testosterone than non-violent alcoholics (Bergman & Brismar, 1994). A study of female inmates found a relationship of testosterone with a history of unprovoked violent crimes compared with those whose violent crimes were defensive in nature or those imprisoned for theft (Dabbs, Ruback, Frady, Hopper, & Sgoritas, 1988). The degree of violence in crimes of delinquent boys (Mattson et al., 1980) and adult male rapists (Rada, Laws, & Kellner, 1976) was related to their levels of testosterone.

Correlational studies, whether of personality or behavioral traits, do not resolve the "chicken-or-egg" priority. Studies of the effects of hormone administration can go further in this regard. Clinical studies of steroid users self-administering androgenic compounds to improve performance in sports or muscle building have shown increased aggressiveness in some of them (Pope & Katz, 1994). In an experimental study, Pope, Kouri, and Hudson (2000) gave testosterone or placebos to normal men, excluding those with clinical disorders, drug users, or weight-lifters. Testosterone increased scores on only one of the Buss-Durkee (1957) Hostility inventory scales: verbal aggression. However, it increased aggression on a laboratory task in which subjects thought they were punishing a competitor. Changes in measures of manic behavior were more impressive in magnitude.

Short-term experimental treatments may have little effect in changing lifelong patterns of aggression based on continuous interactions between hereditary tendencies and life experiences. Longitudinal studies may make some contribution to this question of causation. A group of boys followed from age 6 to 13 found that although testosterone predicted social dominance in adolesence only body mass predicted physical aggression (Tremblay et al., 1998). This result suggests that testosterone may influence aggression through its effect on body mass. Simply put, bigger muscular adolescent males can be aggressive with a better chance of success than smaller, weaker ones. In monkeys, as well as humans, weight and size correlate with aggressiveness (Higley et al., 1992; Mehlman et al., 1994).

Continuity of aggressive behavior from childhood is also a factor in the relationship with testosterone. Men who were aggressive in childhood and adult life and those who became aggressive as adults had higher testosterone levels than those who were aggressive only in childhood or those who were never aggressive (Windle & Windle, 1995). Perhaps only postpubertal testosterone is related to aggression in adolescence and adulthood. The effect of testosterone may depend on the social context. Testosterone was low in aggressive boys at ages 13 and 14, when they were more likely to be rejected by their peers, but a follow-up of the same boys at age 16, after many had dropped out of school, found high testosterone levels (Tremblay et al., 1998). Aggression is probably more adaptive and popular on the street than in the school.

Testosterone among normal adolescents is related to a normal kind of aggressive competitiveness, as in sports, and popularity because of its enhancement of leadership, assertiveness, sociability, and interest in sex. Among delinquents and criminals, however, testosterone is related to a more antisocial kind of aggressiveness often leading to violent crimes.

High levels of cortisol are associated with stress and severe kinds of depression (Traskman et al., 1980), but low levels of this hormone are found in prisoners with histories of psychopathic and violent behavior (Virkkunen, 1985). In contrast, high levels of cortisol are positively associated with hostility as measured by questionnaires (Keltikangas, Räikkönen, & Adlercreutz, 1997; Pope & Smith, 1991). The more psychopathic kinds of aggression are only associated with brief spurts of anger, whereas the festering kind of hostility is associated with anger and depression. Cortisol is probably a symptom of the latter kind of reaction.

Neurotransmitters
A relationship between low levels of CSF 5-HIAA (serotonin metabolite) or reduced reactivity to challenges by serotonin agonists and impulsive aggression is a well-replicated finding (see Åsberg, 1994; Coccaro, 1998; Mann, 1995; Zalsman & Apter, 2002 for reviews). This is consistent with general comparative findings across many species (Soubrié, 1986). CSF 5-HIAA in free-ranging rhesus monkeys is low in monkeys who have many

aggressive encounters, as testified by scars and direct observations (Higley et al., 1992). The rating for aggression was correlated negatively with CSF 5-HIAA ($r = -.58$) and positively with indicators of stress in the HYPAC system including ACTH and norepinephrine (NE). The findings of low 5-HIAA were replicated in a second study for the more serious expressions of aggression, but in this study ACTH and NE were not related to aggression and the dopamine metabolite HVA was negatively related to only one aspect of aggression, the presence of wounds (Mehlman et al., 1994).

Coccaro (1998) reviewed human studies of the relationship between CSF 5-HIAA and aggression in humans. About two thirds of the 20 studies showed reduced 5-HIAA in aggressive subjects or a negative correlation between the serotonin metabolite and measures of aggression. Five studies found no significant differences or correlations, and two studies actually found a positive correlation. Coccaro noted that several of the failures of replication included subjects who were not as severely aggressive as those in the successful replication studies. The latter studies used patients or criminals with a history of violence. Coccaro tends to use patients with personality disorders.

Low serotonin is found in various disorders including violent suicide attempters and completers, major depression, anxiety states, disruptive behavior disorders (in children), and alcoholism (particularly the type II alcoholic characterized by antisocial traits). Some of these seem incompatible, for instance, suicide and homicide. However, among psychiatric patients many of these traits are positively related to each other (Apter, van Praag, Sevy, Korn, & Brown., 1990). Apter et al. compared violent patients, selected for actual assaults on staff or other patients, with nonviolent patients on various trait measures. Apart from general violence risk, the violent patients were higher than the nonviolent patients on anger, suicide risk, and impulsivity, although they did not differ on trait or state anxiety, or sadness. Suicidal patients were higher on violence risk as well as suicide risk. Across all patients, suicidal and violent risk were substantially correlated ($r = .53$), and both of these correlated with impulsivity, state and trait anxiety, and anger. Impulsivity and emotional arousal, anger, or depression and anxiety, seem to be traits in common among those who turn aggression inward to themselves or outward to others. The association between aggression and serotonergic dysfunction may be mediated by negative mood states (Heinz, Mann, Weinberger, & Goldman, 2001). Emotional arousal may increase the impulsive type of aggression.

Coccaro (1998) also reviewed studies that assessed responses to pharmacological challenges to the serotonergic system. As with the studies of

5-HIAA, a preponderance of the studies found a reduced response of serotonin to agonists or reuptake inhibitors in more aggressive subjects.

Coccaro et al. (1989) used a fenfluramine challege, measuring peak prolactin response to the challenge, among patients with major affective disorders and those with only personality disorders. The peak response was lower in both of these groups than in controls, but differences between subgroups showed specificity. Patients with a history of suicide attempts had lower peak responses than those with no suicide attempts. Within the personality disorder group, those with borderline personality disorder had lower peak response than those without this type of personality disorder. Strong inverse correlations between prolactin response and a history of impulsive aggression and scale measures of aggression and impulsivity were found in the personality disorder group but not in the major depression group. The lack of serotonergic responsivity was related not only to inward-turned aggression in the depression group but to both inward and outward directed types of aggression in the personality disorder group.

Coccaro and his colleagues showed that reduced prolactin response to the fenfluramine challenge in a sample of personality disorders was related to an increased risk of impulsive-aggressive personality in their first-degree relatives (Coccaro, Silverman, Klar, Horvath, & Siever (1994). Their results suggest that inheritance of a disposition toward impulsive aggression is mediated by genetic transmission of a weak serotonergic reactivity.

Coccaro (1998) reviewed studies of the platelet 5-HT transporter binding. Three of the four studies of adults reported inverse correlations with aggression or impulsivity.

If serotonergic underactivity is a causal factor in impulsive aggression, then a drug that enhances serotonin reactivity should reduce aggression. Coccaro and Kavoussi (1997) used fluoxetine, a serotonin reuptake inhibiter, to test its possible antiaggression properties in a group of personality disorders with prominent histories of impulsive-aggressive behavior. Potential subjects with current major mood disorder or histories of mania, schizophrenia, or alcoholism were excluded from the study. Compared to those given a placebo, the patients taking fluoxetine showed reductions in behavioral aggression and irritability. The aggression was mainly of the verbal and indirect types. Actual physical aggression against others was noted in the histories of less than half of the group compared to verbal aggression, which was common in all of the subjects, and indirect (against objects) aggression, which was found in more than three quarters of the group. The treatment did not affect questionnaire trait measures of aggression. A 12-week treatment may affect immediate behavior but cannot change traits based on self-concepts.

Serotonin reuptake inhibiters often are used in the treatment of depression, but do they also reduce the angry and hostile feelings often accompanying depression? A study of SSRI therapy showed a signficant decrease in angry-hostility as well as neuroticism (Bagby, Levitan, Kennedy, Levitt, & Joffe, 1999). The decrease in neuroticism was correlated with the decrease in depression, but the decrease in anger-hostility was independent of the reduction of depression, suggesting a direct effect rather than one mediated by the drug induced reduction in depression.

Tryptophan is a precursor of serotonin production in the brain; therefore tryptophan depletion should decrease available serotonin and increase aggression. Using laboratory behavioral tests several investigators have found that rapid tryptophan depletion does increase aggressive responses and subjective feelings of anger and hostility (Cleare & Bond, 1995; Dougherty, Bjork, Marsh & Moeller, 1999; Finn, Young, Pihl, & Ervin, 1998). However, this effect is limited to persons who are high in trait measures of hostility.

In the study by Higley et al. (1992) discussed earlier, in which ratings of aggression in free-ranging monkeys were negatively related to the serotonin metabolite, CSF 5-HIAA, aggression was positively and strongly related ($r =$ .58) to CSF MHPG, the norepinephrine (NE) metabolite. NE in the brain mediates an arousal system and elevated NE could represent the emotional component of aggression (anger). NE is also associated with blood pressure reactivity characteristic of hostile and angry persons as discussed previously. In the study by Ballenger et al. (1983) plasma MHPG was negatively correlated with neuroticism but positively and highly correlated (.64) with the assault subscale of the BDHI. Coccaro et al. (1991) found a positive correlation between the response to the alpha2 NE agonist Clonidine and self-reported irritability. However, Kruesi et al. (1990) reported a negative correlation between CSF MHPG and life history of aggression in children with disruptive behavior disorders. Coccaro (1998, from unpublished study) also reported a modest inverse correlation between plasma free MHPG and life history of aggression. Coccaro reconciles these differences in direction of findings by proposing a variable dysregulation of presynaptic (MHPG) and postsynaptic (Clonidine) responses in some aggressive subjects.

Animal studies suggest a positive relationship between dopamine and aggressiveness. Increasing levels of brain dopamine increase aggressive responding in rats, although it takes a great deal of dopamine depletion to reduce aggressive behavior (Volavka, 1995). Some studies have found negative relationships between the dopamine metabolite HVA and aggression or lower levels in violent offenders. But HVA and 5-HIAA in CSF have strong correlations, perhaps because of serotonin regulation of dopamine release in the frontal cortex (Agren, Mefford, Rudorfer, Linnoila, & Potter, 1986).

CSF HVA may not be a good indicator of brain dopamine levels in other areas. Serotonin regulates dopamine release in the frontal cortex.

The stimulant drugs, amphetamine and cocaine, are associated with easily provoked aggression and hostile paranoid reactions in some chronic drug abusers. These drugs release both NE and dopamine, so it is difficult to say which is involved in the aggressive reactions.

The strongest evidence for a monoamine connection with aggression is the predominant finding of lowered serotonergic activity. The finding is consistent across species. The question is how much of this is the predisposition to antisocial behavior in general, because of the lack of strength of inhibition of approach behavior from frontal cortical areas. Some of the inconsistent findings in the field may be due to the lack of differentiation between two types of aggression: the low arousal type, common in psychopathic personalities, and the impulsive-angry type. Netter, Hennig, and Rohrmann (1999) claim to distinguish between the two types on the basis of selective types of challenges to the monoamine systems. Eysenck's P scale was used as a measure of psychopathy along with an aggression scale. Subjects scoring high on the psychoticism scale showed a strong cortisol response to a drug with dopamine agonist properties. Those scoring high on the aggression scale showed a blunted prolactin response to a drug that is an uptake inhibitor for serotonin. This study should be repeated using behavioral criteria rather than self-report scales by dividing a diagnosed psychopathic group into those who have histories of aggression and those who do not.

NEUROPSYCHOLOGY

Given the role of aggression in evolutionary adaptation it would be surprising if there were not evidence for "hard-wired" loci for the trait. Brain stimulation studies have largely been confined to nonhuman species. Stimulation of some medial sites in the hypothalamus in cats produces predatory type responses (Isaacson, 1982; Linnolia & Charney, 1999). This type of response is called "sham rage," because the animal will attack nearly any object in its environment at the time of stimulation and the response subsides rapidly with the cessation of stimulation.

Stimulation of the lateral hypothalamus in cats elicits angry aggressive reactions like the defensive aggression seen in natural behavior in response to threat or provocation, including emotional arousal, growling, and hissing with paw strikes at the provoking animal or object. It is interesting that this area is also one in which electrical brain self-stimulation can be easily elicited. Aggression for some human males is a kind of recreational sensation seeking and a source of pleasure (Joireman et al., 2003; Joseph, 1996). This kind of reaction in cats is also elicited by stimulation of the medial, anterior, and basomedial nuclei of the amygdala. Stimulation of other areas of the amygdala, the central and lateral nuclei, inhibits defensive rage. Stimulation of septal areas and the prefrontal cortex also suppresses rage and aggressive reactions in cats. Lesions of the amygdala reduce aggressiveness and rage, and emotional reactions in general, in cats, monkeys, and other species (Joseph, 1996). There is also an associated loss of dominance status and increase in submissiveness in several species. Aggression is closely linked to dominance in most species.

The animal studies suggest that certain areas of the amygdala and hypothalamus are "wired" to produce aggressive responses, whereas other areas in these structures and the prefrontal cortex inhibit or modulate rage and aggression. The first studies of brain substrates for aggression were clinical case studies of brain-damaged individuals. The case of Phineas Gage, a railworker whose prefrontal cortices were destroyed in an accident, was discussed in the previous chapter with regard to disinhibition and impulsivity. Gage also showed angry, verbally (but not physically) aggressive reactions after the accident, as part of his general disinhibition of behavior (Damasio et al., 1994). Other case studies of lesions in the orbital frontal cortex and adjacent prefrontal regions, reveal personalities characterized by both impulsivity and aggression (Davidson, Putnam, & Larsen, 2000).

Charles Whitman was a more direct case of brain damage and aggressive expression (Joseph, 1996; Sweet, Ervin, & Mark, 1969). After killing his wife and mother, Whitman went to a tower on the campus at the University of Texas with a hunting rifle and killed 14 more persons and wounded 38, all strangers shot at random. An autopsy of his brain showed a tumor compressing the amygdaloid nucleus. Documents discovered later revealed that he experienced his violent impulses as irrational but overwhelming. He himself requested the autopsy to explain his murderous behavior, mentioning intense headaches in the past.

Animal studies of amygdala removal show a diminution of emotional responses. Perhaps, this is in some part a function of the inability to recognize emotional expressions in conspecifics. A study of a woman with nearly complete bilateral destruction of the amydala, but with intact neocortical and hippocampal structures, showed a loss of ability to recognize intense expressions of fear, anger, and surprise (Adolphs, Tranel, Damasio, & Damasio, 1994).

Beyond the case study approach, visual imaging studies have been done on small samples of violent prisoners using MRI, CT, or PET methods. Mills and Raine (1994), reviewing 15 studies of such groups, found that 9 of the 15 showed some types of structural abnormalities, about evenly divided between frontal and temporal or frontotemporal deficits in activation. Frontal abnormalities were particularly characteristic of violent offenders as compared to sexual, but not necessarily violent, offenders. Another review also found a preponderance of frontal and temporal lobe dysfunction but not always both in the same samples (Soderstrom, Tulberg, Wikkelsö, Ekholm, & Forsman, 2000). In their own study of impulsive violent prisoners using both PET and MRI, Soderstrom et al. found some hypoperfusion in frontal and temporal lobes, but the MRI showed no structural damage in these areas. Reductions in CBF were found in the right angular and medial temporal gyri, in the bilateral hippocampus, and left white frontal matter.

Structural damage was found in two other studies. Tonkonogy (1990) found temporal lobe lesions in 5 of 14 violent patients and Wong et al. (1994) report that 75% of abnormal CT findings in the most violent group were in the temporal lobes.

Experimental laboratory studies have been used to attempt localization of aggressive brain reactions in humans. Exposure of normal subjects to angry facial expressions showed activations of right orbitofrontal cortex (Blair, Morris, Frith, Perrett, & Dolan, 1999). This area was not activated by presentations of sad expressions. Both sad and angry expressions activated the cingulate cortex. The authors suggest that the orbitofrontal response to angry expressions acts to suppress or inhibit aggressive behavior.

Dougherty et al. (1999) used narrative scripts, based on subjects' recall of extreme anger-provoking experiences in their lives, to provoke angry emotional states, while PET recordings were made of their brain activities. Anger provoked activation in the left orbitofrontal cortex, the right anterior temporal cortex, the anterior cingulate cortex, and the bilateral anterior temporal poles. Activation was not detected in the amygdala, perhaps because emotional arousal was not intense enough to overcome inhibition from the orbitofrontal and anterior cingulate cortices. There were no significant changes in heart rate, skin conductance, or frontal electromyograph responses during the anger condition, evidence of a lack of autonomic arousal.

In a study using a similar methodology to induce emotional states with cerebral blood flow measures from PET, both anxiety and aggression induced increased activation of left inferior frontal cortex and left temporal poles, whereas the anger induction specifically increased right inferior and medial frontal lobe activity, and right temporal pole, thalamus, and brain stem activity (Kimbrell et al., 1999).

Davidson, Putnam, and Larson (2000) and Emery and Amaral (2000) propose that negative emotions, like anger, are suppressed and behavioral reactions are inhibited by connections from the orbitofrontal, and other regions of the prefrontal cortex, to the amygdala. Threats that can provoke aggression are conveyed to the lateral nucleus of the amygdala, and then transmitted to the basal nuclei, where information about the social context coming from prefrontal connections is integrated with the perceptual threat information. Aggressive responses are instigated through the projections from the basal nuclei to various higher cortical centers. Physiological responses, like those connected with anger, are produced by projections from the basal nuclei of the amygdala to the central nucleus and then to the hypothalamus and brain stem. The key structures involved in this circuitry of emotion and impulsive aggression are shown in schematic (Figure 6-1) and MRI anatomic (Figure 6-2) forms. The schematic (Figure 6-1) describes the instigation of aggression in a primate from various types of external stimuli. The MRI (Figure 6-2) shows the key structures in the human brain.

Obstetric and Birth Complications

The findings on brain structure and function in subjects showing violent behavior could be due to genetic or prenatal brain damage. In fact, the two sources are somewhat confounded in twin and adoption genetic studies because the biological birth mother is the source of both and the adoptive mother contributes neither genetic or birth factors to the child. Identical twins are more likely to share a single placenta and chorion and therefore more likely to have similar prenatal environmental influences, although birth complications could occur for one and not the other.

The presence of an association between minor physical abnormalities and increased antisocial and violent behavior in children suggests a possible influence of prenatal and birth complications, because these kinds of physical differences often have such origins (Raine, 2002). A large study ($N = 4269$) of a male total cohort from Denmark showed an interaction between a record of birth complications and maternal rejection at one year of age in the predisposition to violent crime at age 18 years (Raine, Brennan, & Medick, 1994). The effect was specific to violent crime and was not found for non-violent crimes. Neither rejection nor birth complications alone increased the rate of violent crime above the rate in those with neither experience, but the combination of the two more than doubled the percentage of subjects with a record of violent crime. The small group with both factors in their background consituted only 4.5% of the population but accounted for 18% of all the violent crimes committed by the entire sample.

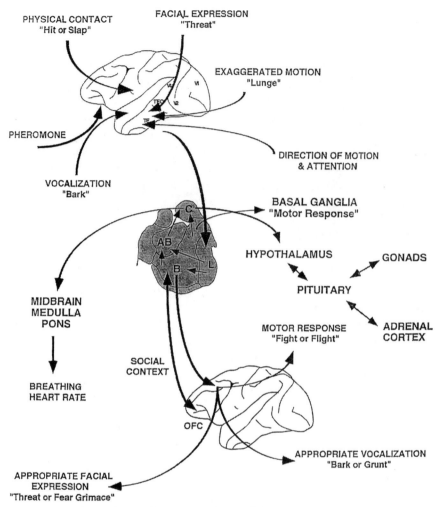

Figure 6-1. Pathways of processing of aggression threatening stimuli in different areas of the brain of a primate. Stimuli may be olfactory (pheromone), somesthetic (physical contact, like a slap), auditory (vocalization, like a "bark"), or visual (like a facial expression of "threat") or exaggerated motion (like a "lunge"). The sensory information is processed in different areas of the neocortex and conveyed to different sensory regions of the lateral nucleus (L) of the amygdala (shown in gray). Polysensory information is passed to the basal nucleus (B) of the amygdala. The significance of the stimuli is determined by the basal nuclei and connections with orbital-frontal cortex (OFC). This information is retrieved by the amygdala and used to produce an appropriate behavioral response according to the social status of the threatening animal. Appropriate behavioral responses may be initiated via projections from the basal nuclei to the basal ganglia and premotor cortex. A challenge from an equal or subordinate would elicit a "threat" facial expresson, a "bark" vocalization, and fighting attack. A challenge from a perceived dominant ape might elicit a "fear grimace" and flight. Increases in testosterone and cortisol may be initiated through projections from

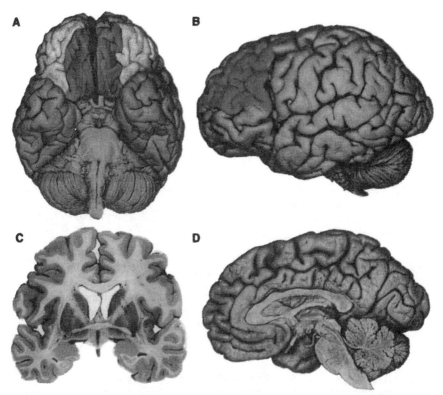

Figure 6-2. Key structures in the circuitry underlying emotion regulation (A) orbital prefrontal cortex [light shade] and the ventromedial prefrontal cortex [dark shade]. (B) Dorsolateral prefrontal cortex. (C) Amygdala. (D) Anterior cingulate cortex. Each of these interconnected structures plays a role in different aspects of emotional regulation, and abnormalities in one or more of these regions and/or in the interconnections among them are associated with failures of emotion regulation and also increased propensity for impulsive aggression and violence. From "Dysfunction in the neural circuitry of emotion regulation – A possible prelude to violence," by R. J. Davidson, K. M. Putnam, & C. L. Larson, 2000, *Science, 289*, p. 592, Copyright 2000 by *Science*. Reprinted by permission.

Figure 6-1 *(continued)*. the central nucleus (C) of the amygdala to the hypothalamus, then via releasing hormones to the pituitary gland, and finally through adrenocorticotropic hormone to the adrenal cortex, releasing cortisol and via gonadotropic hormone to the gonads in the male releasing testosterone. The appropriate physiological responses to fear or anger such as heart rate changes are initiated via projections from the central nucleus (C) of the amygdala to the brainstem increasing or decreasing breathing and heart rates. From "The role of the amygdala in primate social cognition," by N. J. Emery & D. G. Amaral, 2000, in *Cognitive neuroscience of emotion*, p. 180, by P. D. Lane & L. Nadal, Eds., New York: Oxford University Press. Copyright 2000 Oxford University Press. Reprinted by permission.

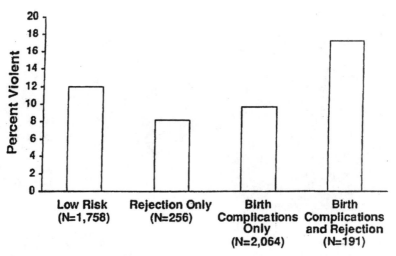

Figure 6-3. Interactions of birth complications with early maternal rejection in pre-disposing individuals to criminal violence at age 34 years. From "Interaction between birth complications and early maternal rejection in predisposing individuals to adult violence: Specificity to serious, early-onset violence," by A. Raine, P. Brennan, & S. A. Mednick, 1997, *American Journal of Psychiatry, 154,* p. 1265. © the American Psychiatric Association, http://AJP Psychiatryonline.org. Reprinted by permission.

A later study of the same sample included the record of crimes by age 34 allowing a closer examination of the age violent offenses began, the types of crimes involved, and the different indices of maternal rejection (Raine, Brennan, & Mednick, 1997). The interaction between birth complications and early maternal rejection was significant for the overall sample as shown in Figure 6-3. The interaction was found for violent crimes, including armed robbery, rape, murder, assault, and domestic violence, but not for threats of violence or weapons violations. The interaction was significant for cases in which the violent offenses began before the age of 18, but not for those with an adult onset after 18. The interaction was significant with the mother's institutionalizing the newborn child and attempts to abort the fetus, but not with not wanting the pregnancy. The presence of a maternal psychiatric illness was not related to birth complications or maternal rejection and did not affect the interaction between the two in producing violent crime, but in another study there was an interaction found between birth complications and mental illness in either parent affecting violent offenses in the child (Brennan, Mednick, & Mednick, 1993).

A study conducted in the United States found an interaction between prenatal and perinatal (birth) problems similar to that found in the

Danish study (Piquero & Tibbetts, 1999). Those with only pregnancy or only poor parenting complications had no higher rate of violent criminal behavior than controls with neither; but those with both types of complication exceeded the controls in adult violence.

An even larger Swedish cohort study of over 15,000 children born in Stockholm in a single year showed an interaction between pregnancy complications and inadequate parenting in producing criminal and violent offenses by age 30 (Hodgins, Kratzer, & McNeil, 2001). Both men and women were included in this study. As in the Danish study birth complications alone did not increase risk for crime or violent crime, nor did complications during pregnancy or neonatal complications independently increase risks for crime. In this study, however, powerful independent effects were found for lower socioeconomic status and inadequate parenting in both nonviolent and violent criminal activity. Inadequate parenting was based on a much broader criterion than in the Danish study where it was just overt maternal rejection indicated by attempts to abort and institutionalize the newborn. In the Swedish study, it was based on investigations by a child welfare committee at periods from birth to age 18. Nearly a third of the violent offenders had poor parenting as compared to 16% of nonoffenders. Pregnancy complications (but not birth or neonatal complications) combined with inadequate parenting slightly increased the risk of offending but more than doubled the risk of violent offending. The interaction between obstetric complications and inadequate parenting was not found for offenders beginning at an early age. The results from this study suggest much more weight for the social environmental factors than for the potential brain damaging factors during pregnancy, birth, or early life in violent and nonviolent crime. The combination of the two kinds of factors is much less common (3–4%) than inadequate parenting alone (28–30%), and only increases the risk for offending slightly.

A study of obstetric complications and psychosocial risk in prediction of childrens' behavior problems at 8 years of age was conducted in Germany (Laught et al., 2000). Newborn infants were rated on the degree of obstretrical complications during birth, including low birth weight. Psychosocial risk was estimated from a parental interview. At 8 years of age, a child behavior checklist was given to the parents to describe their childrens' behavior problems. Biological risk was related to social and attention problems but not to delinquent or aggressive behaviors. Psychosocial risk was related to a much larger range of problems including social and attention problems, but also delinquent and aggressive behaviors, somatic, and broad band externalizing and internalizing problems.

In this study, there was little interaction between biological and social risk factors.

A large scale study conducted in Finland looked at the effects of perinatal, parental, and being an only child on violent and nonviolent criminal behavior by age 32 (Kemppainen, Jokelainen, Järvelin, Isohanni, & Räsänen, 2001). Only children had a higher risk for violent crime than those with siblings. Perinatal risk combined with being an only child doubled the risk factor, and negative maternal attitudes toward the pregnancy and father absence increased the risk factors even more. Paternal absence was the strongest risk factor. When combined with being an only child it increased the risk for committing a violent crime eightfold, with a much smaller increase for nonviolent crime. This could suggest that the absence of a male role model, either a father or a sibling, may be a factor in violent crime. Of course, it is also possible that the absentee fathers were also more criminal and violent and that the connection is a genetic one.

It should be noted that none of the above researches were adoption studies so that there may have been confounding between some of the obstetrical and parental factors. Only the Danish and American studies showed pure interactions with no independent effects of social-environmental factors. Perhaps some of these factors are partly genetic, but they do seem to outweigh the simple prenatal or perinatal biological factors in their influence in any additive type of interaction.

SUMMARY

Aggression is obviously linked to anger and hostility but the emotional and attitudinal components are often located in different trait factor dimensions than aggression itself. In the Alternative-Five factorial model, all three constitute the fourth dimension, somewhat related to Agreeableness in the major Five-Factor model. From a comparative-evolutionary viewpoint, aggression is a major trait in most species of animals.

Heritabilities for aggression (or hostility or agreeableness) range from .3 to .5 depending on the particular type of measure used and gender and age of subjects. Some studies suggest effects of shared environment, particularly in children. One adoption study found an interaction between genetic background and adverse family environment as well as independent effects of these factors. Parents with antisocial personalities tend to have children with antisocial traits, including aggression, and an unstable home environment increases the likelihood of this outcome. But children in the same family may react differently to stress in the home, some becoming antisocial and aggressive, and others developing internalizing problems, or none at all.

At the molecular genetic level, the gene associated with MAO-type A has been related to aggressiveness in mice and humans. In humans, there is evidence of an interaction between the vulnerability produced by one allele of the gene and childhood maltreatment. Childhood maltreatment tends to produce violent criminals in those with the form of the gene producing low MAO-A activity, but not in those with the form related to high MAO-A activity.

The serotonin transporter gene seems to have a role in anger and hostility just as it does in anxiety and neuroticism. In monkeys, the same form is related to aggressive behavior in competitive situations. Dopamine receptor genes DRD4 and DRD5 account for a small percentage of the variance in hostility and aggression just as they do in sensation seeking and impulsivity. This common genetic mechanism may account for some of the phenomenological overlap between aggression and sensation seeking. Polymorphisms of the COMT gene have been related to anger in humans and aggression in mice.

Low resting heart rate and electrodermal signs of low autonomic/sympathetic system activity predict criminal behavior in later life. High levels of activity in these psychophysiological measures seem to have a protective function against such outcomes. Impulsive-aggressive types among alcoholic, prisoner, and college populations show weaker cortical evoked potentials.

Brain imaging studies suggest lower brain activity, particularly in the prefrontal and temporal lobes. Low metabolism in the corpus callosum in murderers is supportive of theories suggesting a lack of hemispheric integration in emotional and verbal functions in psychopathic personalities. The PET studies show results in violent criminals, which are similar to those in nonviolent criminals but more quantitatively extreme. Hypofrontal function may indicate a lack of executive control and consequent impulsivity in violent criminals.

The gonadal hormone testosterone is associated with normal competitive aggression, in a bidirectional manner, being increased by successful competition and reduced by losing. But it also has trait characteristics that may predispose toward enjoyment of this type of aggression. Testosterone is also elevated in delinquents and prisoners with histories of violent crimes.

Studies of humans and other primates show a connection between aggression and low levels of the serotonin metabolite 5-HIAA. Low levels of serotonin are also characteristic in many types of disorders and in violent and impulsive suicides. The common factor in all cases is a lack of control over emotions and behavior. Impulsive aggression may be turned outward or inward or both ways as in homicide and suicide. Drugs that potentiate serotonergic function reduce feelings of anger as well as depression, and reduce verbal hostility. Drugs that deplete serotonin in the brain increase feelings of anger and hostility, at least in persons who are already high in such expressions. There is some evidence of elevated levels of dopamine and norepinephrine related to aggression, but findings are mixed. The stimulant drugs amphetamine and cocaine can sometimes provoke aggressive reactions and paranoid feelings in chronic users. Both of these drugs release catecholamines in the brain.

Aggression in animals can be elicited by direct stimulation of areas in the hypothalamus and amygdala. Lesioning of these areas usually reduces rage and aggression in animals together with a loss of dominance status. Prefrontal regions, particularly the orbitofrontal area of the brain, act to inhibit or suppress aggression and anger. Two-way interconnections between amygdala and prefrontal cortex regulate the expression of aggression.

Obstetric and birth complications causing brain damage may be one source of early appearing and persistent aggression. Some studies suggest an interaction between pregnancy and birth complications and maternal rejection or inadequate parenting in children who later become violent criminals. Pregnancy and birth complications do not in themselves result in violent behavior but may increase the risk in those additionally suffering from parental rejection or neglect. These kinds of parental reactions may have direct environmental effects on the child or may be indicative of a shared genetic effect, such as impulsive and antisocial tendencies. The adoption studies discussed in the previous chapter suggest an important role for genetic factors passed on by antisocial parents who had no direct social influence on the child. Brain damage produced by prenatal or postnatal neglect, alcoholism, drug abuse, smoking, or premature birth or damage during the birth process, may predispose toward a violent antisocial outcome by reducing the brain's potential for inhibition or by limiting cognitive resources such as intelligence and planning ability. Emotional regulation is probably both a biological capacity and a learned ability.

CHAPTER 7

Consilience

> In nature hybrid species are usually sterile, but in science the reverse is often true. Hybrid subjects are often astonishingly fertile, whereas if a scientific discipline remains too pure it usually wilts.
>
> (Crick, 1988, p. 150)

Wilson (1998) used the term *consilience*, defined as that quality of science that combines knowledge across disciplines, to create a common background of explanation. More complex levels of phenomena can be described in terms of simpler phenomena. Personality psychology extends from social phenomena and what we call "personality traits" at the most complex end down to genes and their variations at the simplest level as shown in Figure 7-1. Of course, there is nothing simple about the genome, and we have only the beginning of a science of molecular behavioral genetics. Wilson sees reductionism as the goal of science:

> The cutting edge of science is reductionism, the breaking apart of nature into its natural constituents. . . . It is the search strategy employed to find points of entry into otherwise impenetrably complex systems. Complexity is what interests scientists in the end, not simplicity. Reductionism is the way to understand it. The love of complexity without reductionism makes art; the love of complexity with reductionism makes science. (pp. 58–59)

Personality constitutes a daunting challenge for this kind of reductionism. It can be analyzed in terms of distal to proximal influences along biological and social pathways as shown in Figure 7-1. Both pathways have their origins in evolutionary history. Evolutionary adaptation selects, eliminates, and sorts genes over long periods of time. Although most genes are similar among the individuals of a species, or even across related species, variations in genes appear in subgroups of the population resulting in variations in the neurology, biochemistry, and physiology of the nervous system. Ultimately,

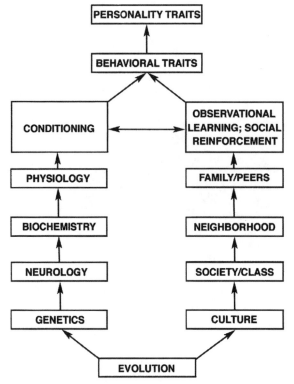

Figure 7-1. Two pathways to individual differences in personality: the biological and the social. From "Biological bases of personality," by M. Zuckerman, 2003, in *Handbook of psychology, Vol. 5, Personality and Social Psychology*, p. 86, T. Millon & M. J. Lerner Eds., I. B. Weiner, Ed.-in-Chief. Hoboken, NJ: Wiley. Copyright 2003 by John Wiley & Sons. Reprinted by permission.

these result in in different propensities for conditioning, as in differential sensitivities to cues for reward and punishment (Gray, 1982, 1987).

The social pathway starts with variations in cultures, representing the collective solutions of the human species to the basic requirements of evolution: survival and reproduction. The comedian Jackie Mason summarized most Jewish holidays: "They tried to kill us, we won, let's eat." We might add to this: "Let's make children and look after them so they can survive and make grandchildren."

Cultural changes can occur much more rapidly than genetic ones, even within the space of a generation. Within culture are variations in society and class which have strong influences on behavior. These are transmitted more directly in the neighborhood and schools through family and peer influences. Family, peers, and other adult models influence the person through observational learning, instrumental learning, and social reinforcement. Of course, what is learned depends on the intraindividual characteristics influenced by the events in the biological pathway. There are many models available to the child, and the selection among them depends on the myriad of biological and social influences shaping personality.

Reductionism across all levels is not a realistic goal for science. At each level the phenomena require new laws and principles of organization that are not reducible to levels below it. One could conceivably find all of the particular genes that contribute to the genetic variance in a personality trait but not be able to account for the complex interactive influences with environment that shaped the trait. Genes and environment interact throughout development and although environment cannot change genes it can affect their expression through releasor genes. Genes do not make personality traits or behavioral traits, they simply make proteins that in turn make neurons, biochemicals, and these affect physiology and ultimately behavior. But environmental events such as stress also affect physiology, neurotransmitters, hormones, and even neurons, sometimes in more than transient ways. The case for irreducible complexity is a strong one. But consilience, or an approach to it, can and does occur at the borders between levels; for example, how does a gene affect a neurotransmitter and behavior under particular environmental conditions?

Evolution has left a particularly cluttered mess in the DNA. The human brain is less like a machine than a jerry-built contraption with new and old mechanisms operating in a variable interactive way. As described by MacLean (1982), the human brain contains structural relics of the "reptillian," paleomammalian, and earlier neomammalian brains, each adding new capacities for more complex behavioral adaptations (Figure 7-2).

After his discovery of DNA with Watson, Crick went on to the study of the brain. His commentary on the difficulties of reductionism in this field is relevant to the consilience idea:

It is thus very rash to use simplicity and elegance as a guide in biological research.... To produce a really good biological theory one must try to see through the clutter produced by evolution to the basic mechanisms lying beneath them, realizing that they are likely to be overlaid by other, secondary mechanisms. What seems to physicists to be a hopelessly complicated process may have been what nature found simplest, because nature could only build on what was there. (Crick, 1988)

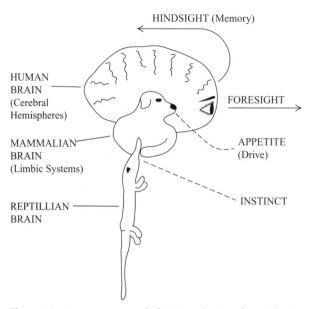

Figure 7-2. A cartoon portrayal of MacLean's *triune brain*. The "reptillian" brain centers on the "striatal complex" (caudate and putamen) and includes the pons, cerebellum, and some parts of the limbic brain such as thalamus and hypothalamus. The "paleomammalian" brain includes the limbic system structures and the "neomammalian" (human brain in the figure) brain consists of the cerebral hemispheres. The reptillian brain functions are governed by fixed action patterns or "instincts" contrasted with the greater plasticity (modification by learning) of appetitive behavior instigated by innate drive mechanisms in mammals. The development of the cerebral hemispheres in the human, with the capacity for language, allows for extended hindsight or memory, and foresight or anticipation of future consequences based on memory. The frontal lobes, in particular, extend the capacity for inhibition of behavior with anticipated negative consequences.

Except in the most rudimentary way, we cannot go back in evolutionary time to study the particular adaptations that led to the behavioral variations we see in our species. There is a way to do this by comparative study of other extant species, particularly with those mammals closest to us in basic behavioral mechanisms. Psychobiological experimental research must depend heavily on animal models in order to find common biological mechanisms underlying *similar* behavior. The catch is in the word "similar." Anthropomorphism is a danger particularly when we go beyond behavioral observations to the inference of humanlike traits. Throughout this book, I have made use of such models. If we assume an evolutionary history for personality traits, then we should see some rudimentary version of them among individual differences in other species. To what extent can we see similar organizations of traits in the behaviors of other species?

PERSONALITY STRUCTURE

Nonhuman Species

Throughout this book, I have used a comparative approach, comparing personality traits in humans with behavioral analogues in other species. To a strict behaviorist, the application of the concept of personality to animals within species is an oxymoron. But ethologists who study colonies of animals recognize individual differences that are fairly stable, often have a genetic basis, and are analogues of human personality differences. Observers' ratings of animals in their natural habitats run the risk of anthropomorphism. Observations of behavior in controlled experimental situations are more reliable but the behavior observed may be specific to the contrived experimental conditions. One must differentiate between species-specific traits and those which are generalizable across species.

Gosling and John (1999) looked for dimensions of personality which might be common across a wide range of species. They reviewed 19 studies of personality factors in 12 nonhuman species using the five-factor (Big-Five) human model as a framework. Fearfulness (N), sociability (E), aggression (A) appeared as factors in most species. Curiosity-exploration, an interest in new situations and novel objects, and playfulness were thought to be analogues of the five-factor trait of openness to experience, although in other models they are considered expressions of sensation seeking (Bardo et al., 1996; Dellu et al., 1993, 1996; Zuckerman, 1979, 1984, 1994). Naturally, the human facets of the openness trait in the Big Five, which include interest in ideas, art, creativity, are irrelevant in species beyond the human. Gosling and John found evidence for analogues of conscientiousness in only one nonhuman species, chimpanzees. Dominance emerged as a separate factor in 7 of the 19 studies, but related to a surgent type of E, physical aggressiveness, and low fearfulness. Assertiveness in the Big Five is only a facet of E. The activity dimension was not consistently found across species and was most prominent in primate infants.

In a second review, focusing on studies of four species (monkey, hyena, cat, and chimpanzee), Gosling (2001) found the most reliable agreement among observers in at least two of the four species on sociability, dominance-submission, anxiety, activity, aggressiveness, and playfulness.

The rat is the most frequently used species in studies of analogues of human personality traits such as anxiety, aggression, and sensation seeking. The open-field test has been used to measure both explorativeness and emotional reactivity or fearfulness in rats and mice. Genetic studies have been done cross-breeding strains, which differ markedly in open-field behavior (Plomin et al., 1997). Factor analyses of behavior in the open field have consistently yielded three factors: exploration (activity), emotional reactivity or fearfulness (defecation) and territorial marking or urination (Royce, 1977). The problem with the usual form of the experiment is that the open-field elicits both fear and exploratory tendencies and the two are negatively related. Another problem is that "exploration of empty spaces" is not necessarily related to exploration of novel stimuli (Simmel, 1984). Garcia-Sevilla (1984) modified the usual open-field situation in a manner that reduced the fear-provoking aspect and found less correlation and a greater discriminant validity between exploration and fearfulness factors in relation to other behavioral criteria of these traits.

Dog owners are familiar with personality differences among domestic dogs. To some degree these differences reflect genetic variations among breeds (Scott & Fuller, 1965), but within-breed variations are also seen. Svartberg and Forman (2002) used a series of behavioral tests given to over 15,000 dogs from 164 different breeds. Factor analyses showed five narrow traits: playfulness, curiosity/fearlessness, sociability, aggressiveness, and chase-proneness. The last of these seems to be a canine species-specific trait. Curiosity and fear are inversely related in a single trait. A higher-order factor analysis showed that four of the traits (excluding aggressiveness) could be organized in a broad factor influencing behavior across a broad range of situations: *shyness versus boldness*. This supertrait is described as a combination of extraversion and neuroticism in the human area. It resembles what has been described as "approach-avoidance" across species.

It is apparent that carnivora species have many personality traits in common with humans testifying to their evolutionary significance in the mammalian line. But the traits of our near cousins in the primate line of evolution are of particular significance because of our common ancestry.

Chamove, Eysenck, and Harlow (1972) observed the interactions of monkeys housed four to a cage and found three basic factors: (1) play, both social and nonsocial; (2) fear, based on inhibition of social exploration, withdrawal from other monkeys, or inappropriate social responses; (3) aggression-hostility, including physical aggression or threat behaviors. Eysenck related these to his own three factor system equating play with E, fear with N, and aggression with P. These factors, however, did not show much consistency across experimental situations, and therefore were of questionable value as traits. A small cage environment is probably not an optimal place to find reliable traits.

Observations of behavior of chimpanzees in their natural environments over long periods of time have revealed clear personality differences

(Goodall, 1986). Although Goodall did no systematic analyses of personality, her detailed descriptions show characteristic traits of sociability, aggression, dominance, and fearfulness among the band she studied over the years. In Chapter 4 of her book, she provides personality descriptions of 30 different adult members of the band.

A more systematic study was made of 100 chimpanzees residing in 12 different zoological parks (King & Figueredo, 1997). Observers made behavior ratings, adapted from those used to assess the Big-Five factors in humans, and factor analyzed the ratings. Six factors were found but these did not correspond in any simple way to the human Big Five.

Factor 1 had its highest loadings on dominance and submission, but the next highest loadings came from emotionality items including "fearful." Dominant chimpanzees were fearless, independent, and aggressive (bullying). Submissive chimps were fearful, timid, dependent, and cautious. The factor is a combination of E and N or surgency versus fearfulness, identified as "boldness" in higher order factor analyses (Svartberg & Forkman, 2002).

Factor 2 contrasted the traits of activity, playfulness, friendly, affectionate, and sociability with solitariness, inactivity, and depression at the other pole. It was called "surgency," but it also included elements of agreeableness as well.

Factor 3 was called "dependability," presumably a prototype of conscientiousness in the human Big-Five. But the four highest loading items, impulsive, defiant, reckless, and erratic, and others including irritable, aggressive, and jealous, suggest it is a combination of aggression-hostility and impulsive sensation-seeking in Zuckerman and Kuhlman's Alternative Five.

Factor 4 was labeled "agreeableness," because it included the terms sympathetic, helpful, sensitive, protective, and gentle. However, other more obviously agreeable terms, friendly and affectionate, were in Factor 2.

Factor 5 was described as "emotionality" because it consisted of three items – stable, excitable, and unemotional – even though other emotionality items were scattered among the first three factors.

Factor 6 consisted of only two items – inventive and inquisitive – and was equated with the human Big-Five factor of openness.

Despite the attempt to fit chimpanzee behavior to the human Big-Five model by using descriptive terms derived from that model, it is obvious that the personality traits of chimpanzees in seminatural surroundings do not correspond in any precise way to that model. Dominance is a major factor among chimpanzees, but it is included as only a secondary one (assertiveness) in E in the human system. In chimpanzees, it combines with fearlessness (N) and aggression (A). Big male chimpanzees dominate through

Table 7-1. Comparison of basic traits derived from animal behavior, children's temperament, and adult personality

Animal behavior	Child temperament	Adult personality
Dominance		(Sociability, aggression, fearlessness)
Sociability	Sociability	Extraversion
Fearfulness	Negative Mood	Neuroticism
Aggression	Anger	Aggression/Agreeableness
Curiosity/Exploration	Approach	Sensation Seeking
	Persistence	Conscientiousness vs. Impulsivity
	(Activity)	(Openness)

aggressiveness and submissive males are realistically fearful and nonaggressive. However, dominance in humans is more complex and not necessarily based on physical aggression or fearlessness. Differences in the organization of traits within animal and human personality may be a function of the transformations produced by cultural evolution rather than biological evolution. But questions remain about the basic structure of traits in the human realm.

Personality Structure in Humans

There are four basic characteristics that are identifiable in studies of nonhuman animals, particularly those who live in social groups, temperament in infants and children, and personality in adolescents and adults, discussed in Chapter 1. Table 7-1 shows the correspondences. Dominance is a major trait in about a third of the animal species, but it seems to be a higher order trait combining surgent extraversion, aggressiveness, and fearlessness. Activity and persistence are found in nearly all analyses of temperament but, with the exception of the inclusion of activity as a primary factor in the Zuckerman-Kuhlman Alternative Five, they are not major factors in most other systems. Persistence could be an early expression of conscientiousness and its lack may be a sign of impulsivity. In the personality realm, conscientiousness is moderately related to psychoticism, impulsive sensation seeking, and constraint, but it is only identifiable in humans and some studies of chimpanzees. Openness is a strictly human trait insofar as it depends on language and culture, but some expressions can be related to curiosity and exploration in animals, infants, and children.

Impulsiveness?

Where does impulsiveness fit into this paradigm? It has behavioral expressions that can be clearly seen in animals, children, and human adults. Undercontrol, which includes impulsivity along with sensation seeking and

aggression, is a higher order trait which is predictive of later antisocial behavior (Caspi, 2000). It is a style of expression rather than a trait limited
to one basic emotion or motivational goal. It is the opposite of inhibition
or constraint and, as we have seen, these have a biological basis in frontal
cortical-amygdala circuits. In view of the above considerations, it should
emerge as a basic temperament and personality factor in its own right.

Buss and Plomin (1975) included impulsivity as a major factor of temperament in their first classification of temperaments but excluded it in the later
version because of questions about its factorial unity and heritability (Buss
& Plomin, 1984). Guilford and Zimmerman (1956) described a major factor called "Restraint," which included impulsivity and demonstrated good
reliability and validity for the scale measuring it (Guilford & Zimmerman,
1956). Eysenck and Eysenck (1964) included impulsivity along with sociability as the two major facets of their earlier extraversion scale, but Carrigan
(1960) and Guilford (1975) argued that the combination of the two traits was
a "shotgun wedding." Sybil Eysenck and Hans Eysenck (1963) defended the
placement of impulsivity in the extraversion factor but also admitted that it
correlated with neuroticism as well. Later, they developed independent impulsivity scales (S. B. G. Eysenck & H. J. Eysenck, 1977). In their final version,
they included two factors: impulsivity and risk taking or venturesomeness
[sensation seeking] (H. J. Eysenck & S. B. G. Eysenck, 1978). Hans Eysenck
and Michael Eysenck (1985) included impulsivity within their major factor
of psychoticism. Costa and McCrae (1992) include impulsivity within their
major factor of neuroticism.

The Eysencks were not the first to link impulsivity and sensation seeking in a common factor. The Buss and Plomin (1975) impulsivity factor
included sensation seeking as well as lack of inhibitory control, quick decision time, and lack of persistence. In the first factor analyses leading to
the development of the ZKPQ we included a number of sensation seeking
and impulsivity scales with the expectation that we would find separate
sensation seeking and impulsivity factors (Zuckerman et al., 1988). Factor
analyses were done with 3, 4, 5, 6, and 7 factors separately for men and
women. At the six-factor level, five of the six factors matched reasonably
well across genders, but the sixth factor, impulsivity, in the men did not
have a clear match in women. However, from the five-factor through the
three-factor analysis, a factor combining impulsivity and sensation seeking
was quite reliable. It also included measures of (non)socialization, autonomy, nonconformity, lack of restraint, and lack of responsibility.

The development of the ZKPQ is described in an article (Zuckerman et al.,
1993) and a recent chapter (Zuckerman, 2002). Item selection based on item
total correlations and factor analysis yielded the scale "Impulsive Sensation

Seeking (ImpSS)." The impulsivity items in this scale describe a lack of planning and a tendency to act quickly on impulse without thinking. ImpSS has a psychobiological model and the concept has been used in comparative studies of other species already described in this book (Zuckerman, 1996). ImpSS is a predictor of risk taking in many different areas (Zuckerman & Kuhlman, 2000).

Barratt (1959) was the first to develop a free-standing impulsivity scale, and he has investigated the nature of the trait at the personality and psychophysiological levels. The fifth version of his scale was based on a factor analysis of items with four orthogonal factors: (1) cognitive impulsivity; (2) lack of impulse control; (3) adventure seeking; and (4) risk taking. The last two of these resemble sensation seeking, but the factors are described as "orthogonal" or uncorrelated. The more recent version of his scale (Barratt, 1983) described only three factors: (1) motor impulsiveness; (2) cognitive impulsiveness; and (3) nonplanning impulsiveness. Motor and nonplanning impulsiveness are the types found in Zuckerman and Kuhlman's ImpSS scale.

Barratt (1994) proposed that impulsivity is related to one form of aggression called "impulsive aggression." Indeed, many others have made this distinction between impulsive and premeditated aggression and it is a factor in legal definitions. The relation with low serotonergic activity described in the previous chapter is specific to the impulsive type of aggression. Psychopathic aggression is usually unplanned and impulsive, but so is aggression in other types based on an inability to control anger expression.

So what is impulsivity and where does it belong within basic dimensions of personality or temperament: extraversion, neuroticism, sensation seeking, aggression, or activity? My answer is "all of the above." The difficulties in defining a pure factor of impulsivity is because different expressions are not necessarily correlated and are primarily related to one or the other of the major personality factors.

The idea that there are different types of impulsivity is not entirely new. Eysenck and Eysenck (1963) suggested that some types are related more to extraversion while others are related more to neuroticism. Dickman (1990) distinguished between functional and dysfunctional impulsivity. Functional impulsivity is the same as cognitive impulsivity in Barratt's classification: the ability to make fast decisions and think quickly and express one's ideas with alacrity. Dysfunctional impulsivity is speaking or acting on impulse without regard for possible negative consequences. The former is probably more related to normal surgent extraversion whereas the latter is related to neuroticism. The two types of impulsivity correlate minimally ($r = .23$).

I would suggest that impulsivity is not a general trait but a style which assumes different forms depending on the associated major trait:

Impulsive Extraversion is related to general speed of response as illustrated by Dickman's item for functional impulsivity: "I like to take part in really fast-paced conversations, where you don't have much time to think before you speak." The opposite extreme verges on obsessiveness: "I don't like to make decisions quickly, even simple decisions such as choosing what to wear, or what to have for dinner."

Impulsive Neuroticism is associated with Dickman's dysfunctional type of impulsivity. Item examples are: "I often do and say things without considering the consequences," and "I often get into trouble because I don't think before I act." The expressions suggest an awareness of the dysfunctional aspects of the behavior as in the last example.

Impulsive Sensation Seeking is associated with Barratt's (1983) Non-Planning type of impulsivity, Examples from the ZKPQ ImpSS items are: "I enjoy getting into new situations where you can't predict how things will turn out," and "I very seldom spend much time on the details of planning ahead," and "I would like to take a trip with no preplanned or definite routes or timetable." Note that none of these examples express any worry about possible negative consequences or regard the behavior as dysfunctional.

Impulsive Aggression is expressed in some items of the Buss–Perry (1992) Hostility Inventory: "Once in a while I cannot control the urge to strike another person," "I can't help getting into arguments when people disagree with me," "When frustrated I let my irritation show," and "I have trouble controlling my temper." All of these items express the inability to inhibit expressions of physical or verbal aggression or anger.

Impulsive Activity is not activity in the pursuit of some work goal, exercise, or sport but simply a general restlessness and need for distraction in activity. An item in the Barratt motor impulsivity scale that illustrates this is, "I find it hard to sit still for long periods of time." The Zuckerman and Kuhlman's activity scale from the ZKPQ contains two subfactors: one is a general need for activity and impatience and restlessness when there is nothing to do. An example is, "I like to keep busy all the time." The other is a preference for challenging or hard work. An example: "When I do things I do them with lots of energy." The first represents the need for activity for its own sake, whereas the second illustrates the nonimpulsive capacity for channelized activity. The Boredom Susceptibility scale of the SSS is related to restlessness because of the lack of stimulation. Hyperactive children and adults are usually also impulsive. Motor behavior provides an escape from boredom for them. Boredom is associated with a state of low arousal or one below the "optimal level of arousal" (Zuckerman, 1979). Physical activity is the most effective way to increase cortical arousal via the reticular activating system.

EVOLUTION AND PERSONALITY

The argument can be made that one extreme of personality is more adaptive to survival and reproduction than another and therefore was selected in the course of human evolution. This case can be easily made for extraversion or sociability. Humans and other primates live in social groups that provide mutual support among their members. Dominance in male chimpanzees is maintained by aggressiveness when confronted with rivals, and also with the formation of alliances with other males (not unlike the human situation). The loner is usually a loser in the sense of being dominated and victimized. Sociability provides the bonds of friendship with the advantages of reciprocity in distribution of food resources and provision of protection when needed. Females who are more popular in a nonsexual context, are the most sought after as mates when they come into estrus (Goodall, 1986).

In the case of impulsive sensation seeking, however, both extremes may be maladaptive and the optimal level of the trait may be somewhere in the middle range. There is a trade-off between risk-taking and the potential advantages in exploration. An organism that ventures too far from home may encounter predators or aggressive members of its own species from other groups. Chimpanzees sometimes kill any strangers from out-groups venturing into their territories (Goodall, 1986). Male chimpanzees generally compete for females in their own groups but they are especially attracted to the "novelty" of immigrant females to the group. Although males generally take the initiative in sexual encounters, adolescent females often take the initiative. Among human tribal groups, males may court females from outside groups or attempt to "kidnap" them at the risk of attack from other males in those groups.

Hunting of large mammals played a major role in the evolution of homo sapiens. Hunting elephants or other large animals is risky. High sensation seekers presumably enjoyed this kind of activity, which made them sources of major resources and attractive to potential mates, but many may have been injured or killed in the hunt. War has been a source of sensation seeking for the human species and high sensation seekers have been attracted to this risky activity. Sensation seeking often involves a trade-off between risk and the reward of "peak-experience" or intense positive arousal.

Aggressiveness is a factor in dominance and combat with outsiders. As such, it has an obvious advantage in resources and mating attractiveness in nonhuman primates. It also may have some advantage in human mating competition. However when men and women in 37 cultures were asked about their preferences for mate selection the highest rated requisite among both genders was "kindness and understanding" (Buss et al., 1990). The personality trait of agreeableness is nearly opposite to aggressiveness.

The second ranked trait for both genders was "intelligent." This is a trait for which there is evidence of *assortative mating*, as measured by correlations between spouses. Intelligence may be most associated with openness in the Big-Five model.

The third ranked trait was described as an "exciting personality." This may correspond to a combination of extraversion and sensation seeking. Most personality traits do not show much evidence of assortative mating (Ahern et al., 1982; Eysenck, 1990). Sensation seeking, however, is an exception with moderate to high correlations between SSS scores of spouses in America, Croatia, Germany, and the Netherlands (Bratko & Butkovic, 2003; Farley & Davis, 1977; Farley & Mueller, 1978; Ficher, Zuckerman, & Neeb, 1981; Ficher, Zuckerman, & Steinberg, 1988; Lesnik-Obserstein & Cohen, 1984). In the case of sensation seeking, like attracts like. Assortative mating suggests the biological importance of this trait and enhances its heritability.

Dependability (Conscientiousness) and emotional stability (low N) were also rated highly by both men and women in the entire international sample (Buss et al., 1992). Despite cultural variations, or between countries differences, there were substantial similarities among the national samples in the ordering of traits. Although there is agreement between genders in the highest rated trait preferences, there were gender differences in two traits in nearly every sample. Men placed a higher value on physical attractiveness in a mate and women valued ambition-industriousness more than men. These differences support Buss's theory of mate selection, which postulates that men place a greater value on looks as a sign of fertility, whereas women are more concerned with the potential of men for supporting their offspring. However, these traits are not the primary ones for either sex in mate selection. Good looks ranked only 10th for men and 13th for women.

Behavioral traits evolve as adaptations to particular kinds of environments and therefore their adaptiveness may change with environmental changes. An example can be drawn from the fate of the green iguana in Mexico, as reported by Browne (1988). Iguanas compete for basking places in the sun on exposed rocks. The choice places are occupied by the larger and more dominant males and females. The subordinate males stay off the open rocks to avoid aggressive encounters with the dominants. As in most species, the more dominant males also are more successful at mating. There is a risk for the large dominants, in that when they are basking in the sun on the rocks they are more exposed to eagles and other predators including humans. Large iguanas are favored by humans as a source of meat. The population of iguanas is shrinking and conservationists are uncertain as to whether they should breed and turn loose the large dominants or the subordinates. If this kind of environmental selection persisted over long periods of time the size of the species members could shrink.

The adaptive value of a trait may change depending on the situation or environment in which it is manifested. Mice, as a species, tend to be wary in open exposed places where they could be seized by predators. However, they must venture out of their burrows to forage for food creating an approach-avoidance conflict. The C57BL strain of mice tends to be relatively fearless and exploratory in the novel environment of an open-field arena. The BALB (B-Albino) mouse strain is fearful and frozen at the periphery of the open-field, although they are more active at night-time than the C57 mice. The C57 has the genetically created advantage for foraging in daytime conditions in open spaces, whereas the BALB avoids the risk of daytime exposure in the open-field and operates at night. If a C57 encounters a BALB in an open lighted arena, it is the more aggressive (Ginsburg & Allee, 1942) and successful in competition for food (Frederickson & Birnbaum, 1954). But if members of the two strains are confined in a small living box for a period of time the BALB emerges as the survivor having killed the C57. The high emotionality of the BALB in his own natural environment makes him the superior warrior.

Speculative extension of this kind of paradigm to the human level might suggest that the high sensation seeker is well adapted to combat and exploration but is at a disadvantage in environments that require stability and order. The author Caputo (1977) was a soldier in Vietnam. He had the opportunity to sit out the war at a desk job but volunteered to return to his front-line company anyway. His account of the reasons for this risky decision shows the strength of his sensation seeking motive:

There were a number of reasons of which the paramount was boredom. The rights or wrongs of the war aside there was a magnetism about combat. You seemed to live more intensely under fire. Every sense was sharper, the mind worked clearer and faster.... You found a precarious emotional edge, experiencing a headiness that no drink or drug could match. (p. 218)

It is a mistake to think of any trait as adaptive or nonadaptive in an invariant sense. In some situations, it might be an advantage and in others a disadvantage. Evolutionary theories of behavior tend to speculate about the role of selection in long distant environments in which the species evolved.

As Buss (1991) describes, humans have many alternative strategies for solving the problems of survival and mating. He suggests that these are heritable and situationally contingent. Some of the major personality traits such as extraversion and agreeableness always may have been adaptive because of their value in the forming of reciprocal alliances and the perception of and respect for the hierarchal positions of others in the social group. However, aggressiveness, that is the near opposite of agreeableness, was certainly an advantage in establishing one's own dominant position in a social hierarchy. Perhaps the intermediate position on a trait continuum is always the most adaptive and the extremes maladaptive.

The postulation of alternative strategies for basic adaptations like mating suggests a role for personality traits in evolution. All personality traits are normally distributed. The idea of alternative strategies implies types with discontinuous or non-normal distributions. Buss (1991) suggests that continuously distributed personality traits may be due to past environments that imposed different adaptive options; for instance, different availability of food resources shifting the balance between the need for risk taking and sensation seeking. The fact is that we can never know the adaptive circumstances in prehistorical environments and that is a fundamental weakness in evolutionary psychology. It is possible that the two extremes of a personality trait once represented alternative strategies, as we see in different strains of mice in their exploratory or fearful reactions to the open-field test (DeFries, Gervais, & Thomas, 1978). At one time different populations of humans, geographically isolated from each other, may have developed particular inbred adaptations to their particular environments. One tribe could have consisted of high sensation seekers and another of low sensation seekers because of different availabilities of resources in their territories. Over time, cross-mating between the populations may have produced the normal distributions like those found in mice cross-bred between two strains with different distributions in open-field behavior.

We can interpret types as simply extremes of traits. If we look at an individual profile on personality traits we usually see that one or two traits are high (or low) for a given individual and therefore represent their most generalized strategies in appropriate situations. Mating strategies are probably a function of personality types. The sociable, sensation seeking, emotionally unstable, or aggressive types have their own styles of courtship and attraction preferences.

Buss et al. (1990) found that the highest rated criterion for mate selection across all cultures was mutual attraction or love. This was true of western countries but not many African countries or China. Even in countries where "love" is of primary importance, the term has different meanings for people. Hendrick and Hendrick (1986) defined six meanings or "styles" of loving. They also could be regarded as "strategies" for mate selection in an evolutionary sense:

> *Eros* is passionate, committed, and romantic love, strongly emotional and needful like that of Romeo and Juliet in Shakespeare's play.
> *Ludus* is a more playful and less committed type of love; a game with more autonomy for partners.
> *Pragma* is based on appraisal of mates based on their potentials for a long-term relationship.
> *Storge* is based on friendship rather than passion.
> *Agape* is a selfless devotion to the loved one.
> *Manic* love is obsessive, dependent, emotionally tense, and possessive.

Men are higher in Ludus type love and women are higher in Pragma, consistent with Buss's hypotheses about mate preferences (Hendrick and Hendrik, 1986). Initially, men tend to be in it for the short-term excitement, women for the long-term security necessary to nurture children. Sensation seeking was positively related to the Ludus type and negatively related to the Pragma type of love (Richardson, Medvin, & Hammock, 1988). Ludus is negative related and Pragma is positively related to the length of relationships and Ludus is positively related to the number of relationships. Thus, personality may be expressed in the strategy of loving and the fate of relationships.

Evolutionary psychology was critically evaluated by Lickliter and Honeycutt (2003). The essential criticism is that evolutionary psychology regards early behavioral adaptions as persistent in the species in the form of genetic modules containing programs for behavioral reactions triggered by current environmental situations. Licklitter and Honeycutt maintain that this thinking ignores the evidence of interaction between genes, biological factors, and environment in the development of the individual. In terms of the ladders shown in Figure 7-1, they assert that evolutionary psychologists go right from evolution to behavioral traits, ignoring the complex biological steps in between, and the social environmental ladder from cultural familial influences on behavioral traits. In other words, explanation is largely in terms of distal behavioral selection rather than proximal biological or social influences.

We believe the persistence of dichotomous thinking in evolutionary psychology is due in large part to the continued acceptance of the distinction between proximate and ultimate causes.... In the general sense, proximate causes are those acting during the life of the organism, whereas ultimate causes are characterized as those acting before the organism was conceived, and that shaped by its genome.... Evolutionary psychology is primarily concerned with the ultimate causation of behavior and therefore focuses on its function or adaptive value with the aim of understanding how the behavior was designed or shaped by natural selection. (Lickliter & Honeycutt, 2003, p. 869)

Proximate causes are obviously of more direct influence than distal causes. Genes undoubtedly influence male and female sexual or mating preferences and behavior, but pre- and postnatal levels of testosterone, differences in brain structures, conditioning by specific experiences during development, and social values, attitudes, and customs are also vital influences and interact with and may even overrule the evolutionary selected preferences. Homosexuals and transsexuals seem to defy the basic aim of evolution, to maximize reproductive potential. Furthermore, given the recent technology of effective birth control, many heterosexuals choose to have sex without ever having children. Throughout history monks and nuns have chosen to abjure sex. One can, of course, devise some convoluted evolutionary explanations for these exceptions to evolutionary selection, but proximate biological and social explanations are more cogent.

Another criticism of evolutionary theory by Lickliter and Honeycut (2003) is the use of hundreds of situation or domain specific cognitive modules or evolved psychological mechanisms to explain behavior. The existence of such modules is usually inferred post hoc from behavior in a situation. Rather than postulating such specific inheritance of narrow behavorial reactions, it might be more parsimonious to regard the behaviors as interactions between personality dispositions and situations. Few claim that personality dispositions are totally genetic, but most admit that they evolve from genetic interactions with experiences during development.

Most evolutionary psychologists do not concern themselves with the details of research in behavioral genetics, but just assume that the genome carries the results of adaptations over countless generations. However, some of the same criticisms that are made of evolutionary psychology could be applied to many behavior geneticists. Until the development of molecular genetics, behavior geneticists have been concerned with the question of how much variance in traits or behaviors is due to environment and how much to genetics, or the infamous "nature versus nurture" problem. This research was based on concepts of genes and environment as independent factors (with the possibility of interactions), and with genes as having a constant influence on behavior. We now know that genes regulate the transcription of other genes in response to immediate effects within the internal and external environments (Plomin et al., 1997). In fact, there may be more DNA in regulatory than in structural genes. Gene expression can change in response to immediate or prolonged stimulation from the environment. This is probably why rats reared in enriched environments have more brain matter than those reared in minimally stimulating environments. Most of the genetic research reviewed in this book came from the traditional twin, adoption, and family studies addressing the nature-nurture question and the questions of genetic mechanisms and shared versus nonshared environment. What have we learned from these?

BEHAVIOR GENETICS

A naive assumption in the earlier days of the nature versus nuture controversy was that some personality traits would turn out to be highly heritable whereas others would be entirely determined by environment. Over the years, it has become apparent that nearly all personality traits have some degree of heritability and the range (.3 to .6) is relatively narrow. Summarizing the data from many studies Loehlin (1992) found a range for the Big-Five of 35 to 49% total (broad) heritability and 22 to 43% for additive (narrow) heritability. About a third of the total is due to nonadditive (dominance or epistasis) genetic mechanisms. The highest total heritabilities were for surgency (.49) and openness (.45) and the lowest were for agreeableness (.35) and conscientiousness (.38). Emotional stability (N) (.41) was intermediate. Shared environment was a low source of variance ranging from 2 to 11%. Surgency was lowest (.02) and agreeableness was highest (.11). The remainder of variance was a function of nonshared environment and error of measurement.

Our own surveys of results show a similar pattern for the alternative-five classification. E-Sociability heritabilities range from .4 to .6, those for N-Anxiety from .4 to .5, those for P-Imp-SS from .3 to .5, and .5 to .6 for sensation seeking. Agreeableness heritabilities range from .3 to .6, but on explicit aggression-hostility scales and ratings they range from 0 to .5., On the latter type of scales, there is a marked gender difference in the heritability of different forms of aggression (Cates et al., 1993; Coccaro et al., 1997). Males show moderate heritability on a scale for direct assault (physical aggression) but low heritability on verbal aggression, whereas females show no heritability for assault and moderate heritability for verbal aggression. Many aggression/hostility scales do not make these distinctions between forms of aggression. Loehlin (1992) notes different heritabilities for impulsivity, dominance, and sociability, regarded as subtraits of extraversion and suggests that genetic analyses should be conducted on a more specific trait level or at both levels. The question is, however, how much of the subtrait is based on a genetic factor common to all of the subtraits, and how much on a genetic factor specific to that subtrait?

The absence of stronger influences of shared environment, which would include family influences, seemingly contradicts most theories of personality, particularly psychodynamic ones, claiming that early parental influences are the basic sources of personality. As a matter of fact, correlations between biological parents and children and siblings are quite low, and between adopted children and their biologically unrelated parents and siblings they are close to zero. Broad heritability from twin studies is usually higher than estimates from nontwin studies, perhaps indicating the influence of nonadditive genetic mechanisms, or stronger influences of identical twins on each other than between fraternal twins. In nontwin studies, age differences between parents and children and between siblings may lower resemblance.

It is possible, of course, that early parental influences are less important in shaping personality than later peer influences. In many families, peers are more readily imitated and used as models for behavior than parents. But both parents and peers do not act on a passive subject. From the time a toddler can move about and increasingly as the child moves away from the home for school and other activities, the child chooses friends and activities. Even role models in the media and books (if any children still read nonassigned books) can be sources of role modeling. This implies a correlative type of interaction between temperament and available models. Differences in temperament between siblings also can elicit different reactions from parents so that the "shared" environment is really not shared by two siblings.

Most twin studies do not actually assess the environment, and the estimate of the genetic and shared environmental influences are made from the differences between identical and fraternal twins using statistical formulae. These population statistics can conceal gene-environment interactions occurring in subpopulations. The study of the heritability of sensation seeking by Boomsma et al. (1999), described in Chapter 5, illustrates this possibility. The heritability for the Disinhibition subscale of the SSS in the total sample was quite high, .62 for males and .60 for females, and there was no indication of an effect of shared environment (Koopmans et al., 1995). But when the sample was divided into those raised in a religious environment and those raised in a nonreligious (presumably more permissive) environment the heritabilities and shared environmental effects were quite different. The twins raised in the nonreligious environment showed the usual results of high heritability and no effect for shared environment. But the twins raised in a religious environment there was no genetic effect for men and a strong effect for shared environment. For women raised in religious families, the two effects were nearly equal. One wonders how many twin studies would show such contrasts if the population samples were subdivided by significant environmental variations.

Adoption studies also have shown interaction effects between congenital and environmental factors. Because there is usually some screening of adopting parents, there is bound to be a smaller range of deviancy in adopting families compared to biological parents but, if samples are large enough, interaction effects can be detected. Some studies of criminality (Ishikawa & Raine, 2002) in children, biological, and adopting parents have shown interactions; criminality in both the adopting and biological parents increases the risk of criminality in the children more than criminality in either the biological or adopting parent alone (Cloninger & Gottesman, 1987; Cloninger et al., 1982; Cadoret et al., 1985). Apart from criminal role models, bad parenting can also interact with genetic predisposition to increase the risk of antisocial behavior in children (Ge et al., 1996). Of course, harsh discipline could be a reaction to misbehavior in children or there could be a reciprocal effect with greater aggressive reaction to harsh discipline in children predisposed to antisocial behavior (Cadoret et al., 1995).

Separating genetic and prenatal environmental effects from those of the social environment is not easy even in adoption studies. Better measures are needed of environmental interactions of parents and children in order to distinguish genetic-environment correlations from interactions of independent genetic and environmental factors. Contrasts of two adopted children in the same family, one with a biological risk factor and the other with none, would be highly informative.

Molecular genetics promises to carry behavior genetics to a more precise level of specificity by identifying genes of major effect underlying personality (Benjamin, Ebstein, & Belmaker, 2002a). The search for genes underlying the major psychiatric disorders has not met with much success in replicable associatons. More significant effects have been found for personality traits, particularly the association between novelty seeking and the DRD4 receptor gene. But even this finding has only been replicated in about 50% of the 21 studies (Prolo & Licino, 2002). Benjamin, Ebstein, and Belmaker (2002b) suggest that interactions between genes may be involved in personality traits as they are in both medical and psychiatric clinical disorders. For instance, in newborns and younger children the DRD4 polymorphism increased approach behavior, consistent with the association with the gene and novelty seeking in adults but only in the presence of short variants of the serotonin transporter promoter-linked polymorphism.

Gottesman (1991) described *endophenotypes* as traits intermediate on the chain of causality from genes to diseases. Such traits and their genes may be contributory or even necessary but not sufficient in producing the full form of the disorder. Benjamin et al. (2002b) proposed that the genes affecting personality traits may constitute endophenotypes for disorders. The DRD4 polymorphisms affect both normal novelty seeking and its expression in heroin users, a group with a high proportion of antisocial personality disorders.

The broad trait of neuroticism has higher heritabilities (.4–.5) than those for diagnosed anxiety disorders (.3–.4) (Zuckerman, 1999). The short form of the serotonin-transporter gene has been associated with high scores on neuroticism, anxiety, anger, and depression scores in general populations and is a likely candidate for an endophenotype for anxiety and mood disorders (Prolo & Lucino, 2002). An understanding of the genetic and neurotransmitter links between personality, personality disorders, and clinical disorders is important for developing rational pharmacotherapeutic treatments for the disorders, as well as a scientific understanding of the psychobiology of personality.

PSYCHOPHYSIOLOGY

Neuroscientists tend to disparage psychophysiology because it deals only with surface recordings of biological activity. The EEG and EP methods are not precise enough in localization of brain activity and the PET and fMRI are replacing them. However, the classical psychophysiological methods have the advantage of more precise temporal location, able to record events in fractions of a second, whereas the imaging methods require longer periods of time to record responses. The classical measures of autonomic activity, heart rate, skin conductance, and blood pressure, are much less intrusive than drawing blood to measure changes in catecholamines or cortisol. The classical psychophysiological methods can track psychological reactions more immediately and therefore are still vital to psychobiology.

The concept of cortical arousal and arousability has been central to Eysenck's theory of extraversion and neo-Pavlovian theories of temperament (Strelau & Eysenck, 1987). EEG studies of introverts and extraverts in resting conditions (reviewed in Gale & Edwards, 1986; O'Gorman, 1984;

Zuckerman, 1991) yielded mixed findings, inconclusive for Eysenck's hypothesis of lower arousal in extraverts than in introverts. Recent studies, including one large one (Matthews & Amelang, 1993), have shown some weak relationships between both extraversion and impulsivity (not sociability) and slow wave activity. Gale's hypothesis that differences would be found only in moderately arousing conditions was not supported. Actually, the differences were found only in the least arousing condition (eyes closed). It is not clear whether it is the broad trait of extraversion or only surgent (impulsive) extraversion, which shows the relationship.

Some believed that the newer PET brain imaging methods would yield more definitive results. Two studies did show negative correlations between CBF in large areas of the brain and extraversion (Mathew et al., 1984; Stenberg et al., 1993), but the results were confined to female subjects only. Other studies found results specific to certain brain areas only, higher arousal in introverts in the temporal lobes or the striate with extraverts showing more arousal in the cingulum. Furthermore, extraverts showed more arousal under stimulating or task involved conditions than introverts. These latter results regarding specificity and interaction with conditions are not clearly predictable from Eysenck's theory. However, Eysenck's theory would predict less arousability in extraverts under low to moderate stimulation but with stronger response than introverts under intense stimulation.

Cortical evoked potentials are appropriate for testing arousability. Stelmack (1990) and Zuckerman (1991) reviewed the EP work. Several investigators found that introverts had higher P300 EP amplitudes than extraverts using the "odd-ball" method or response to an infrequently presented stimulus. However, under conditions of increased auditory stimulus intensity or high rates of stimulus presentation, the extraverts showed high EP amplitudes, consistent with Eysenck's theory.

Stelmack extended EP studies to subcortical levels of the central nervous system (CNS) finding longer latencies of the brainstem auditory EPs and reduced motoneuronal excitability in a reflex leg reaction in extraverts. If such findings are replicated, they may indicate that the low arousability of extraverts under low to moderate stimulation is a characteristic of neural activity in the entire CNS rather than just the cerebral cortex.

A number of studies that looked at the components of extraversion, then regarded as impulsivity and sociability, found that impulsivity was related to conditioning and cortical arousal whereas sociability was not. Sensation seeking was initially based on the same optimal level of arousal theory as extraversion (Zuckerman, 1979; Zuckerman et al., 1964), therefore the first

EEG studies made the same kind of predictions for cortical arousal and arousability. No differences were found between high and low sensation seekers in arousal in nonstimulating conditions. However, the EP paradigm called "augmenting-reducing" by Buchsbaum (1971) revealed a highly replicable association with sensation seeking (Zuckerman, 1990). With increasing levels of intensity of visual or auditory stimulation, the high sensation seekers showed an augmenting pattern and the lows showed a reducing pattern, suggesting cortical inhibition at high intensities of stimulation. The findings were particularly significant for the subscale of sensation seeking called "disinhibition." This is the subscale most highly related to impulsivity. Barratt et al. (1987) showed that direct measures of impulsivity trait were also related to augmenting/reducing. The augmenting pattern also was found in delinquents, crimimals, and drug users, groups characterized by impulsivity and disinhibition.

Most interesting, from an evolutionary comparative viewpoint, is the finding that EP augmenting/reducing could be identified in cats and rats. Siegel and his colleagues showed that the EP paradigm in the cat was associated with impulsive or restrained behaviors in response to novel stimuli or reinforcement paradigm tests of capacity to delay responding for reward.

A study of two strains of rats, one characterized by EP augmenting, the other by EP reducing, showed many strain-related behavioral, physiological, and biochemical differences beween the two strains (Siegel et al., 1993). The behavioral differences on explorativeness, aggression, maternal behavior, and brain self-stimulation were consistent with the human model of impulsive sensation seeking. The greater tolerance for high intensity brain self-stimulation is analogous to the preference of human sensation seekers for drugs and pleasure-producing stimulation of many kinds. Differences in dopaminergic and serotonergic and corticotropin releasing hormone responses to stress point to the psychopharmacological foundation for sensation seeking. Investigators in another laboratory showed that rats who are novelty seekers also show more self-administration of the stimulant drug amphetamine than those who are not reactive to novelty (Dellu et al., 1996). The taste for novelty in high reactive rats was directly correlated with levels of the metabolite of dopamine in the nucleus accumbens, the major site of drug reinforcement effects.

Thus, this psychophysiological paradigm provides a connection between personality and disinhibited forms of psychopathology in humans, and direct analogues of these in other species. It also shows consistent associations between the various levels in Figure 7-1: the personality, behavioral trait, psychophysiological, biochemical, neurological, and genetic levels.

Measures of cortical reactivity such as the evoked potential have yielded more consistent results than measures of arousal using EEG spectrum analysis. However, in the case of neuroticism, neither basal nor stress reaction measures of autonomic arousal are related to the trait levels. There is some increased fast-wave (beta) activity, particularly in the temporal lobe in high N normals. In contrast, clinical anxiety disorders, particularly panic, agoraphobic, and obsessive-compulsive disorders, tend to have elevated basal heart rate levels (Zuckerman, 1991, 1999). As a consequence of high basal levels, patients with anxiety disorders show less response (measured relative to basal levels) than normals to standard laboratory stress tests. However, during panic attacks or provoked with stimuli related to their phobic situational fears patients with anxiety disorders show large increases from their baseline levels of arousal. The difference between normals with high levels of N trait and patients with anxiety disorders suggests a discontinuity in the physiological aspects of the trait. Although neuroticism is part of the predisposition for anxiety and mood disorders, physiological changes may occur only after some threshold is crossed.

In patients with generalized anxiety disorder (GAD), trait anxiety is expressed primarily in cognition (worry) and in muscle tension and fatigue. Normals with high levels of N may be more like the persistent GAD disorder than the disorders in which autonomic arousal is chronic. Their high level of EEG beta activity may be symptomatic of the cognitive element of GAD. Heart rate arousal may be evidence of a chronic threat expectancy or a state of heightened sensitivity to signals of punishment.

The defensive conditioned eye-blink startle response (SR) is closer to the muscle tension found in GAD. Reaction of the eye-blink SR response during the presentation of fear provoking stimuli has been associated with N as a trait in normals. The fear-potentiated SR also has been useful in animal studies of anxiety designed to identify brain areas mediating anxiety response.

Very low as well as high heart rate may be a risk factor for psychopathology. But, in the case of low basal HR, the risk is for antisocial types of disorders and may represent an insensitivity to threat of punishment. However, low basal HR or skin conductance level (SCL) is not associated with sensation seeking. In HR and SCL, indices of the orienting reflex (OR) in response to novel stimuli indicate a stronger OR is found in high sensation seekers than in lows, but this difference quickly habituates when the stimulus is no longer novel. These measures of interest or positive arousal are even stronger when the content of the stimulus is more exciting to the high sensation seeker. Sensation seeking does not fit the low arousal model but instead shows a positive but transient responsivity to novelty.

PSYCHOPHARMACOLOGY

I have described how analyses of animal behavior tend to show a higher order factor that has been called "boldness" (vs. fearful inhibition), or approach versus inhibition and avoidance. Predator species tend to be higher on the former and species that are vegetarian tend to be higher on the latter. The human primate and closely related apes tend to be both predators and prey during the longest parts of their evolutionary histories and therefore had to develop the mechanisms underlying both attack and defense.

Neurotransmitter systems serve many functions, so it is difficult to characterize their behavioral functions in any simple way. However, several theorists have formed some general conclusions about the roles of the three monoamine systems in behavior. Ebstein and Auerbach (2002) have succinctly summarized the broad hypotheses concerning two of these systems:

Our provisional findings are consistent with both human and animal studies that activation of dopaminergic pathways promote exploratory and impulsive behavior, whereas serotonergic pathways are generally inhibitory and advance avoidance behavior. (p. 145)

They go on to say that the DRD4 long allele form promotes the exploratory and impulsive behavior [impulsive sensation seeking], which is opposed by the serotonin transporter short form that tends to inhibit behavior and promote negative emotions and distress [neuroticism-anxiety].

Figure 7-3 shows a psychopharmacological model based on a three-factor theory (Zuckerman, 1994, 1995). Dopamine is related to the generalized approach mechanism, serotonin to the inhibition mechanism, and norepinephrine to the arousal mechanism. Personality traits represent a combination of mechanisms. P-ImpUSS, for instance, is a combination of strong approach [to novelty], weak inhibition [impulsiveness], and weak arousability [fearlessness]. Going to the level of neurotransmitters, this would mean high sensitivity or reactivity of dopamine receptors and low sensitivity of serotonergic and noradrenergic receptors. Previously, these relationships were framed in terms of levels of neurotransmitters. Although receptor sensitivity may be inversely related to levels of intraneuronal transmitter it also can be related to levels of transmitter synthesis or receptor densities. What is important is the reactivity of the system to environmental conditions rather than the basal level of activity in the system during nonstimulating conditions.

The enzymes regulating the systems also play a vital role. There is ample evidence that MAO type B is preferentially related to regulation of dopaminergic systems, the approach behavior affected by these systems, and

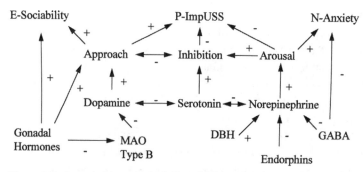

Figure 7-3. A psychopharmacological model for extraversion-sociability (E-Sociability, impulsive unsocialized sensation seeking (P-ImpUSS), and neuroticism-anxiety (N-Anxiety) showing underlying behavioral mechanisms (approach, inhibition, and arousal) and neurotransmitters, enzymes, and hormones involved. Agonistic interactions between factors are indicated by a plus sign and antagonistic interactions are indicated by a minus sign. MAO = monoamine oxidase; DBH = dopamine-ß-hydroxylase; GABA = gamma-aminobutyric acid. From "Good and bad humors: Biochemical bases of personality and its disorders," by M. Zuckerman, 1995, *Psychological Science, 6*, p. 331. Copyright 1995 by American Psychological Society. Reprinted by permission.

personality traits such as impulsive sensation seeking and sociability. Low levels of this enzyme affect approach behavior by dysregulation of dopaminergic systems. Dopamine deamination is mainly a function of MAO-B in human and nonhuman primate brain (Murphy et al., 1987). More recently, it has been discovered that MAO type A and the gene producing it, preferentially affect the serotonergic system (Azmitia & Whitaker-Azmitia, 1995) and are related to antisocial and aggressive behavior traits.

Hormones are involved in a broad variety of behavioral and personality traits. Testosterone, for instance, may account in some major part for the personality differences between men and women and the changes in behavior that occur as a function of age. This hormone is related to dominance, surgency, sensation seeking, sociability, rebelliousness, energy and activity, and aggressiveness. In a word, it is related to *boldness* or the approach motive seen in humans as well as other species.

Cortisol is one of the end products of activation of the hypothalamic-pituitary adrenocortical (HYPAC) stress system and is associated with stress reactivity in depressive and anxiety disorders. The HYPAC system is highly reactive in a strain of rats showing the fearful, nonexploratory, nonaggressive characteristics that are characteristic of generalized inhibition and the cortical evoked potential characteristics of human sensation seekers (Siegel & Driscoll, 1996). In animals, the biological traits underlying behavior are general across a broad spectrum of traits like fear and bold exploration. This also may be the case with humans. Low levels of cortisol and epinephrine and high levels of testosterone are related to impulsive sensation seeking and antisocial personality, whereas the opposite configuration of hormones is found in neuroticism and anxiety.

There is the "chicken-and-egg" problem with hormones and neurotransmitters, in that they are responsive to environmental experiences and their outcomes. Testosterone, for instance, may rise with victorious outcomes and fall with defeats in competiton. Stress may increase cortisol and decrease testosterone levels. However, there are reliable individual differences in average levels and they are in part genetically controlled. In the language of psychometrics, the immediate levels of these biochemicals reflect both traits and states.

Speaking of particular neurotransmitter systems such as the dopaminergic ones as if they were all functionally equivalent ignores the functional differences between the systems. Dopamine is the neurotransmitter for two major systems: (1) the nigrostriatal system originating in the substantia nigra and projecting to the neostriatum including the putamen and caudate nucleus; and (2) the mesocorticolimbic system beginning in the ventral tegmentum and projecting to the nucleus accumbens and limbic areas including the amygdala and septum, and the forebrain including lateral and medial prefrontal cortex. Most of the hypotheses concerning personality concern the second system, because it involves the limbic areas concerned with reward motivation, and emotions whereas the nigrostriatal system is primarily a motor regulation system (although it also may have some motivational functions).

Diffferences within the structures of the mesocorticolimbic system have been demonstrated in two strains of rats, one highly responsive to novelty and the other lowly reactive to or inhibited by novel situations (Dellu et al., 1996). These French scientists have used this animal model as an analogue of human sensation seeking trait. Under basal conditions (autopsy) the highly responsives were found to have lower levels of dopaminergic activity in the prefrontal cortex but higher levels than the lowly reactives in the nucleus accumbens (LeMoal, 1995). The same differences were found after exposure to novelty: The amount of dopaminergic activity in the accumbens was positively related to locomotor reactivity to novelty whereas the dopaminergic activity in the prefrontal cortex was negatively related to exploratory activity. Similar differences were found in rats showing high and low levels of amphetamine self-administration. The opposite relation of dopaminergic activity in the two areas of the brain are consistent with evidence that dopamine release in prefrontal cortex inhibits dopamine transmission in subcortical structures such as the nucleus accumbens. The accumbens is a major site for brain self-stimulation, theorized to be a model for sensation seeking and drug use.

Such specificity of localization is difficult to show in studies of humans in which only an indirect measure of overall dopamine reactivity is usually used. This is why animal models for human personality traits must be used in conjunction with less precise studies of human psychopharmacology to understand the functions of neurotransmitters.

NEUROPSYCHOLOGY

Even more than psychopharmacology, neuropsychology has required integration of findings from research on animals with clinical neuropsychology. However, a new era began with the development of brain imaging techniques, allowing observation of both structural and functional characteristics of all parts of the brain.

Structural differences in brain between personality types is a remote possibility, reminiscent of the pseudoscience of phrenology which assigned traits arbitrarily to various parts of the outer brain. Total brain volume has shown a small but significant correlation with intelligence, and loss of brain volume has been observed in schizophrenic and mood disorders (Elkis, Friedman, Wise, & Meltzer, 1995). The entire brain volume was found to be negatively related to neuroticism alone among the Big-Five personality factors (Knutson et al., 2001). This could be a function of stress reducing brain neurons rather than a causal factor in neuroticism. Volume of the right hippocampus was reduced in patients suffering from posttraumatic stress disorder (Bremmer et al., 1995) and prolonged social stress damages the hippocampus in mice (Blanchard et al., 1995). These deficits could have something to do with the memory problems in PTSD. In the case of the reduction of prefrontal gray matter in persons with antisocial personality disorder (Raine et al., 2000) the structural deficit may play a role in the personality disorder itself, accounting in part to the lack of control and impulsivity characteristic in psychopathy. The deficit also correlates with a lack of autonomic response to social stress, which could account for the impairment in learning to avoid punishment and absence of empathy in the antisocial personality.

Functional brain imaging, using PET and fMRI, is more likely to reveal personality differences. Eysenck's (1967) historical arousal hypothesis suggested that introverts were more arousable that extraverts throughout the entire cortex. PET studies, although not entirely consistent, have suggested a more localized kind of arousal in the temporal lobes, the striate (putamen and caudate) area mediated by one of the dopaminergic systems. Introverts showed greater arousal (blood flow) in these areas. Extraverts had greater arousal in the cingulum, the major pathway between the frontal cortex and the limbic system.

Studies of neuroticism have used emotional induction techniques to study changes in brain function. Earlier theories suggested localization of fear reactions in the entire limbic system (Eysenck, 1967), the Papez (1937) circuit, and the septo-hippocampal system (Gray, 1982), and suggested special sensitivities of this system in persons high in neuroticism or suffering from actual anxiety disorders. More recent theories (Davidson, 2002; Le Doux, 1987, 1998) have emphasized the amygdala as the comparator receiving stimuli from the thalamus and prefrontal cortex and organizing emotional reactions according to the context of the stimuli. Davidson also has suggested that negative emotions are lateralized in the right prefrontal cortex and right amygdala. Imaging studies have shown that negative emotional stimuli do activate the amygdala as well as the temporal cortex and the parahippocampal gyri lying under the temporal lobe (Hariri et al., 2002; Phan et al., 2003). In patients with panic disorders, the right parahippocampal gyri are activated prior to the induction of a panic attack (Reiman, 1990). During the panic attack, there is an increased blood flow in the anterior ends of the temporal lobe.

The neuroimaging studies are beginning to show the actual brain localization of fear reactions in the brain, but thus far few have atttempted to show the connection between these reactions and personality traits like neuroticism. The clinical studies of anxiety disorders suggest that studies of personality dimensions will show positive results, but such studies will require larger numbers of subjects than are typically used in brain imaging studies.

THE WAY AHEAD

The basic personality traits have evolved from the basic mechanisms involved in survival, reproduction, and protection of progeny. Foraging and hunting in the search for food needs exploration or sensation seeking. Facing threats from the environment requires appraisal of the threat (inhibition of ongoing behavior and orienting toward the source), and fight or flight (aggression or anxiety and avoidance). Animals living in social groups depend on alliances with mates or peers for procreation and protection, the basis of sociability. Quick reactions are sometimes necessary for survival but can lead to errors of judgment that are fatal (functional or dysfunctional impulsivity). Social evolution has changed the nature of these basic mechanisms so that their expression in contemporary society is a far cry from their origins in bands of primates and early hominids. But the biological mechanisms underlying personality traits may be quite similar, if not the same, as those for the behavioral mechanisms evolved in our mammalian ancestry.

Most of the basic personality traits are closely associated with emotions: sociability and sensation seeking with positive affects, neuroticism with fear and depression, and aggression with anger (Zuckerman et al., 1999). Emotions have a longer history in human evolution than ideas and are hard-wired. Our understanding of personality, therefore, must depend on future work on the biological basis of emotions. Much of the current work involves the study of psychopathology, particularly anxiety and mood disorders, in which we see emotions in their extremes. Studies of the psychopharmacology of these disorders before and after treatment are important in understanding variations in personality in the normal range.

Movement forward in the psychobiology of personality is a troika pulled by three forces: comparative neuropsychology using animal models, the genetic/biological bases of normal personality traits, and the neurobiology of human psychopathology. Progress will depend on integration of results from all of these fields.

References

Adams, R. D., Victor, M., & Ropper, A. H. (1997). *Principles of neurology*, (6th ed.). New York: McGraw-Hill.

Adolfsson, R., Gottfries, C. G., Oreland, L., Roos, B. E., & Winblad, B. (1978). Monoamine oxidase activity and serotonergic turnover in human brain. *Progress in Neuropsychopharmacology, 2*, 225–230.

Adolphs, R., Tranel, D., Damasio, H., & Damasio, A. (1994). Impaired recognition of emotion in facial expressions following bilateral damage to the human amygdala. *Nature, 372*, 669–672.

Aggleton, J. P., & Mishkin, M. (1986). The amygdala: Sensory gateways to the emotions. In R. Plutchik & H. Kellerman (Eds.) *Emotion: Theory, research, and experience* (Vol. 3, pp. 281–299). New York: Academic Press.

Aggleton, J. P., & Young, A. W. (2000). The enigma of the amygdala: On its contribution to human emotion. In R. D. Lane & L. Nadal (Eds.), *Cognitive neuroscience of emotions* (pp. 106–128). New York: Oxford University Press.

Ågren, H., Mefford, I. N., Rudorfer, M. V., Linnoila, M., & Potter, W. Z. (1986). Interacting neurotransmitter systems: A non-experimental approach to the 5HIAA-HVA correlation in human CSF. *Journal of Psychiatric Research, 20*, 175–193.

Ahern, F. M., Johnson, R. C., Wilson, J. R., McClearn, G. E., & Vandenberg, S. G. (1982). Family resemblance in personality. *Behavior Genetics, 12*, 261–280.

Alm, P. O., Alm, M., Humble, K., Leppert, J., Sörenson, S., Lidberg, L., & Oreland, L. (1994). Criminality and platelet monoamine oxidase activity in former juvenile delinquents as adults. *Acta Psychiatrica Scandinavica, 89*, 41–45.

Aluja, A., & Torrubia, R. (in press) Hostility, aggressiveness, sensation seeking, and sexual hormones in men: reexploring their relationship. *Neuropsychobiology*.

Andreassi, J. L. (1989). *Psychophysiology*. Hillsdale, NJ: Erlbaum.

Andreassi, J. L. (2000). *Psychophysiology human behavior and physiological response*, 4th ed. Mahwah, NJ: Erlbaum.

Angleitner, A., Riemann, R., Spinath, F. M., Hempel, S., Thiel, W., & Strelau, J. (1995). *The Bielefeld-Warsaw Twin Project: First report of the Bielefeld samples*. Workshop on Genetic studies on temperament and personality, Pultusk, Poland.

Apter, A., van Praag, H. M., Sevy, S., Korn, M., & Brown, S. (1990). Interrelationships among anxiety, aggression, impulsiveness and mood. A serotonergically linked cluster? *Psychiatric Research, 32*, 191–199.

Arana, G. W. & Baldessarini, R. J. (1987). Clinical use of the dexamethasone suppression test in psychiatry. In H. Y. Meltzer (Ed.) *Psychopharmacology: The third generation of progress* (pp. 609–615). New York: Raven Press.

Archer, J. (1991). The influence of testosterone on human aggression. *British Journal of Psychology, 82,* 1–28.

Archer, J., Birring, S. S., & Wu, F. C. W. (1998). The association between testosterone and aggression in young men: Empirical findings and a meta-analysis. *Aggressive Behavior, 24,* 411–420.

Arqué, J. M., Ungeta, M., & Torrubia, R. (1988). Neurotransmitter systems and personality variables. *Neuropsychobiology, 19,* 149–157.

Åsberg, M. (1994). Monoamine neurotransmitters in human aggressiveness and violence: A selected review. *Criminal Behaviour and Mental Health, 4,* 303–327.

Åsberg, M. Träskman, L., & Thorén, P. (1976). 5-HIAA in the cerebrospinal fluid – A biochemical suicide predictor? *Archives of General Psychiatry, 33,* 1193–1197.

Azmitia, E. C., & Whitaker-Azmitia, P. M. (1995). Anatomy, cell biology and plasticity of the serotonergic system: *Neuropharmacology: The fourth generation of progress* (pp. 443–449). New York: Raven Press.

Bagby, R. M., Levitan, R. D., Kennedy, S. H., Levitt, A. J., & Joffe, R. T. (1999). Selective alteration of personality in response to noradrenergic and serotonergic antidepressant medication in a depressed sample: Evidence on non-specificity. *Psychiatry Research, 86,* 211–216.

Bailey, J. M., & Pillard, R. C. (1991). A genetic study of male sexual orientation. *Archives of General Psychiatry, 50,* 217–223.

Ball, S. A., & Zuckerman, M. (1990). Sensation seeking, Eysenck's personality dimensions and reinforcement sensitivity in concept formation. *Personality and Individual Differences, 11,* 343–353.

Ballenger, J. C., Post, R. M., Jimerson, D. C., Lake, C. R., Murphy, D. L., Zuckerman, M., & Cronin, C. (1983). Biochemical correlates of personaity traits in normals: An exploratory study. *Personality and Individual Differences, 4,* 615–625.

Bard, P. (1929). The central representation of the sympathetic nervous system: As indicated by certain physiological observations. *Archives of Neurology and Psychiatry, 22,* 230–246.

Bardo, M. T., Donohew, R. L., & Harrington, N. G. (1996). Psychobiology of novelty seeking and drug seeking behavior. *Behavioural Brain Research, 77,* 23–43.

Barratt, E. S. (1959). Anxiety and impulsiveness related to psychomotor efficiency. *Perceptual and Motor Skills, 9,* 191–198.

Barratt, E. S. (1971). Psychophysiological correlates of classical differential eyelid conditioning among subjects selected on the basis of impulsivity and anxiety. *Biological Psychiatry, 3,* 339–346.

Barratt, E. S. (1983). The biological basis of impulsiveness: The significance of timing and rhythm disorders. *Personality and Individual Differences, 4,* 387–391.

Barratt, E. S. (1994). Impulsiveness and aggression. In J. Monahan & H.J. Steadman (Eds.) *Violence and mental disorder* (pp. 61–79). Chicago, IL: University of Chicago Press.

Barratt, E. S., Pritchard, W. S., Faulk, D. M., & Brandty, M. E. (1987). The relationship between impulsiveness subtraits, trait anxiety, and visual N100 augmenting-reducing: A topographic analysis. *Personality and Individual Differences, 8,* 43–51.

Barratt, E. S., Stanford, M. S., Kent, T. A., & Falthous, A. (1997). Neuropsychological and cognitive psychophysiological substrates of impulsive aggression. *Biological Psychiatry, 41,* 1045–1061.

Bartussek, D., Becker, G., Diedrich, O., Neumann, E., & Maier, S. (1996). Extraversion, neuroticism, and event-related brain potentials in response to emotional stimuli. *Personality and Individual Differences, 20,* 301–312.

Bartussek, D., Diedrich, O., Neumannn, E., & Collet, W. (1993). Introversion-extraversion and event related potentials (ERP): A test of J. A. Gray's theory. *Personality and Individual Differences, 14,* 565–574.

Bayley, N. (1969). *Bayley scales of infant development.* New York: Psychological Corporation.

Benjamin, J., Ebstein, R. P., & Belmaker, R. H. (Eds.). (2000a). *Molecular genetics and the human personality.* Washington, DC: American Psychiatric Publishing.

Benjamin, J., Ebstein, R. P., & Belmaker, R. H. (2000b). Genes for human personality traits: Endophenotypes of psychiatric disorders? In J. Benjamin, R. P. Ebstein, & R. H. Belmaker (Eds.), *Molecular genetics and the human personality* (pp. 333–344). Washington, DC: American Psychiatric Publishing.

Benjamin, J., Li. L., Patterson, C., Greenberg, B. D., Murphy, D. L., & Hamer, D. H. (1996). Population and familial association between the D4 dopamine receptor gene and measures of sensation seeking. *Nature Genetics, 12,* 81–84.

Benkelfat, C., Ellenbogen, M. A., Dean, P., Palmour, R. M., & Young, S. N. (1994). Mood-lowering effect of tryptophan depletion: Enhanced susceptibility in young men at genetic risk for major affective disorders. *Archives of General Psychiatry, 51,* 687–697.

Bennett, A. J., Lesch, K. P., Long, J. C., Lorenz, J. G., Shoaf, S. E., Champoux, M., Suomi, S. J., Linnoila, M. V., & Higley, J. D. (2001). Early experience and serotonin transporter gene variation interact to influence primate CNS function. *Molecular Psychiatry, 7,* 118–172.

Bergeman, C. S., Chipuer, H. M., Plomin, R., Pederson, N. L., McClearn, G. E., Nesselroade, J. R., Costa, P. T. Jr., & McCrae, R. R. (1993). Genetic and environmental effects on openness to experience, agreeableness, and conscientiousness: An adoption/twin study. *Journal of Personality, 61,* 159–179.

Bergeman, C. S., Seroczynski, A. D. (1998). Genetic and environmental influences on aggression and impulsivity. In M. Maes & E. G. Coccaro (Eds.), *Neurobiology and clinical views on aggression and impulsivity* (pp. 63–80). Chichester, UK: Wiley.

Bergman, B., & Brismar, B. (1994). Hormone levels and personality traits in abusive and suicidal male alcoholics. *Alcoholism: Clinical and Experimental Research, 18,* 311–316.

Berry, M. D., Juorio, A. V., & Paterson, I. A. (1994). The functional role of monoamine oxidases A and B in the mammalian central nervous system. *Progress in Neurobiology, 42,* 375–391.

Berry, M. D., Scarr, E., Zhu, M. X., Paterson, I. A., & Juorio, A. V. (1994). The effects of administration of monoamine oxidase-B inhibitors on rat striatal neuron responses to dopamine. *British Journal of Pharmacology, 113,* 1159–1166.

Blair, R. J. R. (2002). Neurocognitive models of acquired sociopathy and developmental psychopathy. In J. Glicksohn (Ed.), *The neurobiology of criminal behavior* (pp. 157–186). Boston, MA: Kluwer.

Blair, R. J. R., Morris, J. S., Frith, C. D., & Dolan, R. (1999). Dissociable neural responses to facial expressions of sadness and anger. *Brain, 122,* 883–893.

Blanchard, C., Spencer, R. L., Weiss, S. M., Blanchard, R., McEwen, B. S., & Sakai, R. (1995). Visible burrow system as a model of chronic social stress. *Behavioral Neuroendocrinology, 20,* 117–139.

Block, J. (1971). *Lives through time.* Berkeley, CA: Bancroft.

Block, J. (1977). P scale and psychosis: Continued concerns. *Journal of Abnormal Psychology, 86,* 431–434.

Block, J. (1995). A contrarian view of the five factor approach to personality description. *Psychological Bulletin, 117,* 187–215.

Block, J. (2001). Millennial contrarianism: The five factor approach to personality description 5 years later. *Journal of Research in Personality, 35,* 98–107.

Block, J. H. & Block, J. (1980). The role of ego-control and ego-resilience in the organization of behavior. In W. A. Collins (Ed.), *The Minnesota symposium on Child Psychology, Vol. 13: Development of cognition, affect and social relations* (pp. 39–101). Hillsdale, NJ: Erlbaum.

Bloninger, D. M., Carlson, S. R., Krueger, R. F., & Patrick, C. J. (2003). A twin study of self-reported psychopathic traits. *Personality and Individual Differences, 35,* 179–197.

Bloom, F. E., & Kupfer, D. J. (Eds.). (1995). *Psychopharmacology: The fourth generation of progress.* New York: Raven Press.

Bogaert, A. F., & Fisher, W. A. (1995). Predictors of university men's number of sexual partners. *Journal of Sex Research, 32,* 119–130.

Boomsma, D. I., de Geus, E. J. C., van Baal, G. C. M., & Koopmans, J. R. (1999). A religious upbringing reduces the influence of genetic factors on disinhibition: Evidence for interaction between genotype and environment on personality. *Twin Research, 2,* 115–125.

Boomsma, D. I., & Plomin, R. (1986). Heart rate and behavior of twins. *Merrill Palmer Quarterly, 32,* 141–151.

Borkenau, P., Rieman, R., Angleitner, A., & Spinath, F. M. (2001). Genetic and environmental influences on observed personality: Evidence from the German observational study of adult twins. *Journal of Personality and Social Psychology, 80,* 655–668.

Bouchard, T. J., Jr. (1993). Genetic and environmental influences on adult personality: Evaluating the evidence. In J. Hettema & I. J. Deary (Eds.), *Foundations of Personality* (pp. 15–44). Dordrecht, Netherlands: Kluwer.

Bouchard, T. J., Jr., & Hur, J.-M. (1998). Genetic and environmental influences on the continuous scales of the Myers-Briggs Type Indicator: An analysis based on twins reared apart. *Journal of Personality, 66,* 135–149.

Bouchard, T. J., Jr., Lykken, D. T., McGue, M., Segal, N. L., & Tellegen, A. (1990). Sources of human psychological differences: The Minnesota study of twins-reared apart. *Science, 250,* 223–228.

Bouchard, T. J., Jr., McGue, M., Hur, Y-M, & Horn, J. M. (1998). A genetic and environmental analysis of the California Psychological Inventory using adult twins reared apart and together. *European Journal of Personality, 12,* 307–320.

Bozarth, M. A. (1987). Ventral tegmental reward system. In J. Engel, L. Oreland, B. Pernor, S. Rössner, & L. A. Pelhorn (Eds.), *Brain reward systems and abuse* (pp. 1–17). New York: Raven Press.

Bradley, M., & Lang, P. J. (2000). Emotion, behavior, feeling, and physiology. In E. Richard & D. Lane (Eds.), *Cognitive neuroscience of emotion.* London: Oxford University Press.

Bradwejn, J., Koszycki, D., & Couetoux-de-Terte, A. (1992). The cholecystokinin hypothesis of panic and anxiety disorders: A review. *Journal of Psychopharmacology, 6,* 345–351.

Branchey, M. H., Buydens-Branchey, L., & Lieber, C. S. (1988). P3 in alcoholics with disordered regulation of aggression. *Psychiatry Research, 25,* 49–58.

Bratko, D., & Butkovic (2003). Family study of sensation seeking. *Personality and Individual Differences, 35,* 1559–1570.

Braungart, J. M., Plomin, R., De Fries, J. C., & Fulker, D. W. (1992). Genetic influence on tester-rated infant temperament as assessed by Bayley's Infant Behavior Record: Nonadoptive and adoptive siblings and twins. *Developmental Psychology, 28,* 40–47.

Breier, A., Buchanan, R. W., Elkashef, A., Munson, R. C., Kirkpatrick, B., & Gellad, F. (1992). Brain morphology and schizophrenia: A magnetic resonance imaging study of limbic prefrontal cortex and caudate structures. *Archives of General Psychiatry, 49,* 921–924.

Bremner, J. D., Randall, P., Scott, T. M., Bronen, R. A., Seibyl, J. P., Southwick, S. M., Delaney, R. C., McCarthy, G., Charney, D. S. & Innis, R. B. (1995). MRI-based measurement of hippocampal volume in patients with combat-related posttraumatic stress disorder. *American Journal of Psychiatry, 152,* 973–981.

Brennan, P. A., Mednick, B. R., & Mednick, S. A. (1993). Parental psychopathology, congenital factors, and violence. In S. Hodgins (Ed.), *Mental disorder and crime* (pp. 244–261). Thousand Oaks, CA: Sage.

Brocke, B., Beauducel, A., John, R., Debener, S., & Heilemann, H. (2000). Sensation seeking and affective disorders: Characteristics in the intensity dependence of acoustic evoked potentials. *Neuropsychobiology, 41,* 24–30.

Brocke, B., Tasche, K. G., & Beauducel, A. (1997). Biopsychological foundations of extraversion: Differential effort reactivity and state control. *Personality and Individual Differences, 22,* 447–458.

Bronson, W. C. (1966). Central organizations: A study of behavior organization from childhood to adolescence. *Child Development, 37,* 125–155.

Browne, M. W. (1988, Oct. 18). For iguanas place in sun may be too bright. *New York Times,* p. C1.

Brunner, H. G., Nelsen, M., Breakefield, X. O., Ropers, H. H., & Van Oost, B. A. (1993). Abnormal behavior associated with a point mutation in the structural gene for monoamine oxidase-A. *Science, 262,* 578–580.

Buchsbaum, M. S. (1971). Neural events and the psychophysical law. *Science, 172,* 502.

Buchsbaum, M. S. (1974). Average evoked response and stimulus intensity in identical and fraternal twins. *Physiological Psychology, 2,* 365–370.

Buckingham, R. M. (2002). Extraversion, neuroticism and the four temperaments of antiquity: An investigation of physiological reactivity. *Personality and Individual Differences, 32,* 225–246.

Buss, A. H., & Durkee, A. (1957). An inventory for assessing different kinds of hostility. *Journal of Consulting Psychology, 21,* 343–349.

Buss, A. H., & Perry, M. (1992). The aggression questionnaire. *Journal of Personality and Social Psychology, 63,* 452–459.

Buss, A. H., & Plomin, R. (1975). *A temperament theory of personality development.* New York: Wiley.

Buss, A. H., & Plomin, R. (1984). *Temperament: Early developing personality traits.* Hillsdale, NJ: Erlbaum.

Buss, D. M. (1991). Evolutionary personality psychology. *Annual Review of Psychology, 42,* 459–491.

Buss, D. M., Abbott, M., & Angleitner, A., et al. (1990). International preferences in selecting mates: A study of 37 cultures. *Journal of Cross-Cultural Psychology, 48,* 247–249.

Cadoret, R. J., O'Gorman, T. W., Troughton, E., & Haywood, E. (1985). Alcoholism and antisocial personality: Interrelationships, genetic and environmental factors. *Archives of General Psychiatry, 42,* 161–167.

Cadoret, R. J., Yates, W. R., Troughton, E., Woodworth, G., & Stewart, M. A. (1995). Adoption study demonstrating two genetic pathways to drug abuse. *Archives of General Psychiatry, 52,* 42–52.

Cameron, O. G., Smith, C. B., Nesse, R. M., Hill, E.M., Hollingsworth, P. J., Abelson, J. A., Hariharan, M., & Curtis, G. C. (1996). Platelet alpha-2-adrenoreceptors, catecholamines, hemodynamic variables and anxiety in panic patients and their asymptomatic relatives. *Psychosomatic Medicine, 58,* 289–301.

Campbell, A., Muncer, S., & Ohber, J. (1997). Aggression and testosterone: Testing a bio-social model. *Aggressive Behavior, 23,* 229–238.

Canli, T., Desmond, J. E., King, E., Gross, J., & Gabrieli, J. D. E. (2001). An fMRI study of personality influences on brain reactivity to emotional stimuli. *Behavioral Neuroscience, 115,* 33–42.

Cannon, W. B. (1929). *Bodily changes in pain, hunger, fear and rage: Vol. 2.* New York: Appleton.

Canter, S. (1973). Personality traits in twins. In G. Claridge, S. Canter, & W. I. Hume (Eds.), *Personality differences and biological variations* (pp. 21–51). New York: Pergamon Press.

Caputo, P. (1977). *Rumor of war.* New York: Ballantine Books.

Carlson, N. R. (1986). *Physiology of behavior,* 3rd edition. Boston, MA: Allyn & Bacon.

Carrigan, P. M. (1960). Extraversion-introversion as a dimension of personality: A reappraisal. *Psychological Bulletin, 57,* 329–360.

Carrilo-de-la-Peña, M. T. & Barratt, E. S. (1993). Impulsivity and the ERP augmenting/reducing. *Personality and Individual Differences, 15,* 25–32.

Carrol, E. N., Zuckerman, M., & Vogel, W. H. (1982). A test of the optimal level of arousal theory of sensation seeking. *Journal of Personality and Social Psychology, 42,* 572–575.

Carver, C. S., & White, T. L. (1994). Behavioral inhibition, behavioral activation, and affective responses to impending reward and punishments: The BIS/BAS scales. *Journal of Personality and Social Psychology, 67,* 319–333.

Caspi, A. (2000). The child is father of the man: Personality continuities from childhood to adulthood. *Journal of Personality and Social Psychology, 78,* 158–172.

Caspi, A., McClay, J., Moffitt, T. E., Mill, J., Martin, J., Craig, I. W., Taylor, A., & Poulton, R. (2002). Role of genotype in the cycle of violence in maltreated children. *Science, 297,* 851–854.

Caspi, A., Moffitt, T. E., Newman, D. L., & Silva, P. A. (1996). Behavioral observations at age 3 years predict adult psychiatric disorders: Longitudinal evidence for a birth cohort. *Archives of General Psychiatry, 53,* 1033–1039.

Castro, I. P., Ibanez, A., Torres, P., Sáiz-Ruiz, J., & Fernández-Piqueras, J. (1997). Genetic association study between pathological gambling and a functional DNA polymorphism at the D4 receptor gene. *Pharmacogenetics, 7,* 345–348.

Cates, D. S., Houston, B. K., Vavak, C. R., Crawford, M. H., & Uttley, M. (1993). Heritability of hostility related emotions, attitudes, and behavior. *Journal of Behavioral Medicine, 18,* 237–256.

Cattell, R. B. (1957). *Personality and motivation structure and measurement.* New York: Harcourt.

Cattell, R. B. (1982). *The inheritance of personality and ability.* New York: Academic Press.

Chamove, A. S., Eysenck, H. J., & Harlow, H. F. (1972). Personality in monkeys: Factor analysis of Rhesus social behavior. *Quarterly Journal of Experimental Psychology, 24,* 496–504.

Champoux, M., Bennett, A., Shannon, C., Higley, J. D., Lesch, K. P., & Suomi, S. J. (2002). Serotonin transporter gene polymorphism, differential early rearing and behavior in Rhesus monkey neonates. *Molecular Psychiatry, 7,* 1058–1013.

Charney, D. S., & Heninger, G. R. (1986). Abnormal regulation of noradrenergic function in panic disorders. *Archives of General Psychiatry, 43,* 1042–1054.

Chess, S., & Thomas, A. (1984). *Origins and evolution of behavior disorders.* New York: Bruner/Mazel.

Chipuer, H. M., Plomin, R., Pederson, N. L., McClearn, G. E., & Nesselroade, J. R. (1993). Genetic influence on family environment: *Developmental Psychology, 29,* 110–118.

Chozick, B. S. (1986). The behavioral effects of lesions of the amygdala: A review. *International Journal of Neuroscience, 29,* 205–221.

Church, A. T., & Burke, P. J. (1994). Exploration and confirmatory tests of the Big Five and Tellegen's three and four-dimensional models of personality structure. *Journal of Personality and Social Psychology, 66,* 93–114.

Cleare, A. J., & Bond, A. J. (1995). The effects of tryptophan depletion and enhancement on subjective and behavioral aggression in normal male subjects. *Psychopharmacology, 118,* 72–81.

Cleckley, H. (1976). *The mask of sanity,* 5th ed. St. Louis, MO: Mosby.

Cloninger, C. R. (1987). A systematic method for clinical description and classification of personality variants. *Archives of General Psychiatry, 44,* 573–588.

Cloninger, C. R., & Gottesman, I. I. (1987). Genetic and environmental factors in antisocial behavior. In S. A. Mednick, T. E. Moffitt, & S. A. Stack (Eds.) *The causes of crime: New biological approaches* (pp. 92–109). Cambridge: Cambridge University Press.

Cloninger, C. R., Przybeck, T. R., Svrakic, D. M., & Wetzel, R. D. (1994). *The Temperament and Character Inventory (TCI): A guide to its development and use.* St. Louis, MO: Center for Psychobiology of Personality.

Cloninger, C. R., Sigvardsson, S., Bohman, M., & von Knorring, A. L. (1982). Predisposition to petty criminality in Swedish adoptees: II. Cross-fostering analysis of genetic environment interaction. *Archives of General Psychiatry, 39,* 1242–1247.

Cloninger, C. R., Svrakic, D. M., Przybeck, T. R. (1993). A psychobiological model of temperament and character. *Archives of General Psychiatry, 50,* 975–990).

Coccaro, E. F. (1998). Central neurotransmitter function in human aggression and impulsivity. In M. Maes & E. F. Coccaro (Eds.), *Neurobiology and clinical views on aggression and impulsivity* (pp. 143–168). Chichester, UK: Wiley.

Coccaro, E. F., Bergeman, C. S., Kavoussi, R. J., & Seroczynski, A. D. (1997). Heritability of aggression and impulsivity: A twin study of the Buss-Durkee aggression scales in adult male twins. *Biological Psychiatry, 41,* 273–284.

Coccaro, E. F., & Kavoussi, R. J. (1997). Fluoxetine and impulsive aggressive behavior in personality disordered subjects. *Archives of General Psychiatry, 54,* 1081–1088.

Coccaro, E. F., Lawrence, T., Trestman, R., Gabriel, S., Klar, H. M., & Siever, L. J. (1991). Growth hormone responses to intravenous clonidine challenge correlates with behavioral irritability in psychiatric patients and health volunteers. *Psychiatry Research, 39,* 129–139.

Coccaro, E. F., & Siever, L. J. (1995). The neuropsychopharmacology of personality disorders. In F. E. Bloom & D. J. Kupfer (Eds.), *Psychopharmacology: The fourth generation of progress* (pp. 1567–1579). New York: Raven Press.

Coccaro, E. F., Siever, L. J., Klar, H. M., Maurer, G., Cochrane, K., Cooper, T. B., Mohs, R. C., & Davis, K. L. (1989). Serotonergic studies in patients with affective and personality disorders. *Archives of General Psychiatry, 46,* 587–599.

Coccaro, E. F., Silverman, J. M., Klar, H. M., Horvath, T. B., & Siever, L. J. (1994). Familial correlates of reduced central serotonergic system function in patients with personality disorders. *Archives of General Psychiatry, 51,* 318–324.

Comings, D. E., Rosenthal, R. J., Lesieur, H. R., Rugle, L. J., Muhleman, D., Chiu, C., Dietz, G., & Gade, R. (1996). A study of the D2 receptor gene in pathological gambling. *Pharmacogenetics, 6,* 223–234.

Comings, D. E., Saucier, G., & MacMurray, J. P. (2002). Role of DRD2 and other dopamine genes. In J. Benjamin, R. P. Ebstein, & R. H. Belmaker (Eds.), *Molecular genetics and the human personality* (pp. 165–191). Washington, DC: American Psychiatric Publishing.

Coplan, J. D., Wolk, S. I., & Klein, D. F. (1995). Anxiety and serotonin IA receptor. In P. E. Bloom & R. J. Kupfer (Eds.), *Psychopharmacology: A fourth generation of progress* (pp. 1301–1310). New York: Raven Press.

Corr, P. J. (1999). Does extraversion predict positive incentive motivation? *Behavioral and Brain Sciences, 22,* 520–521.

Corr, P. J., Kumari, V., Wilson, G. D., Checkley, S., & Gray, J. A. (1997). Harm avoidance and affective modulation of the startle reflex: A replication. *Personality and Individual Differences, 22,* 591–593.

Corr, P. J., Wilson, G. D., Fotiadou, M., Kumari, V., Gray, N. S., Checkley, S., & Gray, J. A. (1995). Personality and affective modulation of the startle reflex. *Personality and Individual Differences, 19,* 543–553.

Costa, P. T., Jr., & McCrae, R. R. (1985). *The NEO Personality Inventory Manual.* Odessa, FL: Psychological Assessment Resources.

Costa, P. T., Jr. & McCrae, R. R. (1988). Personality in adulthood: A six-year longitudinal study of self-reports and spouse ratings on the NEO Personality Inventory. *Journal of Personality and Social Psychology, 54,* 853–863.

Costa, P. T., Jr. & McCrae, R. R. (1992a). *NEO-PI-R: Revised NEO Inventory (NEO-PI-R).* Odessa, FL: Psychological Assessment Resources.

Costa, P. T., Jr. & McCrae, R. R. (1992b). Four ways five factors are basic. *Personality and Individual Differences, 13,* 653–665.

Costa, P. T., Jr, McCrae, R. R., & Arenberg, D. (1980). Enduring dispositions in adult males. *Journal of Personality and Social Psychology, 38,* 793–800.

Costa, P. T., Jr., McCrae, R. R., Martin, T. A., Oryol, V. E., Senin, G., Rukavishnikon, A. A., Shimonnaka, Y., Kakazato, K., Gondo, Y., Takayema, T., & Realo, A. (2000).

Personality development from adolescence through adulthood: Further cross-cultural comparisons of age differences. In V. J. Molfese & D. Molfese (Eds.), *Temperament and personality development across the life span* (pp. 235–252). Hillsdale, NJ: Erlbaum.

Costa, P. T., Jr., Terracciano, A., & McCrae, R. R. (2001). Gender differences in personality traits across cultures. Robust and surprising findings. *Journal of Personality and Social Psychology, 81*, 322–342.

Cosyns, P. (1998). Aggression, impulsivity and compulsivity in male sexual abusers. In M. Maes & E. F. Coccaro (Eds.), *Neurobiology and clinical views on aggression and impulsivity* (pp. 15–27). Chichester, UK: Wiley.

Coursey, R. D., Buchsbaum, M. S., & Murphy, D. L. (1979). Platelet MAO activity and evoked potentials in the identification of subject biologically at risk for psychiatric disorders. *British Journal of Psychology, 134*, 372–381.

Cox, D. N. (1977). *Psychophysiological correlates of sensation seeking and socialization during reduced stimulation.* Unpublished doctoral dissertation, University of British Columbia.

Cox-Fuenzalida, L-E, Gilliland, K., & Swickert, R. J. (2001). Congruency of the relationship between extraversion and the brain-stem evoked response based on the EPI versus the EPQ. *Journal of Research in Personality, 35*, 117–126.

Crick, F. (1988). *What mad pursuit.* New York: Basic Books.

Croft, R. J., Klugman, A., Baldeweg, T., & Gruzelier, J. H. (2001). Electrophysiological evidence of serotonergic impairment in long term MDMA ("ecstacy") users. *American Journal of Psychiatry, 158*, 1667–1692.

Crow, T. J. (1977). Neurotransmitter related pathways: The structure and function of central monoamine neurons. In A. N. Davison (Ed.), *Biochemical correlates of brain structure and function* (pp. 137–174). New York: Academic Press.

Dabbs, J. M., Jr. (2000). *Heroes, rogues, and lovers.* New York: McGraw-Hill.

Dabbs, J. M., Jr., Carr, T. S., Frady, R. L., & Riad, J. K. (1995). Testosterone, crime, and misbehavior among 692 prison inmates. *Personality and Individual Differences, 18*, 627–633.

Dabbs, J. M., Jr., Hopper, C. H., & Jurkovic, B. V. (1990). Testosterone and personality among college students and military veterans. *Personality and Individual Differences, 11*, 1263–1269.

Dabbs, J. M., Jr., Ruback, R. B., Frady, R. L., Hopper, C. H., & Sgoritas, D. S. (1988). Saliva testosterone and criminal violence among women. *Personality and Individual Differences, 9*, 269–275.

Daitzman, R. J., & Zuckerman, M. (1980). Disinhibitory sensation seeking, personality, and gonadal hormones. *Personality and Individual Differences, 1*, 103–110.

Dakof, G. A., & Mendelsohn, G. A. (1986). Parkinson's disease: The psychological aspects of a chronic illness. *Psychological Bulletin, 99*, 375–387.

Damasio, H., Grabouski, T., Frank, R., Calaburda, A. M., & Damasio, A. R. (1994). The return of Phineas Gage: Clues about the brain from the skull of a famous patient. *Science, 264*, 1102–1105.

Daruna, J. H., Karrer, R., & Rosen, A. J. (1985). Introversion, attention, and the late positive component of event-related potentials. *Biological Psychology, 20*, 249–259.

Davidson, R. J. (1992). Emotion and affective style: Hemispheric substrates. *Psychological Science, 3*, 39–43.

Davidson, R. J. (2002). Anxiety and affective style: Role of prefrontal cortex and amygdala. *Biological Psychiatry, 51*, 68–80.

Davidson, R. J., Putnam, K. M., & Larson, C. L. (2000). Dysfunction in the neural circuitry of emotion regulation: A possible prelude to violence. *Science, 289,* 591–594.

Davis, M. (1986). Pharmacological and anatomical analysis of fear conditioning using the fear-potentiated startle paradigm. *Behavioral Neuroscience, 100,* 814–824.

Davis, M., Hitchhock, J. M., & Rosen, J. B. (1987). Anxiety and the amygdala: Pharmacological and anatomical analysis of the fear-potentiated startle paradigm. J. M. Hitchcock & J. B. Rosen (Eds.), *The psychology of learning and motivation, vol. 21* (pp. 268–305) New York: Academic Press.

DeFries, J. C., Gervais, M. C., & Thomas, E. A. (1978). Response to 30 generations of selection for open-field activity in laboratory mice. *Behavior Genetics, 8,* 3–13.

Delgado, P. L., Charney, D. S., Price, L. H., Aghajanian, G. K., Landis, H., & Heninger, G. R. (1990). Serotonin function and the mechanism of antidepressant action. *Archives of General Psychiatry, 47,* 411–418.

Dellu, F., Mayo, W., Le Moal, M., & Simon, H. (1993). Individual differences in behavioral responses to novelty in rats. Possible relationship with the sensation seeking trait in man. *Personality and Individual Differences, 15,* 411–418.

Dellu, F., Piazza, P. V., Mayo, W., Le Moal, M., & Simon, H. (1996). Novelty-seeking in rats-Biobehavioral characteristics and possible relationships with the sensation-seeking trait in man. *Neuropsychobiology, 34,* 136–145.

De Pascalis, V., Fiore, A. D., & Sparita, A. (1996). Personality, event-related potential (ERP) and heart rate (HR): An investigation of Gray's theory. *Personality and Individual Differences, 20,* 733–746.

Depue, R. A. (1995). Neurobiological factors in personality and depression. *European Journal of Personality, 9,* 413–439.

Depue, R. A., & Collins, P. F. (1999). Neurobiology of the structure of personality: Dopamine facilitation of incentive motivation and extraversion. *Behavioral and Brain Sciences, 22,* 491–569.

Depue, R. A. & Iacono, W. G. (1989). Neurobehavioral aspects of affective disorders. *Annual Review of Psychology, 40,* 457–492.

Depue, R. A., Luciana, M., Arbisi, P., Collins, P., & Leon, A. (1994). Dopamine and the structure of personality: Relationship of agonist induced dopamine activity to positive emotionality. *Journal of Personality and Social Psychology, 67,* 485–498.

Dickman, S. J. (1990). Functional and dysfunctional impulsivity. *Journal of Personality and Social Psychology, 58,* 95–102.

DiLalla, D. L., Carey, G., Gottesman, I. I., & Bouchard, T. J. Jr. (1996). Heritability of MMPI personality indicators of psychopathology. *Journal of Abnormal Psychology, 105,* 491–499.

DiTraglia, G. M., & Polich, J. (1991). P300 and introverted-extraverted personality types. *Psychophysiology, 28,* 177–184.

Dolan, R. J., & Morris, J. S. (2000). The functional anatomy of innate and acquired fear: Perspectives from neuroimaging. In P. D. Lane & L. Nadal (Eds.), *Cognitive neuroscience of emotion* (pp. 225–241). New York: Oxford University Press.

Dougherty, D. D., Shin, L. M., Alpert, N. M., Pitman, R. K., Orr, S. P., Lasko, M., Mecklin, M. L., Fischman, A. J., & Rauch, S. L. (1999). Anger in healthy men: A PET study using script-driven imagery. *Biological Psychiatry, 46,* 466–472.

Dougherty, D. M., Bjork, J. M., Marsh, D. M., & Moeller, F. G. (1999). Influence of trait hostility on tryptophan depletion-induced laboratory aggression. *Psychiatry Research, 88,* 227–232.

Du, L. Bakish, D., Ravindran, A. V., & Hrdina, P. D. (2002). Does fluoxetine influence major depression by modifying five-factor personality traits. *Journal of Affective Disorders, 71*, 235–241.

Duaux, E., Gorwood, P., Griffon, N., Bourdel, M. C., Sautel, F., Sokoloff, P., Schwartz, J. C., Ades, J., Lôo, H., & Poirier, M. F. (1998). Homozygosity at the dopamine D3 receptor gene is associated with opiate dependence. *Molecular Psychiatry, 3*, 333–336.

Eaves, L. J., & Eysenck, H. J. (1975). The nature of extraversion: A genetical analysis. *Journal of Personality and Social Psychology, 32*, 102–112.

Eaves, L. J., & Eysenck, H. J. (1977). A genotype-environmental model for psychoticism. *Advances in Behaviour Research and Therapy, 1*, 5–26.

Eaves, L. J., Eysenck, H. J., & Martin, N. G. (1989). *Genes, culture, and personality.* London, UK: Academic Press.

Eaves, L. J., Martin, N. G., & Eysenck, S. B. G. (1977). An application of the analysis of covariance structure to the psychological study of impulsiveness. *British Journal of Mathematical and Statistical Psychology, 30*, 185–187.

Ebmeier, K. P., Deary, I. J., Carroll, R. E., Prentice, N, Moffoot, A. P. R., & Goodwin, G. M. (1994). Personality associations with the uptake of the cerebral blood flow marker 99MTc-Exametazime estimated with single photon emission tomography. *Personality and Individual Differences, 17*, 587–595.

Ebstein, R. P., & Auerbach, J. G. (2002). Dopamine D4 receptor and serotonin transporter polymorphisms and temperament in early childhood. In J. Benjamin, R. P. Ebstein, & R. H. Belmaker (Eds.), *Molecular genetics and the human personality* (pp. 137–149). Washington, DC: American Psychiatric Publishing.

Ebstein, R. P., & Kotler, M. (2002). Personality, substance abuse, and genes. In J. Benjamin, R. P. Ebstein, & R. H. Belmaker (Eds.), *Molecular genetics and the human personality* (pp. 151–163). Washington, DC: American Psychiatric Publishing.

Ebstein, R. P., Levine, L., Geller, V., Auerbach, J., Gritsenko, I., & Belmaker, R. H. (1998). Dopamine D4 receptor and serotonin transporter promoter in the determination of neonatal temperament. *Molecular Psychiatry, 3*, 238–246.

Ebstein, R. P., Novick, O., Umansky, R., Priel, B., Osher, Y., Blaine, D., Bennett, E. R., Nemanov, L., Katz, M., & Belmaker, R. H. (1996). Dopamine D4 receptor (D4DR) exon III polymorphism associated with the human personality trait of novelty seeking. *Nature Genetics, 12*, 78–80.

Eley, T. C. (1997). General genes: A new theme in developmental psychopathology. *Current Directions in Psychological Science, 6*, 90–95.

Elkis, H., Friedman, L., Wise, A., & Meltzer, H. Y. (1995). Meta-analyses of studies of ventricular enlargement and cortical sulcal prominence in mood disorders. *Archives of General Psychiatry, 52*, 735–746.

Emery, N. J. & Amaral, D. G. (2000). The role of the amygdala in primate social cognition. In P. D. Lane & L. Nadal (Eds.), *Cognitive neuroscience of emotion* (pp. 156–191). New York: Oxford University Press.

Epstein, S. (1979). The stability of behavior: I. On predicting most of the people much of the time. *Journal of Personality and Social Psychology, 37*, 1097–1126.

Eysenck, H. J. (1947). *Dimensions of personality.* New York: Praeger.

Eysenck, H. J. (1955). Psychiatric diagnosis as a psychological and statistical problem. *Psychological Reports, 1*, 3–17.

Eysenck, H. J. (1957). *The dynamics of anxiety and hysteria.* New York: Praeger.

Eysenck, H. J. (1967). *The biological basis of personality.* Springfield, IL: Charles C. Thomas.

Eysenck, H. J. (1983). A biometrical-genetical analysis of impulsive and sensation seeking behavior. In M. Zuckerman (Ed.), *Biological bases of sensation seeking, impulsivity, and anxiety* (pp. 1–27). Hillsdale, NJ: Erlbaum.

Eysenck, H. J. (1990). Genetic and environmental contributions to individual differences: Three major dimensions of personality. *Journal of Personality, 58,* 245–261.

Eysenck, H. J. (1992). Four ways five factors are not basic. *Personality and Individual Differences, 13,* 667–673.

Eysenck, H. J. (1994). The big five or giant three: Criteria for a paradigm. In G. A. Kohnstamm & R. P. Martin (Eds.), *The developing structure of temperament and personality from infancy to adulthood* (pp. 53–68). Hillsdale, NJ: Erlbaum.

Eysenck, H. J., Barrett, P., Wilson, G., & Jackson, C. (1992). Primary trait measurement of the 21 components of the PEN system. *European Journal of Psychological Assessment, 8,* 109–117.

Eysenck, H. J., & Eysenck, M. W. (1985). *Personality and Individual Differences: A natural science approach.* New York: Plenum Press.

Eysenck, H. J., & Eysenck, S. B. G. (1975). *Manual of the Eysenck Personality Questionnaire (junior and adult).* London: Hodder and Stoughton.

Eysenck, H. J. & Eysenck, S. B. G. (1976). *Psychoticism as a dimension of personality.* London: Hodder and Stoughton.

Eysenck, H. J. & Levey, A. (1972). Conditioning, introversion-extraversion, and the strength of the nervous system. In V. D. Nebylitsyn & J. A. Gray (Eds.), *Biological bases of individual behavior* (pp. 206–220). New York: Academic Press.

Eysenck, S. B. G. (1956). Neurosis and psychosis: An experimental analysis. *Journal of Mental Science, 102,* 517–529.

Eysenck, S. B. G. & Eysenck, H. J. (1963). On the dual nature of extraversion. *British Journal of Social and Clinical Psychology, 2,* 46–55.

Eysenck, S. B. G., & Eysenck, H. J. (1977). The place of impulsiveness in a dimensional system of personality description. *British Journal of Social and Clinical Psychology, 16,* 57–68.

Eysenck, S. B. G., & Eysenck, H. J. (1978). Impulsiveness and venturesomeness: Their position in a dimensional system of personality description. *Psychological Reports, 43,* 1247–1255.

Eysenck, S. B. G., Eysenck, H. J., & Barrett, P. (1985). A revised version of the psychoticism scale. *Personality and Individual Differences, 6,* 21–29.

Fahrenberg, J. (1987). Concepts of activation and arousal in the theory of emotionality (neuroticism). A multivariate conceptualization. In J. Strelau & H. J. Eysenck (Eds.), *Personality dimensions and arousal* (pp. 99–120). New York: Plenum.

Falconer, D. S. (1981). *Introduction to quantitative genetics,* 2nd ed. London: Longman.

Farde, L., Gustavson, J. P., & Jönsson, E. (1997). D2 dopamine receptors and personality traits. *Nature, 385,* 590.

Farley, F. H., & Davis, S. A. (1977). Arousal, personality, and assortative mating in marriage. *Journal of Sex and Marital Therapy, 3,* 122–127.

Farley, F. H., & Mueller, C. B. (1978). Arousal, personality, and assortative mating in marriage: Generalizability and cross-cultural factors. *Journal of Sex and Marital Therapy, 4,* 50–53.

Farrington, D. P. (1997). The relationship between low resting heart rate and violence. In A. Raine, P. A. Brennan, D. P. Farrington, & S. A. Mednick (Eds.), *Biosocial bases of violence* (pp. 89–106). New York: Plenum Press.

Feij, J. A., Orlebeke, J. F., Gazendam, A., & van Zuilen, R. (1985). Sensation seeking: Measurement and psychophysiological correlates. In J. Strelau, F. Farley, & A. Gale (Eds.), *Biological bases of personality and behavior, Vol 1* (pp. 195–210). Washington, DC: Hemisphere.

Feldman, R. S., Meyer, J. S., & Quenger, L. F. (1997). *Principles of neuropsychopharmacology.* Sunderland, MA: Sinauer Associates.

Ficher, I. V., Zuckerman, M., & Neeb, M. (1981). Marital compatibility in sensation seeking trait as a factor in marital adjustment. *Journal of Sex and Marital Therapy, 7*, 60–69.

Ficher, I. V., Zuckerman, M., & Steinberg, M. (1988). Sensation seeking in couples as a determinant of marital adjustment: A partial replication and extension. *Journal of Clinical Psychology, 44*, 803–809.

Fink, A., Schrausser, D. G., & Neubauer (2002). The moderating influence of extraversion on the relationship between IQ and cortical activation. *Personality and Individual Differences, 33*, 311–326.

Finn, P. R., Young, S. N., Pihl, R. O., & Ervin, F. R. (1998). The effect of acute plasma tryptophan manipulation on hostile mood: The influence of trait hostility. *Aggressive Behavior, 24*, 173–185.

Fischer, H., Wik, G., & Frederickson, M. (1997). Extraversion, neuroticism and brain function: A PET study of personality. *Personality and Individual Differences, 23*, 345–352.

Fiske, D. W. (1949). Consistency of factorial structures for personality ratings from different sources. *Journal of Abnormal and Social Psychology, 44*, 329–344.

Flor-Henry, P. (1976). Lateralized temporal-limbic dysfunction and psychopathology. *Annals of the New York Academy of Sciences, 280*, 777–797.

Fox, N. A. (1991). If it's not left it's right. *American Psychologist, 46*, 863–872.

Frederickson, E., & Birnbaum, E. A. (1954). Competititve fighting between mice with different hereditary backgrounds. *Journal of Genetic Psychology, 85*, 271–280.

Freud, S. (1922/1961). *Beyond the pleasure principle.* Translated and edited by J. Strachey, 1961. New York: Norton.

Fridland, A. J., Schwartz, G. E., & Fowler, S. C. (1984). Pattern recognition of self-reported emotional state from multiple-site facial EMG activity during affective imagery. *Psychophysiology, 21*, 622–637.

Frith, U., & Frith, C. (2001). The biological basis of social interaction. *Current Directions in Psychological Science, 10*, 151–155.

Fulker, D. W., Eysenck, S. B. G., & Zuckerman, M. (1980). A genetic and environmental analysis of sensation seeking. *Journal of Research in Personality, 14*, 261–281.

Fuster, J. M. (1997). *The prefrontal cortex: Anatomy, physiology, and neuropsychology of the frontal lobe, 3rd edition.* Philadelphia, PA: Lippincott-Raven.

Gadow, K. D. (2001). Attention-deficit/hyperactivity disorder in adults. *Archives of General Psychiatry, 58*, 784–785.

Gale, A. (1983). Electroencephalographic studies of extraversion-introversion: A case study in the psychophysiology of individual differences. *Personality and Individual Differences, 4*, 371–380.

Gale, A., & Edwards, J. A. (1986). Individual differences. In M. G. H. Coles, E. Donchin, & S. W. Porges (Eds.), *Psychophysiology: Systems, processes and applications* (pp. 431–507). New York: Guilford.

Gallagher, J. E., Yarnell, J. W., Sweetman, P. M., Elwood, P. C., & Stansfield, S. A. (1999). Anger and incident heart disease in the Caerphilly study. *Psychosomatic Medicine, 61*, 446–453.

Garcia-Sevilla, L. (1984). Extraversion and neuroticism in rats. *Personality and Individual Differences, 5*, 511–532.

Gatzke-Kopp, L. M., Raines, A., Buchsbaum, M. S., & La Casse, L. (2001). Temporal lobe deficits in murderers: EEG findings undetected by PET. *Journal of Neuropsychiatry and Clinical Neuroscience, 13*, 486–491.

Ge, X., Cadoret, R. J., Conger, R. D., Neiderhiser, J. M., Yates, W., Troughton, E., & Stewart, M. A. (1996). The developmental interface between nature and nurture: A mutual influence model of child antisocial behavior and parent behaviors. *Developmental Psychology, 32*, 574–589.

Geer, J. H. (1975). Direct measurement of genital responding. *American Psychologist, 30*, 415–419.

Geer, J. H., O'Donohue, W. T., & Schorman, R. H. (1986). Sexuality. In M. G. H. Coles, E. Donchin, & S. W. Porges (Eds.), *Psychophysiology: Systems, processes and applications* (pp. 559–564). New York: Guilford.

Gerra, G., Zaimovic, A., Timpano, M., Zambelli, U., Delsignore, R., & Brambilla, F. (2000). Neuroendocrine correlates of temperamental traits in humans. *Psychoneuroendocrinology, 25*, 479–496.

Gerstle, J. E., Mathias, C. W., & Stanford, M. S. (1998). Auditory P300 and self-reported impulsive aggression. *Progress in Neuropsychopharmacology and Biological Psychiatry, 22*, 575–583.

Ghodsian-Carpey, J., & Baker, L. A. (1987). Genetic and environmental influences on aggression in 4- to 7-year old twins. *Aggressive Behavior, 13*, 173–186.

Ginsburg, B., & Allee, W. C. (1942). Some effects of conditioning on social dominance and subordination in inbred strains of mice. *Physiological Zoology, 15*, 485–506.

Glennon, R. A., & Dukat, M. (1995). Serotonin receptor subtypes. In F. E. Bloom & D. J. Kupfer (Eds.), *Psychopharmacology: The fourth generation of progress* (pp. 415–430). New York: Raven Press.

Goldberg, L. R. (1990). An alternative description of personality: The Big-Five factor structure. *Journal of Personality and Social Psychology, 59*, 1216–1229.

Goldberg, L. R. (1994). The big five factor structure as an integrating framework: An empirical comparison with Eysenck's P-E-N model. In C. Halverson, D. Kohnstamm, & R. Martin (Eds.), *The developing structure of temperament and personality from infancy to adulthood* (pp. 7–35). Hillsdale, NJ: Erlbaum.

Goldring, J. F., & Richards, M. (1985). EEG spectral analysis, visual evoked potentials and photic-driving correlates of personality and memory. *Personality and Individual Differences, 6*, 67–76.

Goldsmith, H. H., & Campos, J. J. (1986). Fundamental issues in the study of early temperament. The Denver Twin Temperament Study. In M. E. Lamb, A. L. Brown, & B. Rogoff (Eds.), *Advances in developmental psychology, Vol.4* (pp. 231–283). Hillsdale, NJ: Erlbaum.

Goldsmith, H. H., & Gottesman, I. I. (1981). Origins of variation in young twins. *Child Development, 52*, 91–103.

Goodall, J. (1986). *The chimpanzees of Gombe.* Cambridge, MA: The Belknap Press of Harvard University.

Gosling, S. D. (2001). From mice to men: What can we learn about personality from animal research? *Psychological Bulletin, 127*, 45–86.

Gosling, S. D., & John, O. J. (1999). Personality dimensions in nonhuman animals: A cross-species review. *Current Directions in Psychological Science, 8*, 69–75.

Gottesman, I. I. (1991). *Schizophrenia genesis: The origins of madness.* New York: W. H. Freeman.

Graham, F. K. (1979). Distinguishing among orienting, defensive, and startle reflexes. In H. D. Kimmel, E. H. van Olst, & J. F. Orlebeke (Eds.), *The orienting reflex in humans.* Hillsdale, NJ: Erlbaum.

Gray, J. A. (1971). *The psychology of fear and stress.* New York: McGraw-Hill.

Gray, J. A. (1973). Causal theories of personality and how to test them. In J. R. Royce (Ed.), *Multivariate analysis and psychological theory* (pp. 409–463). New York: Academic Press.

Gray, J. A. (1982). *The neuropsychology of anxiety: An enquiry into the function of the septohippocampal system.* New York: Oxford University Press.

Gray, J. A. (1986). Discussions arising from Cloninger, C. R.: A unified biosocial theory of personality and its role in the development of anxiety states. *Psychiatric Developments, 3*, 167–226.

Gray, J. A. (1987). The neuropsychology of emotion and personality. In S. M. Stahl, S. D. Iverson, & E. C. Goodman (Eds.), *Cognitive neurochemistry* (pp. 171–190). Oxford: Oxford University Press.

Gray, J. A. (1991). The neuropsychology of temperament. In J. Strelau & A. Angleitner (Eds.) *Explorations in temperament: International perspectives on theory and measurement* (pp. 105–128) London: Plenum Press.

Gray, J. A. (1999). But the schizophrenic connection. . . . *Behavioral and Brain Sciences, 22*, 523–524.

Gray, J. A., Pickering, A. D., & Gray, J. A. (1994). Psychoticism and dopamine D2 binding in the basal ganglia using single photon emission tomography. *Personality and Individual Differences, 17*, 431–434.

Grillon, C., Dierker, L., & Merikangas, K. R. (1998). Fear potentiated startle in adolescent offspring of parents with anxiety disorders. *Biological Psychiatry, 44*, 990–997.

Guerra, R. J., O'Donnell, B. F., Nestor, P. G., Gainski, J., & McCarley, R. W. (2001). The P3 auditory event-related brain potential indexes major personality traits. *Biological Psychiatry, 49*, 922–929.

Guilford, J. P. (1975). Factors and factors of personality. *Psychological Bulletin, 82*, 802–814.

Guilford, J. P., & Zimmerman, W. S. (1956). Fourteen dimensional temperament factors. *Psychological Monographs, 70*, No. 10, 1–26.

Haan, N. (1981). Common dimensions of personality development: Early adolescence to middle-life. In D. H. Eichorn (Ed.), *Present and past in middle life* (pp. 117–151). New York: Academic Press.

Haier, R. J. (1998). Brain scanning/neuroimaging. In H. S. Friedman (Ed.), *Encyclopedia of mental health, Vol. 1* (pp. 317–329). New York: Academic Press.

Haier, R. J., Sokolski, K., Katz, M., & Buchsbaum, M. S. (1987). The study of personality with positron emission tomography. In J. Strelau & H. J. Eysenck (Eds.), *Personality dimensions and arousal* (pp. 251–267). New York: Plenum.

Hall, R. A., Rappaport, M., Hopkins, H. K., Griffin, R. B., & Silverman, J. (1970). Evoked response and behavior in cats. *Science, 170*, 998–1000.

Hallman, J., von Knorring, A. L., von Knorring, L., & Oreland, L. (1990). Clinical characteristics of female alcoholics with low platelet monoamine oxidase activity. *Alcoholism: Clinical and Experimental Research, 14*, 227–231.

Halperin, J. M., & Newcorn, J. H. (1998). Impulsivity and aggression in children with ADHD. In M. Maes & E. F. Coccaro (Eds.), *Neurobiology and clinical views on aggression and impulsivity* (pp. 47–61). Chichester, UK: Wiley.

Hamer, D. H., Greenberg, B. D., Sabol, S. Z., & Murphy, D. L. (1999). Role of the serotonin transporter gene in temperament and character. *Journal of Personality Disorders, 13,* 312–328.

Hamer, D. H., Hu, S., Magnuson, V. L., Hu, N., & Pattatucci, A. M. L. (1993). A linkage between DNA markers on the X chromosone and male sexual orientation. *Science, 261,* 321–327.

Hansenne, M., Pinto, E., Pitchot, W., Reggers, G. S., Moor, M., & Ansseau, M. (2002). Further evidence on the relationship between dopamine and novelty seeking: A neuroendocrine study. *Personality and Individual Differences, 33,* 967–977.

Hansenne, M., Pitchot, W., Moreno, A. G., Reggers, J., Machurot, P-Y, & Ansseau, M. (1997). Harm avoidance dimension of the tridimensional personality questionnaire and serotonin-1A activity in depressed patients. *Biological Psychiatry, 42,* 959–961.

Hare, R. D. (1973). Orienting and defensive responses to visual stimuli. *Psychophysiology, 10,* 453–464.

Hare, R. D. (1978). Electrodermal and cardiovascular correlates of psychopathy. In R. D. Hare & D. Schalling (Eds.), *Psychopathic behaviour: Approaches to research* (pp. 107–143). Chichester, UK: Wiley.

Hare, R. D., & Cox, D. N. (1978). Clinical and empirical conceptions of psychopathy and the selection of subjects for research. In R. D. Hare & D. Schalling (Eds.), *Psychopathic behaviour: Approaches to research* (pp. 1–22). Chichester, UK: Wiley.

Hare, R. D. & McPherson, L. M. (1984). Violent and aggressive behavior by criminal psychopaths. *International Journal of Law and Psychiatry, 7,* 35–50.

Hariri, A. R., Mattay, V. S., Tessitore, A., Kotachena, B., Fera, F., Goldman, D., Egan, M. F., & Weinberger, D. R. (2002). Serotonin transporter, genetic variation and the response of the human amygdala. *Science, 297,* 400–403.

Harpur, T. J., & Hare, R. D. (1994). Assessment of psychopathy as a function of age. *Journal of Abnormal Psychology, 103,* 604–609.

Harpur, T. J., Hare, R. D., & Hakstian, R. (1989). Two-factor conceptualization of psychopathy: Construct validity and assessment implications. *Psychological Assessment, 1,* 6–17.

Harris, J. A., Rushton, J. P., Hampson, E., & Jackson, D. N. (1996). Salivary testosterone and self-report aggression and pro-social personality characteristics in men and women. *Aggressive Behavior, 22,* 321–331.

Harris, J. A., Vernon, P. A., & Boomsma, D. I. (1992). The heritability of testosterone: A study of Dutch adolescent twins and their parents. *Behavior Genetics, 28,* 165–171.

Hart, S. D., Hare, R. D., & Forth, A. E. (1994). Psychopathy as a risk marker for violence: Validation of a screening version of the revised psychopathy checklist. In J. Monohan & H. J. Steadman (Eds.), *Violence and mental disorder* (pp. 81–98). Chicago: University of Chicago Press.

Hassett, J. (1978). *A primer of psychophysiology.* San Francisco, CA: W. H. Freeman & Company.

Hebb, D. O. (1955). Drives and the C. N. S. (conceptual nervous system). *Psychological Review, 62,* 243–254.

Heimburger, R. F., Whitlock, C. C., & Kalsbeck, J. E. (1966). Stereotaxic amygdalotomy for epilepsy with aggressive behavior. *Journal of the American Medical Association, 198,* 741–745.

Heinz, A., Jones, D. W., Mazzanti, C., Goldman, D., Ragan, P., Hammer, D., Linnoila, M., & Weinberger, D. R. (1999). A relationship between serotonin transporter genotype and in vivo protein expression and alcohol neurotoxicity. *Biological Psychiatry, 47,* 643–649.

Heinz, A., Mann, K., Weinberger, D. R., & Goldman, D. (2001). Serotonergic dysfunction, negative mood states, and response to alcohol. *Alcoholism: Clinical and Experimental Research, 25,* 487–495.

Heinz, A., Weingarten, H., George, D., Hammer, D., Wolkowitz, O. M., & Linnoila, M. (1999). Severity of depression in abstinent alcoholics is associated with monoamine metabolites and dehydroepiandrosterone-sulfate concentrations. *Psychiatry Research, 89,* 97–106.

Hendrick, C., & Hendrick, S. S. (1986). A theory and method of love. *Journal of Personality and Social Psychology, 50,* 392–402.

Heninger, G. R. (1999). Special challenges in the investigation of the neurobiology of mental illness. In D. S. Charney, E. J. Nestler, & B. S. Bunney (Eds.), *Neurobiology of mental illness* (pp. 89–99). New York: Oxford University Press.

Hennig, J., Kroeger, A., Meyer, B., Prochaska, H., Krien, P., Huwe, S., & Netter, P. (1998). Personality correlates of $+/-$ pinodol induced decreases in prolactin. *Pharmacopsychiatry, 31,* 19–24.

Higley, J. D., Mehlman, D. M., Taub, S. B., Higley, S. J., Suomi, M., Linnoila, M., & Vickers, J. H. (1992). Cerebrospinal fluid and adrenal correlates of aggression in free ranging Rhesus monkeys. *Archives of General Psychiatry, 49,* 436–441.

Higley, J. D., Suomi, S. J., & Linnoila, M. (1992). A longitudinal study of CSF monoamine metabolite and plasma cortisol concentrations in young Rhesus monkeys. *Biological Psychiatry, 32,* 127–145.

Hirshfeld, D. R., Rosenbaum, J. F., Biederman, J., Bolduc, E., Faraone, S. V., Snidman, N., Reznick, J. S., & Kagan, J. (1992). Stable behavioral inhibition and its association with anxiety disorder. *Journal of the American Academy of Child and Adolescent Psychiatry, 31,* 103–111.

Hodges, W. F. (1976). The psychophysiology of anxiety. In M. Zuckerman & C. D. Spielberger (Eds.), *Emotions and anxiety: New concepts, methods, and applications.* Hillsdale, NJ: Erlbaum.

Hodgins, S., Kratzer, L., & McNeil, T. F. (2001). Obstetric complications, parenting, and risk of criminal behavior. *Archives of General Psychiatry, 58,* 746–752.

Hogan, R. (1982). A socioanalytic theory of personality. In M. M. Page (Ed.), *Personality: Current theory and Research: 1982 Nebraska Symposium on Motivation* (pp. 55–89). Lincoln: University of Nebraska Press.

Holsboer, F. (1995). Neuroendocrinology of mood disorders. In F. E. Bloom & D. J. Kupfer (Eds.), *Psychopharmacology: The fourth generation of progress* (pp. 957–969). New York: Raven Press.

Hull, C. L. (1943). *Principles of behavior.* New York: Appleton.

Hur, Y-M., & Bouchard, T. J. Jr. (1995). Genetic influences on perceptions of childhood family environment: A reared apart twin study. *Child Development, 66,* 330–345.

Hur, Y-M., & Bouchard, T. J. Jr. (1997). The genetic correlation between impulsivity and sensation seeking traits. *Behavior Genetics, 27,* 455–463.

Hutchinson, W. D. (1999). Pain-related neurons in the human cingulate. *Nature Neuroscience, 2,* 403–405.

Hutchison, K. E., Wood, M. D., & Swift, R. (1999). Personality factors moderate subjective and psychophysiological responses to d-amphetamine in humans. *Experimental and Clinical Psychopharmacology, 7,* 493–501.

Huttunen, M. O., & Nyman, G. (1982). On the continuity, change, and clinical value of infant temperament in a prospective epidemiological study. In Ciba Foundation symposium 89. *Temperament differences in infants and young children* (pp. 240–247). London: Pitman.

Hyman & E. J. Nestler (1993). *The molecular foundations of psychiatry.* Washington, DC: American Psychiatric Publishing.

Insel, T. R. (1997). A neurobiological basis of social attachment. *American Journal of Psychiatry, 154,* 726–735.

Isaacson, R. L. (1982). *The limbic system,* 2nd ed. New York: Plenum.

Ishikawa, S. S., & Raine, A. (2002). Behavior genetics and crime. In J. Glicksohn (Ed.), *The neurobiology of criminal behavior* (pp. 81–110). Boston, MA: Kluwer Publishers.

Ishikawa, S. S., Raine, A., Lencz, T., Bihrle, S., & Lacasse, L. (2001). Autonomic stress reactivity and executive functions in successful and unsuccessful criminal psychopaths from the community. *Journal of Abnormal Psychology, 110,* 423–432.

Ivashenko, O. V., Berus, A. V., Zhuravlev, A. B., & Myamlin, V. V. (1999). Individual and typological features of basic personality traits in norms and their EEG-correlates. *Human Physiology, 25,* 162–170.

Izard, C. E. (1993). *The psychology of emotions.* New York: Plenum.

James, W. (1884). What is emotion? *Mind, 9,* 188–205.

Janet, P. (1907). *Major symptoms of hysteria.* New York: Macmillan.

Jang, K. L., Hu, S., Livesley, W. J., Angleitner, A., Riemann, R., Ando, J., Ono, Y., Vernon, P. A, & Hamer, D. H. (2001). Covariance structure of neuroticism and agreeableness: A twin and molecular genetic analysis of the role of the serotonin transporter gene. *Journal of Personality and Social Psychology, 81,* 295–304.

Jang, K. L., Livesley, W. J., & Vernon, P. A. (1996). Heritability of the big five personality dimensions and their facets: A twin study. *Journal of Personality, 64,* 575–591.

Jang, K. L., McCrae, R. R., Angleitner, A., Rieman, R., & Livesley, W. J. (1998). Heritability of facet-level traits in a cross-cultural twin sample: Support for a hierarchal model of personality. *Journal of Personality and Social Psychology, 74,* 1556–1565.

Jinks, J. L., & Fulker, D. W. (1970). Comparison of the biometrical genetical MAVA, and the classical approaches to the analysis of human behavior. *Psychological Bulletin, 73,* 311–349.

Johnson, D. L., Wiebe, J. S., Gold, S. M., Andreasen, N. C., Hichwa, R. D., Watkins, G. L., & Ponto, L. L. B. (1999). *American Journal of Psychiatry, 156,* 252–257.

Joireman, J., Anderson, J., & Strathman (2003). The aggression paradox: Understanding links among aggression, sensation seeking, and the consideration of future consequences. *Journal of Personality and Social Psychology, 84,* 1287–1302.

Jönsson, E., Sedvall, G., Brené, S., Gustafsson, J. P., Geijer, T., Terenius, L., Crocq, M. A., Lannfett, T., Tyke, A., Sokoloff, P., Schwartz, C., & Wiesel, F. A. (1996). Dopamine-related genes and their relationship to monoamine metabolites in CSF. *Biological Psychiatry, 40,* 1032–1043.

Joseph, R. (1996). *Neuropsychiatry, neuropsychology, and clinical neuroscience,* 2nd ed. Baltimore, MD: Williams & Wilkins.

Jung, C. G. (1933). *Psychological types.* New York: Harcourt.

Kagan, J. (1989). Temperamental contributions to social behavior. *American Psychologist, 44,* 668–674.

Kagan, J. (1994). *Galen's prophecy: Temperament in human nature.* New York: Basic Books.

Kagan, J. & Moss, H. A. (1962). *Birth to maturity.* New York: Wiley.

Kagan, J., Reznick, J. S., & Snidman, N. (1988). Biological bases of childhood shyness. *Science, 240*, 167–171.

Kagan, J., & Snidman, N. (1999). Early childhood predictors of adults anxiety disorders. *Biological Psychiatry, 46*, 1536–1541.

Kalin, N. H., Larson, C., Shelton, S. E., & Davidson, B. J. (1998). Asymmetric frontal brain activity, cortisol, and behavior associated with fearful temperament in rhesus monkeys. *Behavioral Neuroscience, 112*, 286–292.

Kalin, N. H., Shelton, S. E., & Davidson, R. J. (2000). Cerebrospinal fluid corticotropin-releasing hormone levels are elevated in monkeys with patterns of brain activity associated with fearful temperament. *Biological Psychiatry, 47*, 579–585.

Kaplan, J. R., Manuck, S. B., Fontenot, B., & Mann, J. J. (2002). Central nervous system monoamine correlates of social dominance in Cynomologus monkeys (Macca fascicularis). *Neuropsychopharmacology, 26*, 431–443.

Kaprio, J., Koshenvuo, M., & Rose, R. J. (1990). Change in cohabitation and intrapair similarity of monozygotic (MZ) cotwins for alcohol use. *Behavioral Genetics, 20*, 265–276.

Keltikangas, J. L., Räckkönen, K., & Adlercreutz, H. (1997). Response of the pituitary adrenal axis in terms of Type A behavior, hostility, and vital exhaustion in healthy middle-aged men. *Psychology and Health, 12*, 533–542.

Kemppainen, L., Jokelainen, J., Jaervelin, M. R., Isohanni, M., & Raessenen, P. (2001). The one-child family and violent criminality. A 31-year follow-up study of the Northern Finland 1966 birth cohort. *American Journal of Psychiatry, 158*, 960–962.

Kimbrell, T. A., George, M. S., Parekh, P. I., Ketter, T. A., Podell, D. M., Danielson, A. L., Repella, J. D., Benson, B. E., Willis, M. W., Herscovich, P., & Post, R. M. (1999). Regional brain activity during transient self-induced anxiety and anger in healthy adults. *Biological Psychiatry, 46*, 454–465.

King, J. E., & Figuerdo, A. J. (1997). The Five-Factor model plus dominance in chimpanzee personality. *Journal of Research in Personality, 31*, 257–271.

King, R. J., Mefford, I. N., Wang, C., Murchison, H., Caligari, E. J., & Berger, P. A. (1986). CSF dopamine levels correlate with extraversion in depressed patients. *Psychiatry Research, 19*, 305–310.

Kish, K. B. (1970). Reduced cognitive innovation and stimulus seeking in chronic schizophrenics. *Journal of Clinical Psychology, 26*, 170–174.

Kling, A., & Stelkis, H. D. (1976). A neural substrate for affiliative behavior in non-human primates. *Brain, Behavior, and Evolution, 13*, 216–238.

Knutson, B., Momenan, R., Rawlings, R. R., Fong, G. W., & Hommer, D. (2001). Negative association of neuroticism with brain-volume ratio in healthy humans. *Biological Psychiatry, 50*, 685–690.

Knutson, B., Wolkowitz, O. M., Cole, S. W., et al. (1998). Selective alteration of personality and social behavior by serotonergic intervention. *American Journal of Psychiatry, 155*, 373–379.

Knyazev, G. G., Slobodskaya, H. R., & Wilson, G. D. (2002). Psychophysiological correlates of behavioural inhibition and activation. *Personality and Individual Differences, 33*, 647–660.

Konner, M. (2002). Two views of human nature: Cultivating nature – including ours. Review of Paul Ehrlich, Human Nature: Genes, Culture, and the Human Prospect. *Contemporary Psychology, 47*, 659–661.

Koopmans, J. R., Boomsa, D. I., Heath, A. C., & Lorenz, J. P. (1995). A multivariate genetic analysis of sensation seeking. *Behavior Genetics, 25*, 349–356.

Korczyn, A. D. (1995). Parkinson's disease. In F. E. Bloom, & D. J. Kupfer (Eds.), *Psychopharmacology: The fourth generation of progress* (pp. 1479–1484). New York: Raven Press.

Kräpelin, E. (1899). *Psychiatrie*. Leipzig: Germany: Barth.

Krueger, R. F., Hicks, B. M., & McGue, M. (2001). Altruism and antisocial behavior: Independent tendencies, unique personality correlates, distinct etiologies. *Psychological Science, 12*, 397–402.

Kruesi, M. J. P., Rapoport, J. L., Hamburger, S., Hibbs, E., Potter, W. Z., Lenane, M., & Brown, G. L. (1990). Cerebrospinal fluid monoamine metabolite expression, and impulsivity in disruptive behavior disorders of children and adolescents. *Archives of General Psychiatry, 47*, 419–426.

Kuperman, S., Kramer, J., & Loney, J. (1988). Enzyme activity in hyperactive children grown up. *Biological Psychiatry, 24*, 375–383.

Lacey, J. I. (1959). Psychophysiological approaches to the evaluation of psychotherapeutic process and outcome. In E. A. Rubenstein, & M. B. Parloff (Eds.), *Research in psychotherapy*. Washington, DC: American Psychological Association.

Laitenen, L. V., & Vílkki, J. (1973). Observations on the transcallosal emotional connections. In L. V. Laitenan & K. E. Livingston (Eds.), *Surgical approaches in psychiatry* (pp. 74–80). Baltimore, MD: University Park Press.

Lang, P. J. (1995). The emotion probe: Studies of motivation and attention. *American Psychologist, 50*, 372–385.

Langinvaino, H., Kaprio, J., Koskenvuo, M., & Lonnqvist, J. (1984). Finnish twins reared apart III: Personality factors. *Acta Geneticase Medicae et Gemillologiae, 33*, 259–264.

Laucht, M., Esser, G., Baving, L., Gerhold, M., Hoesch, I., Ihle, W., Steigleder, P., Stock, B., Stoehr, R. M. Weindrich, D., & Schmidt, M. H. (2000). Behavioral sequelae of perinatal insults and early family adversity at 8 years of age. *Journal of the American Academy of Child and Adolescent Psychiatry, 39*, 1229–1237.

Leckman, J. F., Gershon, E. S., Nichols, A. S., & Murphy, D. L. (1977). Reduced MAO activity in first degree relatives of individuals with bipolar affective disorders. *Archives of General Psychiatry, 34*, 601–606.

Le Doux, J. E. (1987). Emotion. In F. Plum (Ed.), *Handbook of physiology: The nervous system* (Vol. 5, pp. 419–459). Bethesda, MD: American Physiological Society.

Le Doux, J. E. (1998). *The emotional brain*. London: Weidenfeld Nicolson.

Le Moal, M. (1995). Mesocorticolimbic dopaminergic neurons. Functional and regulatory roles. In F. E. Bloom, & D. J. Kupfer (Eds.), *Psychopharmacology: The fourth generation of progress* (pp. 283–294). New York: Raven Press.

Lesch, K. P., Bengel, D., Heils, A., Sabol, S. Z., Greenberg, B. D., Petri, S., Benjamin, J., Müller, C. R., Hamer, D. H., & Murphy, D. L. (1996). Association of anxiety-related traits with a polymorphism in the serotonin transporter gene regulation region. *Science, 274*, 1527–1531.

Lesch, K. P., Greenberg, B. D., Higley, J. D., Bennett, A., & Murphy, D. L. (2002). Serotonin transporter, personality and behavior: Towards dissection of gene-gene and gene-environment interaction. In J. Benjamin, R. P. Ebstein, & R. H. Belmaker (Eds.), *Molecular genetics and the human personality* (pp. 109–135). Washington, DC: American Psychiatric Publishing.

Lesnik-Oberstein, M., & Cohen, L. (1984). Cognitive style, sensation seeking, and assortative mating. *Journal of Personality and Social Psychology, 46*, 112–117.

Lickliter, R., & Honeycutt, H. (2003). Developmental dynamics: Toward a biologically plausible evolutionary psychology. *Psychological Bulletin, 120,* 819–835.

Lidberg, L., Modlin, I., Oreland, L., Tuck, J. R., & Gillner, A. (1985). Platelet monoamine oxidase and psychopathy. *Psychiatry Research, 16,* 339–343.

Lim, K. O., Rosenbloom, M., & Pfefferbaum, A. (1995). In vivo structural brain assessment. In F. E. Bloom & D. J. Kupfer (Eds.), *Psychopharmacology: The fourth generation of progress* (pp. 881–894). New York: Raven Press.

Limson, R., Goldman, D., Roy, A., Lamparski, D., Ravitz, B., Adinoff, B., & Linnoila, M. (1991). Personality and cerebrospinal monoamine metabolites in alcoholics and normals. *Archives of General Psychiatry, 48,* 437–441.

Lindsley, D. B., Bowden, J., & Magoun, H. W. (1949). Effect upon EEG of acute injury to the brain stem activating system. *Electroencephalography and Clinical Neurophysiology, 1,* 475–486.

Linnoila, M., & Charney, D. S. (1999). The neurobiology of aggression. In D. S. Charney, E. J. Nestler, & B. S. Bunney (Eds.), *Neurobiology of Mental Illness* (pp. 872–879). New York: Oxford University Press.

Linström, L. H. (1985). Low HVA and normal 5HIAA CSF levels in drug-free schizophrenic patients compared to healthy volunteers: Correlations to symptomatology and family history. *Psychiatry Research, 14,* 265–273.

Loehlin, J. C. (1992). *Genes and environment in personality development.* Newbury Park, CA: Sage Publications.

Loehlin, J. C., & Martin, N. G. (2001). Age changes in personality traits and their heritabilities during the adult years. Evidence from Australian twin registry samples. *Personality and Individual Differences, 30,* 1147–1160.

Loehlin, J. C., McCrae, R. R., Costa, P. T. Jr., & John, O. P. (1998). Heritabilities of common and measure-specific components of the Big Five personality factors. *Journal of Research in Personality, 32,* 431–453.

Loehlin, J. C., Neiderhiser, M., & Reiss, D. (2003). The behavior genetics of personality and the NEAD study. *Journal of Research in Personality, 37,* 373–377.

Loehlin, J. C., Willerman, L., & Horn, I. M. (1985). Personality resemblances in adoptive families when the children are late adolescent or adult. *Journal of Personality and Social Psychology, 48,* 376–392.

Loehlin, J. C., Willerman, L., & Horn, J. M. (1987). Personality resemblance in adoptive families. A 10-year follow up. *Journal of Personality and Social Psychology, 53,* 961–969.

van Londen, L., Goekoop, J. C., van Kempen, G. M. J., Frankhuijzen-Sierevogel, A. C., Wiegart, V. M., van der Velde, E. A., & De Wied, D. (1997). Plasma levels of arginine vasopressin elevated in patients with major depression. *Neuropsychopharmacology, 17,* 284–292.

Lubin, B., & Zuckerman, M. (1999). *MAACL-R: Manual for the multiple affect adjective check list.* San Diego, CA: Educational and Industrial Testing Service.

Lucas, R. E., & Diener, E. (2001). Understanding extravert's enjoyment of social situations: The importance of pleasantness. *Journal of Personality and Social Psychology, 81,* 343–356.

Lukas, J. H., & Siegel, J. (1977). Cortical mechanisms that augment or reduce evoked potentials in cats. *Science, 196,* 73–75.

Lykken, D. T. (1982). Research with twins: The concept of emergenesis. *Psychophysiology, 25,* 4–15.

Lykken, D. T., Iacono, W. G., Harocan, K., McGue, M., & Bouchard, T. J. (1988). *Psychophysiology, 25*, 4–15.

Lyons, M. J., True, W. R., Eisen, S. A., Goldberg, J., Meyer, J. M., Faraone, S. V., Eaves, L. J., & Tsuang, M. T. (1995). Differential heritability of adult and juvenile antisocial traits. *Archives of General Psychiatry, 52*, 906–915.

MacDonald, K. (1999). What about sex differences? An adaptationist perspective on "the lives of causal influence" of personality systems. *Behavioral and Brain Sciences, 22*, 530–531.

MacLean, P. D. (1982). On the origin and progressive evolution of the triune brain. In C. Armstrong & D. Falk (Eds.), *Primate brain evolution. Methods and concepts* (pp. 291–316). New York: Plenum Press.

Maes, M., & Meltzer, H. J. (1995). The serotonin hypothesis of major depression. In F. E. Bloom & D. J. Kupfer (Eds.), *Psychopharmacology: The fourth generation of progress* (pp. 933–944). New York: Raven Press.

Magnusson, D. (1987). Individual development in an interactional perspective. In D. Magnusson (Ed.), *Paths through life*. Hillsdale, NJ: Erlbaum.

Magnusson, D. (1996). The patterning of antisocial behavior and autonomic reactivity. In D. M. Stoff & R. B. Cairns (Eds.), *Aggression and violence. Genetic, neurobiological, and biosocial perspectives.* (pp. 291–308).

Major, L. F., & Murphy, D. L. (1978). Platelet and plasma amine oxidase activity in alcoholic individuals. *British Journal of Psychiatry, 132*, 548–554.

Mann, J. J. (1995). Violence and aggression. In F. E. Bloom & D. J. Kupfer (Eds.), *Psychopharmacology: The fourth generation of progress* (pp. 1919–1928). New York: Raven Press.

Manuck, S. B., Flory, J. D., McCaffery, B. A., Mathews, K. A., Mann, J. J., & Muldoon, M. F. (1998). Aggression, impulsivity, and central nervous system serotonergic responsivity in a nonpatient sample. *Neuropsychopharmacology, 19*, 287–299.

Mark, V. H., Sweet, W. H., & Erbin, F. R. (1972). The effect of amygdalotomy on violent behavior in patients with temporal lobe epilepsy. In E. Hitchcock, L. Laitinen, & K. Vaernet (Eds.), *Psychosurgery* (pp. 139–155). Springfield, IL: Charles C. Thomas.

Matheny, A. P., Jr. (1980). Bayley's Infant Record: Behavioral component and twin analyses. *Child Development, 51*, 1157–1167.

Matheny, A. P., Jr., & Dolan, A. B. (1980). A twin study of personality and temperament during middle childhood. *Journal of Research in Personality, 14*, 224–234.

Mathew, R. J., Weinman, M. L., & Barr, D. L. (1984). Personality and regional blood flow. *British Journal of Psychiatry, 144*, 529–532.

Matthews, G., & Amelang, M. (1993). Extraversion, arousal theory and performance: A study of individual differences in EEG. *Personality and Individual Differences, 14*, 347–363.

Matthysse, S. (1973). Antipsychotic drug actions: A clue to the neuropathology of schizophrenia? *Federation Proceedings, 32*, 200–205.

Mattson, A., Schalling, D., Olweus, D., Low, H., & Svensson, J. (1980). Plasma testosterone, aggressive behavior, and personality dimensions in young male delinquents. *Journal of the American Academy of Child Psychiatry, 19*, 476–490.

McCleery, J. M., & Goodwin, G. M. (2001). High and low neuroticism predict different cortisol responses to the combined dexamethasone-CRH test. *Biological Psychiatry, 49*, 410–415.

McCrae, R. R., & Costa, P. T., Jr. (2003). *Personality in adulthood: A five-factor theory perspective* (2nd ed.). New York: Guilford Press.

McCrae, R. R., Zonderman, A. B., Costa, P. T., Jr., Bond, M. H., & Paunonen, S. V. (1996). Evaluating replicability of factors in the revised NEO personality inventory: Confirmatory factor analysis vs. Procrustes rotation. *Journal of Personality and Social Psychology, 70,* 552–566.

McGuffin, P., Owen, M. J., Donovan, M. C., Thapar, A., & Gottesman, I. I. (1994). *Seminars in Psychiatric Genetics.* London: Gaskell.

McManis, M. H., Kagan, J., Snidman, N. C., & Woodward, S. A. (2002). EEG asymmetry, power, and temperament in children. *Developmental Psychobiology, 41,* 169–177.

Mednick, S. A., Gabrelli, W. F., & Hutchings, B. (1987). Genetic factors in the etiology of criminal behavior. In S. A. Mednick, T. E. Moffitt, & S. A. Stack (Eds.), *The causes of crime: New biological approaches* (pp. 74–91). New York: Cambridge University Press.

Mednick, S. A., Moffitt, T., Gabrielli, W. J., & Hutchings, B. (1986). Genetic factors in criminal behavior. In D. Olweus, J. Block, & M. Radke-Yarrow (Eds.), *Development of antisocial and prosocial behavior* (pp. 33–50). New York: Academic Press.

Mehlman, P. T., Higley, J. D., Faucher, I., Lilly, A. A., Taub, D. M., Vickers, J., Suomi, S. J., & Linnoila, M. (1994). Low CSF-HIAA concentrations and severe aggression and impaired impulse control in nonhuman primates. *American Journal of Psychiatry, 151,* 1485–1491.

Mejia, J. M., Erwin, F. R., Baker, G. B., & Palmour, R. M. (2002). Monoamine oxidase inhibition during brain development induces pathological aggressive behavior in mice. *Biological Psychiatry, 52,* 811–822.

Mendelsohn, G., Darley, G. A., & Shaff, M. (1995). Personality change in Parkinson's disease patients: Chronic disease and aging. *Journal of Personality, 63,* 233–257.

Menza, M. A., Golbe, L. I., Cody, R. A., & Forman, N. E., (1993). Dopamine-related personality traits in Parkinson's disease, *Neurology, 43,* 505–508.

Merikangas, K. R., Avenevolli, S., Dierker, L., & Grillon, C. (1999). Vulnerability factors among children at risk for anxiety disorders. *Biological Psychiatry, 46,* 1523–1535.

Miles, D. R., & Carey, G. (1997). Genetic and environmental architecture of human aggression. *Journal of Personality and Social Psychology, 72,* 207–217.

Miller, E. (2002). Brain injury as a contributory factor in offending. In J. Glicksohn (Ed.), *The neurobiology of criminal behavior* (pp. 137–153). Boston, MA: Kluwer.

Mills, S., & Raine, A. (1994). Neuroimaging and aggression. *Journal of Offender Rehabilitation, 21,* 145–158.

Mischel, W. (1968). *Personality and assessment.* London: Wiley.

Mischel, W., Shoda, Y., & Peake, P. K. (1988). The nature of adolescent competencies predicted by preschool delay of gratification. *Journal of Personality and Social Psychology, 54,* 687–696.

Mitchell-Heggs, N., Kelly, D., & Richardson, A. (1976). Stereotaxic limbic leucotomy: A follow-up at 16 months. *British Journal of Psychiatry, 128,* 226–240.

Montgomery, S. A. (1995). Selective serotonin reuptake inhibitors in the acute treatment of depression. In F. E. Bloom & D. J. Kupfer (Eds.), *Psychopharmacology: The fourth generation of progress* (pp. 1043–1051). New York: Raven Press.

Moruzzi G., & Magoun H. W. (1949). Brain stem reticular formation and activation of the EEG. *EEG Clinical Neurophysiology, 1,* 455–473.

Murphy, D. L., Aulakh, C. S., Garrich, N. A., & Sunderland, T. (1987). Monoamine oxidase inhibitors as antidepressants: Implications for the mechanism of antidepressants and the psychobiology of the affective disorders. In H. Y. Meltzer (Ed.), *Psychopharmacology: The third generation of progress* (pp. 545–552).

Murphy, D. L., & Weiss, R. (1972). Reduced monoamine oxidase in blood platelets from bipolar depressed patients. *American Journal of Psychiatry, 128,* 1351–1357.

Murphy, D. L., Wright, C., Buchsbaum, M. S., Nichols, A., Costa, J. L., & Wyatt, R. J. (1976). Platelet and plasma amine oxidase activity in 680 normals: Sex and age differences and stability over time. *Biochemical Medicine, 16,* 254–265.

Murphy, G. (1947). *Personality: A biosocial approach to origins and structure.* New York: Harper.

Muscettola, G., Casiello, M., Giannini, C. P., & Bosi, L. (1986). Pilot study of Progabide in depression. In G. Bartholini, J. C. Friedman, S. Z. Langer, P. L. Morselli, & A. Wick (Eds.), *GABA and mood disorders* (pp. 113–118). New York: Raven Press.

Myrtek, M. (1984). *Constitutional psychophysiology.* London: Academic Press.

Naveteur, J. & Baque, E. F. (1987). Individual differences in electrodermal activity as a function of subjects' anxiety. *Personality and Individual Differences, 8,* 615–626.

Neary, R. S., & Zuckerman, M. (1976). Sensation seeking, trait and state anxiety, and the electrodermal orienting reflex. *Psychophysiology, 13,* 205–211.

Netter, P., Hennig, J., & Roed, I. S. (1996). Serotonin and dopamine as mediators of sensation seeking behavior. *Neuropsychobiology, 34,* 155–165.

Netter, P., Hennig, J., & Rohrmann, S. (1999). Psychobiological differences between the aggression and psychoticism dimension. *Pharmacopsychiatry, 32,* 5–12.

Netter, P., Toll, C., Reuter, M., & Hennig, J. (2003). Impulse control as related to noradrenergic and serotonergic responsivity. Paper presented at the 11th Biennial Meeting of the International Society for the Study of Individual Differences, Graz, Austria.

New, A. S., Goodman, M., Mitropoulou, M. A., & Siever, L. (2002). Genetic polymorphisms and aggression. In J. Benjamin, R. P. Ebstein, & R. H. Belmaker (Eds.), *Molecular genetics and the human personality* (pp. 231–244). Washington, DC: American Psychiatric Publishing.

New, A. S., Novotny, S. L., Buchsbaum, M. S., & Siever, L. J. (1998). Neuroimaging in impulsive-aggressive personality disorder. In M. Maes & E. F. Coccaro (Eds.), *Neurobiology and clinical views on aggression and impulsivity* (pp. 81–93). Chichester, UK: Wiley.

Noble, E. P. (1998). The D2 dopamine receptor gene: A review of association studies in alcoholism and phenotypes. *Alcohol, 16,* 33–45.

Noble, E. P., Blum, B., Khalsa, M. E., Ritchie, T., Montgomery, A., Wood, R. C., Fitch, R. J., Ozkaragoz, T., Sheridan, P. J., Anglin, M. D., Paredes, A., Treiman, L. J., & Sparkes, R. S. (1993). Allelic association of the D2 dopamine receptor gene with cocaine dependence. *Drug and Alcohol Dependence, 33,* 211–285.

Norman, W. T. (1963). Toward an adequate taxonomy of personality attributes: Replicated factor structure. *Journal of Abnormal and Social Psychology, 66,* 574–583.

Nutt, D. J., Glue, P., Lawson, C. W., & Wilson, S (1990). Flumazenil provocation of panic attacks: Evidence for altered benzodiazepine receptor sensitivity in panic disorder. *Archives of General Psychiatry, 47,* 917–925.

O'Carroll, R. E. (1984). Androgen administration to hygonadal and eugonadal men: Effects on measures of sensation seeking, personality, and spatial ability. *Personality and Individual Differences, 5,* 595–598.

O'Connor, M., Foch, T. T., Sherry, T., & Plomin, R. (1980). A twin study of specific behavioral problems of socialization as viewed by parents. *Journal of Abnormal Child Psychology, 8,* 189–199.

O'Gorman, J. G. (1984). Extraversion and the EEG I: An evaluation of Gale's hypothesis. *Biological Psychology, 19,* 95–112.

O'Gorman, J. G., & Lloyd, J. E. M. (1987). Extraversion, impulsiveness and EEG alpha activity, *Personality and Individual Differences, 8,* 169–174.

O'Gorman, J. G., & Mallis, L. R. (1984). Extraversion and the EEG II: A test of Gale's hypothesis. *Biological Psychology, 19,* 113–127.

O'Hara, B. F., Smith, S. S., Bird, G., Persico, A. M., Suaref, B. K., Cutting, G. R., & Uhl, G. R. (1993). Dopamine D2 receptor RFLPs, haplotypes and their association with substance use in black and caucasian research volunteers. *Human Heredity, 43,* 209–218.

Olweus, D. (1987). Testosterone and adrenaline: Aggressive antisocial behavior in normal adolescent males. In S. A. Mednick, T. E. Moffitt, & S. A. Stack (Eds.), *The causes of crime: New biological approaches* (pp. 263–282) Cambridge: Cambridge University Press.

Oreland, L., Wiberg, A., & Fowler, C. J. (1981). Monoamine oxidase activity as related to monoamine oxidase activity and monoaminergic function in the brain. In B. Angrist (Ed.), *Recent advances in neuropsychopharmacology* (Vol. 31). Oxford: Pergamon Press.

Orlebeke, J. F., & Feij, J. A. (1979). The orienting reflex as a personality correlate. In E. H. Van Holst & J. F. Orlebeke (Eds.), *The orienting reflex in humans* (pp. 567–585). Hillsdale, NJ: Erlbaum.

Owens, M. J., & Ritchie, J. C. (1999). Clinical neurochemistry. In D. S. Charney, E. J. Nestler, & B. S. Bunney (Eds.), *Neurobiology of mental illness* (pp. 132–148). New York: Oxford University Press.

Packard, M. G., Schroeder, J. P., & Gerianne, M. A. (1998). Expression of testosterone conditioned place preference is blocked by peripheral or intra-accumbens injection of alpha-flupenthixol. *Hormones and Behavior, 34,* 39–47.

Panksepp, J. (1982). Toward a general psychobiological theory of emotions. *The Behavioral and Brain Sciences, 5,* 407–422.

Papez, J. W. (1937). A proposed mechanism of emotion. *Archives of Neurology and Psychiatry, 38,* 725–743.

Parker, T. (1989, June). *Television viewing and aggression in four and seven year old children.* Paper presented at Summer Minority Access to Research Training meeting, University of Colorado, Boulder.

Partanen, J., Bruun, K., & Markkenen, T. (1966). *Inheritance of drinking behavior: A study on intelligence, personality and use of alcohol in adult twins.* Helsinki, Finland: Keskushirjapaino.

Paul, S. M. (1995). GABA glycine. In P. E. Bloom & R. J. Kupfer (Eds.), *Psychopharmacology: A fourth generation of progress* (pp. 87–94). New York: Raven Press.

Pavlov, I. P., (1927/1960). *Conditioned reflexes, An investigation of the physiological activity of the cerebral cortex* (G. V. Anrep, Trans. and Ed.). New York: Dover Publications.

Pederson, N. L., Plomin, R., McClearn, G. E., & Friberg, L. (1988). Neuroticism, extraversion, and related traits in adult twins reared apart and reared together. *Journal of Personality and Social Psychology, 55,* 950–957.

Peirson, A. R., Heuchert, J. W., Thomala, L., Berk, M., Plein, H., & Cloninger, C. R. (1999). Relationship between serotonin and the Temperament and Character Inventory. *Psychiatry Research, 89*, 29–37.

Perkins, K. A., Gerlach, D., Broge, M., Grobe, J. E., & Wilson, A. (2000). Greater sensitivity to subjective effects of nicotine in nonsmokers high in sensation-seeking. *Experimental and Clinical Psychopharmacology, 8*, 462–471.

Persson, M. L., Wasserman, D., Geijer, T., Frisch, A., Rockah, R., Michaelovsky, E., Apter, A., Weizman, A., Joensson, E. G., & Bergman, H. (2000). Dopamine D4 receptor gene polymorphism and personality traits in healthy volunteers. *European Archives of Psychiatry and Clinical Neuroscience, 250*, 203–206.

Petrie, A., Collins, W., & Solomon, P. (1958). Pain sensitivity, sensory deprivation and susceptibility to satiation. *Science, 128*, 1431–1433.

Phan, K. L., Taylor, S. F., Welsh, R. C., Decker, L. R., Noll, D. C., Nichols, T. E., Britton, J. C., & Liberzon, I. (2003). Activation of the medial prefrontal cortex and extended amygdala by individual ratings of emotional arousal: A fMRI study. *Biological Psychiatry, 53*, 211–215.

Pickering, A. D. (1999). Personality correlates of the dopaminergic facilitation of incentive motivation. Impulsive sensation seeking rather than extraversion? *Behavioral and Brain Sciences, 22*, 534–535.

Pickering, A. D., Corr, P. J., Powell, J. H., Kumari, V., Thornton, J. C., & Gray, J. A. (1997). Individual differences in reactions to reinforcing stimuli are neither black nor white: To what extent are they Gray? In H. Nyborg (Ed.), *The scientific study of human nature: Tribute to Hans Eysenck at eighty* (pp. 36–67). Oxford: Elsevier Science.

Piquero, A., & Tibbetts, S. (1999). The impact of pre/perinatal disturbances and disadvantaged familial environment in predicting criminal offending. *Studies on crime and crime prevention, 8*, 52–70.

Pivik, R. T., Stelmack, R. M., & Bylsma, F. W. (1988). Personality and individual differences in spinal motoneuronal excitability. *Psychophysiology, 25*, 16–24.

Plomin, R., Coon, H., Carey, G., De Fries, J. C., & Fulker, D. W. (1991). Parent-offspring and sibling adoption analyses of parental ratings of temperament in infancy and childhood. *Journal of Personality, 59*, 705–732.

Plomin, R., De Fries, J. C., McClearn, G. E., & Rutter, M. (1997). *Behavioral genetics* (3rd ed.) New York: W. H. Freeman & Co.

Plomin, R., Foch, T. T., & Rowe, D. C. (1981). Bobo clown aggression in childhood: Environment not genes. *Journal of Research in Personality, 15*, 331–342.

Plomin, R., Reiss, D., Hetherington, E. M., & Howe, G. (1994). Nature and nurture: Genetic influences on measures of the family environment. *Developmental Psychology, 30*, 32–43.

Plouffe, L., & Stelmack, R. M. (1986). Sensation seeking and the electrodermal orienting response in young and elderly females. *Personality and Individual Differences, 7*, 119–120.

Pope, H. G., & Katz, D. L. (1994). Psychiatric and medical effects of anabolic-androgenic steroid use: A controlled study of 160 athletes. *Archives of General Psychiatry, 51*, 375–382.

Pope, H. G., Kouri, E. M., & Hudson, J. I. (2000). Effects of supraphysiologic doses of testosterone on mood and aggression in men: A randomized controlled study. *Archives of General Psychiatry, 57*, 133–140.

Pope, M. K., & Smith, T. W. (1991). Cortisol secretion in high and low cynically hostile men. *Psychosomatic Medicine, 53*, 386–392.

Powell, G. E. (1981). A survey of the effects of brain lesions upon personality. In H. J. Eysenck (Ed.) *A model for personality.* Weildelberg, Germany: Springer-Verlag.

Preston, S. D., & de Waal, F. B. M. (2002). Empathy: Its ultimate and proximate bases. *Behavioral and Brain Sciences, 25*, 1–144.

Prolo, P., & Licinio, J. (2002). DRD4 and novelty seeking. In J. Benjamin, R. P. Ebstein, & R. H. Belmaker (Eds.), *Molecular genetics and the human personality* (pp. 91–107). Washington, DC: American Psychiatric Publishing.

Rada, R. T., Laws, D. R., & Kellner, R. (1976). Plasma testosterone levels in the rapist. *Psychosomatic Medicine, 38*, 257–258.

Raine, A. (1993). *The psychopathology of crime: Criminal behavior as a clinical disorder.* San Diego, CA: Academic Press.

Raine, A. (1996). Autonomic nervous system activity and violence. In D. M. Stoff & R. B. Cairns (Eds.), *Aggression and violence: Genetic, neurobiological, and biosocial perspectives* (pp. 145–168) Mahwah, NJ: Erlbaum.

Raine, A. (2002). Biosocial studies of antisocial and violent behavior in children and adults: A review. *Journal of Abnormal Child Psychology, 30*, 311–326.

Raine, A., Brennan, P., & Mednick, S. A. (1994). Birth complications combined with early maternal rejection at age 1 predispose to violent crime at 18 years. *Archives of General Psychiatry, 51*, 984–988.

Raine, A., Brennan, P., & Mednick, S. A. (1997). Interaction between birth complications and early maternal rejection in predisposing individuals to adult violence: Specificity to serious, early-onset violence. *American Journal of Psychiatry, 154*, 1265–1271.

Raine, A., Buchsbaum, M. S., & La Casse, L. (1997). Brain abnormalities in murderers indicated by positron emission tomography. *Biological Psychiatry, 42*, 495–508.

Raine, A., Ishikawa, S. S., Arce, E., Lencz, T., Knuth, K. H., Bihrle, S., La Casse, L., & Colleti, P. (2004). Hippocampal structural asymmetry in unsuccessful psychopaths. *Biological Psychiatry, 55*, 185–191.

Raine, A., Lencz, T., Bihrle, S., & La Casse, L. (2000). Reduced prefrontal gray matter volume and reduced autonomic activity in antisocial personality disorder. *Archives of General Psychiatry, 57*, 119–127.

Raine, A., Reynolds, C., Venables, P. H., Mednick, S. A., & Farrington, D. P. (1998). Fearlessness, stimulation-seeking and large body size at age 3 years as early predispositions to childhood aggression at age 11 years. *Archives of General Psychiatry, 55*, 745–751.

Raine, A., Stoddard, J., Bihrle, S., & Buchsbaum, M. S. (1998). Prefrontal deficits in murderers lacking psychosocial deprivation. *Neuropsychiatry, Neuropsychology, and Behavioral Neurology, 11*, 1–7.

Raine, A., & Venables, P. H. (1990). Evoked potential augmenting-reducing in psychopaths and criminals with impaired smooth-pursuit eye-movements. *Psychiatry Research, 31*, 85–88.

Raine, A., Venables, P. H., & Mednick, S. A. (1997). Low resting heart rate at age 3 years predisposes to aggression at age 11 years: Findings from the Mauritius Joint Child Health Project. *Journal of the American Academy of Child and Adolescent Psychiatry, 36*, 1457–1464.

Ramboz, S., Oosting, R., Amara, D. A., Kung, H. F., Blier, P., Mendelsohn, M., Mann, J. J., Bruner, D., & Hen, R. (1998). Serotonin, 1A knockout: An animal model of anxiety-related disorder. *Proceedings of the National Academy of Science, 95,* 14476–14481.

Rammsayer, T. H. (1998). Extraversion and dopamine: Individual differences in response to changes in dopaminergic activity as a possible biological basis of extraversion. *European Psychologist, 3,* 37–50.

Rammsayer, T. H., Netter, P., & Vogel, W. (1993). A neurochemical model underlying differences in reaction times between introverts and extraverts. *Personality and Individual Differences, 14,* 701–712.

Rao, D. C., & Gu, C. (2002). Principles and methods in the study of complex phenotypes. In J. Benjamin, R. P. Ebstein, & R. H. Belmaker (Eds.), *Molecular genetics and the human personality* (pp. 1–32). Washington, DC: American Psychiatric Publishing Company.

Rawlings, D. (2003). Personality correlates of liking for 'unpleasant' paintings and photographs. *Personality and Individual Differences, 34,* 395–410.

Redmond, D. E., Jr. (1985). Neurochemical basis for anxiety and anxiety disorders: Evidence from drugs which decrease human fear or anxiety. In A. H. Tuna & J. D. Maser (Eds.), *Anxiety and the anxiety disorders* (pp. 533–555). Hillsdale, NJ: Erlbaum.

Redmond, D. E., Jr. (1987). Studies of locus coeruleus in monkeys and hypotheses for neuropsychopharmacology. In H. Y. Meltzer (Ed.), *Psychopharmacology: The third generation of progress* (pp. 967–975). New York: Raven Press.

Redmond, D. E., Jr., Katz, M. M., Maas, J. W., Swann, A., Casper, R., & Davis, J. M. (1986). Cerebrospinal fluid amine metabolites: Relationships with behavioral measurements in depressed, manic, and healthy control subjects. *Archives of General Psychiatry, 43,* 938–947.

Redmond, D. E., Jr., Murphy, D. L., & Baulu, J. (1979). Platelet monoamine oxidase activity correlates with social affiliative and agonistic behaviors in normal rhesus monkeys. *Psychosomatic Medicine, 41,* 87–100.

Reiman, E. M. (1990). PET, panic disorder, and normal anticipatory anxiety. In J. C. Ballenger (Ed.), *Neurobiology of panic disorder* (pp. 245–270). New York: Wiley-Liss.

Reiman, E. M., Lane, R. D., Ahern, G. L., Schwartz, G. E., & Davidson, R. J. (2000). Positron emission tomography in the study of emotion, anxiety and anxiety disorders. In P. D. Lane & L. Nadal (Eds.), *Cognitive neuroscience of emotion* (pp. 389–406). New York: Oxford University Press.

Reist, C., Haier, R. J., De Met, E., & Cicz-De Met, A. (1990). Platelet MAO activity in personality disorders and normal controls. *Psychiatry Research, 30,* 221–227.

Reuter, M., Netter, P., Toll, C., & Hennig, J. (2002). Dopamine agonist and antagonist responders as related to types of nicotine craving and facets of extraversion. *Progress in Neuro-Psychopharmacology and Biological Psychiatry, 26,* 845–853.

Richards, M., & Eves, F. F. (1991). Personality, temperament and the cardiac defense response. *Personality and Individual Differences, 12,* 999–1007.

Richardson, D. R., Medvin, N., & Hammock, G. (1988). Love styles, relationship experience and sensation seeking: A test of validity. *Personality and Individual Differences, 9,* 645–651.

Ridgeway, P., & Hare, R. D. (1981). Sensation seeking and psychophysiological responses to auditory stimulation. *Psychophysiology, 18,* 613–618.

Riemann, R., Angleitner, A., & Strelau, J. (1997). Genetic and environmental influences on personality: A study of twins reared together using the self- and peer report NEO-FFI scales. *Journal of Personality, 65,* 449–475.

Roberts, B. W., & Del Vecchio, W. F. (2000). The rank-order consistency of personality traits from childhood to old age: A quantitative review of longitudinal studies. *Psychological Bulletin, 126,* 26–77.

Robins, L. N., & Regier (1991). *Psychiatric disorders in America: The epidemiologic catchment area study.* New York: Free Press.

Robinson, D. L. (2001). How brain arousal systems determine different temperament types and the major dimensions of personality. *Personality and Individual Differences, 31,* 1233–1259.

Robinson, D. S., Davis, J. M., Nies, A., Ravaris, C. L., & Sylvester, D. (1971). Relation of sex and aging to monoamine oxidase activity of human brain, plasma, and platelets. *Archives of General Psychiatry, 24,* 536–539.

Robinson, T. N. Jr., & Zahn, T. P. (1983). Sensation seeking, state anxiety and cardiac and EDR orienting reactions. *Psychophysiology, 20,* 465. [Abstract]

Rose, R. J., Koskenvuo, M., Kaprio, J., Sarna, S., & Langinvainio, H. (1988). Shared genes, shared experiences, and similarity of personality. *Journal of Personality and Social Psychology, 54,* 161–171.

Rothbart, M. K., & Derryberry, D. (1981). Development of individual differences in temperament. In M. E. Lamb & A. L. Brown (Eds.), *Advances in developmental psychology, Vol 1* (pp. 37–86). Hillsdale, NJ: Erlbaum.

Rothbart, M. K., Derryberry, D., & Posner, M. I. (1994). A psychobiological approach to the development of temperament. In J. E. Bates & T. D. Wachs (Eds.), *Temperament: Individual differences at the interface of biology and behavior* (pp. 83–116). Washington, DC: American Psychological Association.

Roy, A. (1999). CSF correlates with neuroticism in depressed patients. *Journal of Affective Disorders, 52,* 247–249.

Royce, J. R. (1977). On the construct validity of open-field measures. *Psychological Bulletin, 84,* 1098–1106.

Ruegg, R. G., Gilmore, J., Ekstrom, R. D., Corrigan, M., Knight, B., Tancer, M., Leatherman, M. E., Carson, S. W., & Golden, R. N. (1997). Clomipramine challenge responses covary with the Multidimensional Personality Questionnaire scores in healthy subjects. *Biological Psychiatry, 42,* 1123–1129.

Rujesai, D., Giegling, I., Gietl, A., Hartmann, A. M., & Möller, H-J (2003). A functional single nucleotide polymorphism (V158M) in the COMT gene is associated with aggressive personality traits. *Biological Psychiatry, 54,* 34–39.

Rushton, J. P., Fulker, J. L., Neale, M. C., Nias, D. K. B., & Eysenck, H. J. (1986). Altruism and aggression: The heritability of individual differences. *Journal of Personality and Social Psychology, 50,* 1192–1198.

Rust, J. (1975). Genetic effects in the cortical auditory evoked potential: A twin study. *Electroencephalography and Clinical Neurology, 39,* 321–327.

Rusting, C. L., & Larsen, R. J. (1997). Extraversion, neuroticism, and susceptibility to positive and negative affect: A test of two theoretical models. *Personality and Individual Differences, 22,* 607–612.

Sackett, G. P. (1966). Monkeys reared in isolation with pictures as visual input: Evidence for an innate releasing mechanism. *Science, 154,* 1468–1473.

Samochowiez, J., Lesch, K. P., Rottmann, M., Smolka, M., Syagailo, Y. U., Okladnova, O., Commelspacher, H., Winterer, G., Schmidt, L. G., & Sander, T. (1999). Association of a regulator polymorphism in the promoter region of the monoamine oxidase A gene with antisocial alcoholism. *Psychiatry Research, 86,* 67–72.

Saudino, K. J., Gagne, J. R., Grant, J., Ibatoulina, A., Marytuina, T., & Ravich-Scherbo, I. (1999). Genetic and environmental influences on personality in adult Russian twins. *International Journal of Behavioral Development, 23,* 375–389.

Saxton, P. M., Siegel, J., & Lukas, J. H. (1987). Visual evoked potential augmenting/reducing slopes in cats 2. Correlations with behavior. *Personality and Individual Differences, 8,* 511–519.

Scarr, S., Webber, P. L., Weinberg, R. A., & Wittig, M. A. (1981). Personality resemblance among adolescents and their parents in biologically related and adoptive families. *Journal of Personality and Social Psychology, 40,* 885–898.

Schalling, D., Åsberg, M., & Edman, G. (1984). Personality and CSF monoamine metabolites. Unpublished manuscript, Department of Psychiatry and Psychology, Karolinska Hospital, and the Department of Psychology, University of Stockholm, Sweden.

Schatzberg, A. F., & Schildkraut, J. J. (1995). Recent studies on norepinephrine systems in mood disorders. In P. E. Bloom & R. J. Kupfer (Eds.), *Psychopharmacology: The fourth generation of progress* (pp. 911–920). New York: Raven Press.

Schinka, J. A., Letsch, E. A., & Crawford, F. C. (2002). DRD4 and novelty seeking: Results of meta-analyses. *American Journal of Medical Genetics, 114,* 643–648.

Schukit, M. A. (1994). Familial alcoholism. In T. A. Widiger, A. J. Francis, H. A. Pincus, M. B. First, R. Ross, & W. Davis (Eds.), *DSM IV-Sourcebook* (Vol. I, pp. 159–167). Washington, DC: American Psychiatric Press.

Schildkraut, J. J. (1965). The catecholamine hypothesis of affective disorders: A review of supporting evidence. *American Journal of Psychiatry, 122,* 509–522.

Schlyer, D. J. (1991). The use of positron-emission tomography in identifying and quantitating receptors involved in schizophrenia. In N. D. Volkow & A. P. Wolf (Eds.), *Positron-emission tomography in schizophrenia research* (pp. 75–100). Washington, DC: American Psychiatric Press.

Schmidt, L. A. (1999). Frontal brain electrical activity in shyness and sociability. *Psychological Science, 10,* 316–320.

Schmidt, L. A., & Fox, N. A. (2002). Molecular genetics of temperamental differences in children. In J. Benjamin, R. P. Ebstein, & R. H. Belmaker (Eds.), *Molecular genetics and the human personality* (pp. 257–272). Washington, DC: American Psychiatric Publishing.

Schmidt, L. A., Fox, N. A., Rubin, K. H., Hu, S., & Hamer, D. H. (2002). Molecular genetics of shyness and aggression in preschoolers. *Personality and Individual Differences, 33,* 227–238.

Schmitz, S., Saudino, K. J., Plomin, R., Fulker, D. W., & De Fries, J. C. (1996). Genetic and environmental influences on temperament in middle childhood: Analyses of teacher and tester ratings. *Child Development, 27,* 409–422.

Scott, J. P., & Fuller, J. L. (1965). *Genetics and the social behavior of dogs.* Chicago: University of Chicago Press.

Seeman, P. (1995). Dopamine receptors. Clinical correlates. In F. E. Bloom & D. J. Kupfer (Eds.), *Psychopharmacology: The fourth generation of progress* (pp. 295–302). New York: Raven Press.

Sen, S., Villafuerte, S., Nesse, R., Stoltenberg, S. F., Hopican, J., Gleiberman, L., Weder A., & Burmeister, M. (2004). Serotonin transporter and GABA(A) Alpha 6 receptor variants are associated with neuroticism. *Biological Psychiatry, 55,* 244–249.

Shader, R. I., & Greenblatt, D. J. (1995). The pharmacotherapy of acute anxiety: A mini-update. In F. E. Blook & D. J. Kupfer (Eds.), *Psychopharmacology: The fourth generation of progress* (pp. 1341–1348). New York: Raven Press.

Sheard, M. H., Marini, J. L., Bridges, C. I., & Wagner, E. (1976). The effect of lithium on impulsive aggressive behavior in man. *American Journal of Psychiatry, 133,* 1409–1413.

Shekim, W. O., Bylund, D. B., Alexson, J., Glaser, R. D., Jones, S. B., Hodges, K., & Perdue, S. (1986). Platelet MAO and measures of attention disorder deficit and hyperactivity. *Psychiatry Research, 18,* 179–188.

Sheldon, W. H. (1942). *The varieties of human temperament.* New York: Harper.

Sher, K. J. (1993). Children of alcoholics and the intergenerational transmission of alcoholism: A biopsychosocial perspective. In J. S. Baer, A. Marlatt, & R. J. McMahon (Eds.), *Addictive behaviors across the life span* (pp. 3–33). Newbury Park, CA: Sage Publications.

Shields, J. (1962). *Monozygotic twins brought up apart and brought up together.* London: Oxford University Press.

Shih, J. C., & Chen, K. (1999). MAO-A and -B gene knock-out mice exhibit distinctly different behavior. *Neurobiology, 7,* 235–246.

Shih, J. C., Chen, K., & Ridd, M. J. (1999). Monoamine oxidase: From genes to behavior. *Annual Review of Neuroscience, 22,* 197–217.

Siegfried, J., & Ben-Shmuel, A. (1972). Neurosurgical treatment of aggressivity. Stereotaxic amygdalotomy versus leukotomy. In E. Hitchcock, L. Laitinen, & K. Vaernet (Eds.), *Psychosurgery* (214–229). Springfield, IL: Charles C. Thomas.

Siegel, J., & Driscoll, P. (1996). Recent developments in an animal model of visual evoked potential augmenting/reducing and sensation seeking behavior. *Neuropsychobiology, 34,* 130–135.

Siegel, J., Sisson, D. F., & Driscoll, P. (1993). Augmenting and reducing of visual evoked potentials in Roman high- and low-avoidance rats. *Physiology and Behavior, 54,* 707–711.

Siever, L. J. & Trestman, R. L. (1993). The serotonin system and aggressive personality. *International Clinical Psychopharmacology, 8,* 33–39.

Simmel, E. C. (1984). Sensation seeking: Exploration of empty spaces or novel stimuli? *Behavioral and Brain Sciences, 3,* 449–450.

Smith, B. D., Davidson, R. A., Smith, D. L., Goldstein, H., & Perlstein, W. (1989). Sensation seeking and arousal: Effects of strong stimulation on electrodermal activation and memory task performance. *Personality and Individual Differences, 10,* 671–679.

Smith, B. D., Perlstein, W. M., Davidson, R. A., & Michael, K. (1986). Sensation seeking: Differential effects of relevant novel stimulation on electrodermal activity. *Personality and Individual Differences, 4,* 445–452.

Smith, S. S., O'Hara, B. F., Persico, A. M., Gorelick, D. A., Newlin, D. B., Vlahov, D., Solomon, L., Pickens, R., & Uhl, G. R. (1992). Genetic vulnerability to drug abuse. *Archives of General Psychiatry, 49,* 723–727.

Smith, T. W., & Gallo, L. C. (1999). Hostility and cardiovascular reactivity during marital interaction. *Psychosomatic Medicine, 61,* 436–445.

Soderstrom, H., Tullberg, M., Wikkelsoe, C., Ekholm, S. & Forsman, A. (2000). Reduced regional cerebral blood flow in non-psychotic violent offenders. *Psychiatry Research: Neuroimaging, 98,* 29–41.

Sokolov, E. N. (1963). *Perception and the conditioned reflex.* New York: Macmillan.

Sostek, A J., Sostek, A. M., Murphy, D. L., Martin, E. B., & Born, W. S. (1981). Cord blood amine oxidase activities relate to arousal and motor functioning in human newborns. *Life Sciences, 28,* 2561–2568.

Soubrié, P. (1986). Reconciling the role of central serotonin neurons in human and animal behavior. *Behavioral and Brain Sciences, 9,* 319–364.

Spivak, B., Vered, Y., Graff, E., Blum, J., Mester, R., & Weizman, A. (1999). Low platelet-poor plasma concentrations of serotonin in patients with combat-related post-traumatic stress disorders. *Biological Psychiatry, 45,* 840–845.

Stallings, M. C., Hewitt, J. K., Cloninger, C. R., Heath, A. C., & Eaves, L. J. (1996). Genetic and environmental structure of the tridimensional questionnaire: Three or four temperament dimensions? *Journal of Personality and Social Psychology, 70,* 127–140.

Stanford, M. S., Houston, R. J., Villemarette-Pittman, N. R., & Greve, K. W. (2003). Pre-meditated aggression: Clinical assessment and cognitive psychophysiology. *Personality and Individual Differences, 34,* 773–781.

Stein, L. (1978). Reward transmitters: Catecholamines and opioid peptides. In M. A. Lipton, A. DiMascio, & K. F. Killam (Eds.), *Psychopharmacology: A generation of progress.* New York: Raven Press.

Stellar, J. R., & Stellar, E. (1985). *The neurobiology of motivation and reward.* New York: Springer-Verlag.

Stelmack, R. M. (1990). Biological bases of extraversion: Psychophysiological evidence. *Journal of Personality, 58,* 293–311.

Stelmack, R. M., Campbell, K. B., & Bell, I. (1993). Extraversion and brainstem auditory evoked potentials. *Personality and Individual Differences, 14,* 447–453.

Stelmack, R. M., & Wilson, K. G. (1982). Extraversion and the effects of frequency and intensity on the auditory brainstem evoked response. *Personality and Individual Differences, 3,* 373–380.

Stenberg, G. (1992). Personality and the EEG: Arousal and emotional arousability. *Personality and Individual Differences, 13,* 1047–1113.

Stenberg, G. (1994). Extraversion and the P300 in a visual classification task. *Personality and Individual Differences, 16,* 543–560.

Stenberg, G., Risberg, J., Warkentin, S., & Rosen, I. (1990). Regional patterns of cortical blood flow distinguish extraverts from introverts. *Personality and Individual Differences, 11,* 663–673.

Stenberg, G., Rosen, I., & Risberg, J. (1990). Attention and personality in augmenting/reducing of visual evoked potentials. *Personality and Individual Differences, 11,* 1243–1254.

Stenberg, G., Wendt, P. E., & Risberg, J. (1993). Regional cerebral blood flow and extraversion. *Personality and Individual Differences, 15,* 547–554.

Stern, G. S., Cox, J., & Shahan, D. (1981). Feedback and divergent affective reactions for high and low sensation seekers. *Biofeedback and Self Regulation, 6,* 315–326.

Stewart, M. E., Deary, I. J., & Ebmeier, K. P. (2002). Neuroticism as a predictor of mood change. The effects of tryptophan depletion. *British Journal of Psychiatry, 171,* 242–247.

Strelau, J. (1983). Temperament, personality, activity. London: Academic Press.

Strelau, J. (1987). Personality dimensions based on arousal theories: Search for integration. In J. Strelau & H. J. Eysenck (Eds.), *Personality dimensions and arousal* (pp. 269–286). New York: Plenum Press.

Strelau, J. (1998). *Temperament: A psychological perspective.* New York: Plenum Press.

Strelau, J., Angleitner, A., Bantelmann, J., & Ruch, W. (1990). The Strelau Temperament Inventory-Revised (STI-R): Theoretical considerations and scale development. *European Journal of Personality, 4*, 209–235.

Strelau, J., & Eysenck, H. J. (Eds.). (1987). *Personality dimensions and arousal.* New York: Plenum Press.

Strelau, J., & Zawadzki, B. (1993). The Formal Characteristics of Behavior-Temperament Inventory (FCB-TI): Theoretical assumptions and scale construction. *European Journal of Personality, 7*, 313–336.

Strobel, A., Debener, S., Schmidt, D., Hünnerkopf, R., Lesch, K. P., & Brocke, B. (2003). Allelic variation in serotonin transporter function associated with the intensity dependence of the auditory evoked potential. *American Journal of Medical Genetics. Part B (Neuropsychiatric Genetics), 118B*, 41–47.

Strobel, A., Wehr, A., Michel, A., & Brocke, B. (1999). Association between the dopamine D4 receptor (DRD4) exon III polymorphism and measures of Novelty Seeking in a German population. *Molecular Psychiatry, 4*, 378–384.

Suarez, E. C., Kuhn, C. M., Schanberg, S. M., Williams, R. B. Jr., & Zimmerman, E. A. (1998). Neuroendocrine, cardiovascular, and emotional responses of hostile men: The role of interpersonal challenge. *Psychosomatic Medicine, 60*, 78–88.

Svartberg, K., & Forkman, B. (2002). Personality traits in the domestic dog (canis familiaris). *Applied Animal Behavior Science, 79*, 133–155.

Sweet, W. H., Ervin, F., & Mark, V. H. (1969). The relationship of violent behavior in focal cerebral disease. In S. Garattini & E. Sigg (Eds.), *Aggressive Behavior.* New York: Wiley.

Tauscher, J., Bagby, R. M., Javanomard, M., Christensen, B. F., Kaspar, S., & Kapur, S. (2001). Inverse relationship between 5HT1A receptor binding and anxiety: A [11C]way-100635 PET investigation in healthy volunteers. *American Journal of Psychiatry, 158*, 1326–1328.

Tellegen, A. (1985). Structures of mood and personality and their relevance to assessing anxiety, with an emphasis on self-report. In A. H. Tuma & J. D. Maser (Eds.) *Anxiety and the anxiety disorders* (pp. 681–706). Hillsdale, NJ: Erlbaum.

Tellegen, A., Lykken, D. T., Bouchard, T. J., Wilcox, K. Segal, N., & Rich, A. (1980). Personality similarity in twins reared together and apart. *Journal of Personality and Social Psychology, 54*, 1031–1039.

Tellegen, A. & Waller, N. G. (in press) *Exploring personality through test construction. Development of the Multidimensional Personality Questionnaire.* Minneapolis: University of Minnesota Press.

Thomas, A., & Chess, S. (1977). *Temperament and development.* New York: Bruner/Mazel.

Thomas, A., & Chess, S. (1986). The New York Longitudinal Study: From infancy to early adult life. In R. Plomin & J. Dunn (Eds.), *The study of temperament: Changes, continuities, and challenges* (39–52). Hillsdale, NJ: Erlbaum.

Thomas, A., Chess, S., & Birch, H. G. (1968). *Temperament and behavior disorders in children.* New York: New York University Press.

Thornquist, M. H., & Zuckerman, M. (1995). Psychopathy, passive-avoidance learning and basic dimensions of personality. *Personality and Individual Differences, 19*, 525–534.

Tomarken, A. J., Davidson, R. J., Wheeler, R. E., & Doss, R. C. (1992). Individual differences in anterior brain asymmetry and fundamental dimensions of emotion. *Journal of Personality and Social Psychology, 62*, 676–687.

Tonkonogy, J. M. (1990). Violence and the temporal lobe lesion. *Journal of Neuropsychiatry, 3*, 189–196.

Torgersen, A. M. (1985). Temperamental differences in infants and 6-year old children: A follow-up study of twins. In J. Strelau, F. H. Farley, & A. Gale (Eds.), *The biological basis of personality and behavior: Theories, measurement techniques and development* (pp. 227–239). Washington, DC: Hemisphere.

Torrey, E. F., Bowler, A. E., Taylor, E. H., & Gottesman, I. I. (1994). *Schizophrenia and manic-depressive disorder*. New York: Basic Books.

Torrubia, R., Avila, C., Moltó, J., & Caserás, X. (2001). The sensitivity to punishment and sensitivity to reward questionnaire (SPSRQ) as a measure of Gray's anxiety and impulsivity dimensions. *Personality and Individual Differences, 15*, 837–862.

Tran, Y., Craig, A., & McIssac, P. (2001). Extraversion-introversion and 8-13 Hz waves in frontal cortical regions. *Personality and Individual Differences, 30*, 205–215.

Traskman, L., Tybring, G., Åsberg, M., Bertilsson, L., Lantis, O., & Schalling, D. (1980). Cortisol in the CSF of depressed and suicidal patients. *Archives of General Psychiatry, 37*, 761–767.

Tremblay, R. E., Schaal, B., Boulerice, B., Arseneault, L., Soussignan, R. G., Paquette, D., & Laurent, D. (1998). Testosterone, physical aggression, dominance, and physical development in early adolescence. *International Journal of Behavioral Development, 22*, 753–777.

Tuchtenhagen, F., Daumann, J., Gobbele, R., Becker, S., Pelz, S., Sass, H., Buchner, H., & Gouzoulis-Mayfrank, E. (2000). High intensity dependence of auditory evoked dipole source activity indicates decreased serotonergic activity in abstinent ecstacy (MDMA) users. *Neuropsychopharmacology, 22*, 608–617.

Tupes, E. C., & Christal, R. E. (1961). Recurrent personality factors based on trait ratings. *USAF ASD Technical Reports (No. 61-970)*.

Twenge, J. M. (2001). Birth cohort changes in extraversion: a cross temporal meta-analysis, 1966–1993. *Personality and Individual Differences, 30*, 735–748.

Uhl, G. R., Persico, A. M., & Smith, S. S. (1992). Current excitement with D2 dopamine receptor gene alleles in substance abuse. *Archives of General Psychiatry, 49*, 157–160.

Ursin, H., & Kaada, B. R. (1960). Function localization within the amygdaloid complex in the cat. *Electroencephalogram Clinical Neurophysiology, 12*, 1–20.

Valentino, R. J., & Aston-Jones, G. S. (1995). Physiological and anatomical determinants of Locus Coeruleus discharge: Behavioral and clinical implications. In F. E. Bloom & D. J. Kupfer (Eds.), *Psychopharmacology: The fourth generation of progress* (pp. 373–385). New York: Raven Press.

Valva, G., Thomas, P., Ducrocq, F., Fontaine, M., Boss, V., Devos, P., Rascle, C., Cottencen, O., Brunet, A., Laffargue, P., & Goudemand, M. (2004). Low posttraumatic GABA plasma levels as a predictive factor in the development of acute posttraumatic stress disorder. *Biological Psychiatry, 55*, 250–254.

Valzelli, L. (1981). *Psychobiology of aggression and violence*. New York: Raven Press.

Vando, A. (1974). The development of the R-A scale: A paper-and-pencil measure of pain tolerance. *Personality and Social Psychology Bulletin, 1*, 28–29

Verona, E., Patrick, C. J., & Lang, A. R. (2002). A direct assessment of the role of state and trait negative emotion in aggressive behavior. *Journal of Abnormal Psychology, 111*, 249–258.

Viken, R. J., Rose, R. J., Kaprio, J., & Koskenvuo, M. (1994). A developmental genetic analysis of adult personality: Extraversion and neuroticism from 18 to 59 years of age. *Journal of Personality and Social Psychology, 66,* 722–730.

Virkkunen, M. (1985). Urinary free cortisol secretion in habitually violent offenders. *Acta Psychiatrica Scandinavica, 72,* 40–44.

Volavka, J. (1995). *Neurobiology of violence.* Washington, DC: American Psychiatric Press.

Volavka, J., & Citrome, L. (1998). Aggression, alcohol, and other substances of abuse. In M. Maes & E. F. Coccaro (Eds.), *Neurobiology and clinical views on aggression and impulsivity* (pp. 29–45). Chichester, UK: Wiley.

Volkow, N. D., Tancredi, L. R., Grant, C., Gillespie, H., Valentine, A., Mullani, N., Wang, G.-J., & Hollister, L. (1995). Brain glucose metabolism in violent psychiatric patients. A preliminary study. *Psychiatry Research: Neuroimaging, 61,* 243–253.

von Knorring, L., Oreland, L., & von Knorring, A. L. (1987). Personality traits and platelet MAO activity in alcohol and drug abusing teenage boys. *Acta Psychiatrica Scandinavica, 75,* 307–314.

von Knorring, L., Oreland, L., & Winblad, B. (1984). Personality traits related to monoamine oxidase activity in platelets. *Psychiatry Research, 12,* 11–26.

Vrana, S. R., Spence, E. L., & Lang, P. J. (1988). The startle probe response: A new measure of emotion? *Journal of Abnormal Psychology, 97,* 487–491.

Walter, W. G., Cooper, R., Aldrige, V. J., McCallum, W. C., & Winter, A. L. (1964). Contingent negative variation: An electrical sign of sensory-motor association and expectancy in the human brain. *Nature, 203,* 380–384.

Wang, S., Mason, J., Charney, D., & Yehuda, R. (1997). Relationships between hormone profile and novelty seeking in combat-related posttraumatic stress disorder. *Biological Psychiatry, 41,* 145–151.

Watson, J. D., Crick, F. H. C. (1953). Genetical implications of the structure of deoxyribonucleic acid. *Nature, 171,* 964–967.

Weizman, R., Tanne, Z., Branek, M., Karp, L., Golomb, M., Tyano, S., & Gavish, M. (1987). Peripheral benzodiazepine binding sites on platelet membranes are increased during diazepam treatment of anxious patients. *European Journal of Pharmacology, 138,* 289–292.

Wenger, M. A. (1941). The measurement of individual differences in autonomic balance. *Psychosomatic Medicine, 3,* 427–434 Wenger, M. A., & Cullen, T. D. (1972). Studies of autonomic balance in children and adults. In N. S. Greenfield & R. A. Sternback (Eds.), *Handbook of psychophysiology* (pp. 535–669). New York: Holt.

Wenger, M. A., & Cullen, T. D. (1972). Studies of autonomic balance in children and adults. In N. S. Greenfield & R. A. Sternback (Eds.), *Handbook of psychophysiology* (pp. 535–569). New York: Holt.

Whyte, W. H. (1956). *The organization man.* New York: Simon & Shuster.

Widiger, T. A. (1991). Personality disorder models proposed for DSM-IV. *Journal of Personality Disorders, 5,* 386–398.

Widiger, T. A. & Sankis, L. M. (2000). Adult psychopathology: Issues and controversy. In S. T. Fiske (Ed.), *Annual Review of Psychology* (pp. 377–404). Palo Alto, CA: Annual Reviews.

Wiesbeck, G. A., Mauerer, C., Thome, J., Jacob, F., & Boening, J. (1995). Neuroendocrine support for a relationship between "novelty seeking" and dopaminergic function in alcohol-dependent men. *Psychoneuroendocrinology, 20,* 755–761.

Willner, P. (1995). Dopaminergic mechanisms in depression. In P. E. Bloom & D. J. Kupfer. (Eds.), *Psychopharmacology: The fourth generation of progress* (pp. 921–931). New York: Raven Press.

Wilson, E. O. (1998). *Consilience: The unity of knowledge.* New York: Vintage Books.

Wilson, G. D., Barrett, P. T., & Gray, J. A. (1989). Human reactions to reward and punishment: A questionnaire examination of Gray's personality theory. *British Journal of Psychology, 80,* 509–515.

Wilson, G. D., Kumari, V., Gray, J. A., & Corr, P. J. (2000). The role of neuroticism in startle reactions to fearful and disgusting stimuli. *Personality and Individual Differences, 29,* 1077–1082.

Wilson, M. A., & Languia, M. L. (1990). A topographic study of differences in the P300 between introverts and extraverts. *Brain Topgraphy, 2,* 269–274.

Windle, M. (1994). Temperamental inhibition and activation: Hormonal and psychosocial correlates and associated psychiatric disorders. *Personality and Individual Differences, 17,* 61–70.

Windle, R. C., & Windle, M. (1995). Longitudinal patterns of physical aggression: Associations with adult social, psychiatric, and personality functioning and testosterone levels. *Development and Psychopathology, 7,* 563–585.

Wong, D. F., & Young, L. T. (1991). Quantification of human neuroreceptors in neuropsychiatric disorders with positron emission tomography. In N. D. Volkow & A. P. Wolf (Eds.), *Positron-emission tomography in schizophrenia* (pp. 101–124). Washington, DC: American Psychiatric Press.

Wong, M. T. H., Lumsden, J., Fenton, G. W., & Fenwick, P. B. C. (1994). Electroencephalography, computed tomography and violence ratings of male patients in a maximum security hospital. *Acta Psychiatrica Scandinavica, 90,* 97–101.

Woodsworth, M., & Porter, S. (2002). In cold blood: Characteristics of criminal homicides as a function of psychopathy. *Journal of Abnormal Psychology, 111,* 436–445.

Zahn, T. P., Schooler, C., & Murphy, D. L. (1986). Autonomic correlates of sensation seeking and monoamine oxidase activity: Using confirmation factor analysis on psychophysiological data, *Psychophysiology, 23,* 521–531.

Zaleski, Z. (1984). Sensation seeking and preference for emotional visual stimuli. *Personality and Individual Differences, 5,* 609–611.

Zalsman, G., & Apter, A. (2002). Serotonergic metabolism and violence/aggression. In J. Glicksohn (Ed.), *Neurobiology of criminal behavior* (pp. 231–250). Boston, MA: Kluwer Academic Publishers.

Zuckerman, M. (1969). Theoretical foundations: I. In J. P. Zubek (Ed.), *Sensory deprivation: Fifteen years of research* (pp. 407–432). New York: Appleton.

Zuckerman, M. (1971a). Dimensions of sensation seeking. *Journal of Consulting and Clinical Psychology, 36,* 45–52.

Zuckerman, M. (1971b). Physiological measures of sexual arousal in the human. *Psychological Bulletin, 75,* 297–329.

Zuckerman, M. (1976). General and situation specific traits and states: New approaches to assessment of anxiety and other constructs. In M. Zuckerman & C. D. Spielberger (Eds.), *Emotions and anxiety: New concepts, methods, and applications* (pp. 133–174). Hillsdale, NJ: Erlbaum.

Zuckerman, M. (1979). *Sensation seeking: Beyond the optimal level of arousal.* Hillsdale, NJ.: Erlbaum.

Zuckerman, M. (1984). Sensation seeking: A comparative approach to a human trait. *Behavioral and Brain Sciences, 7,* 413–434, 453–471.

Zuckerman, M. (1986). Sensation seeking and augmenting-reducing: Evoked potentials and/or kinesthetic aftereffects. *Behavioral and Brain Sciences, 9*, 749–754.

Zuckerman, M. (1989). Personality in the third dimension: A psychobiological approach. *Personality and Individual Differences, 10*, 391–418.

Zuckerman, M. (1990). The psychophysiology of sensation seeking. *Journal of Personality, 58*, 313–345.

Zuckerman, M. (1991). *Psychobiology of personality*. Cambridge: Cambridge University Press.

Zuckerman, M. (1992). What is a basic factor and which factors are basic? Turtles all the way down. *Personality and Individual Differences, 13*, 675–681.

Zuckerman, M. (1993). Sensation seeking and impulsivity: A marriage of traits made in biology? In W. G. McCown, J. L. Johnson, & M. B. Shure (Eds.), *The impulsive client: Theory, research and treatment* (pp. 71–91). Washington, DC: American Psychological Association.

Zuckerman, M. (1994a). Behavioral expressions and biosocial bases of sensation seeking. New York: Cambridge University Press.

Zuckerman, M. (1994b). An alternative five-factor model for personality. In C. F. Halverson Jr., G. A. Kohnstamm, & R. P. Martin (Eds.), *The developing structure of temperament and personality from infancy to adulthood* (pp. 53–68). Hillsdale, NJ: Erlbaum

Zuckerman, M. (1995). Good and bad humors: Biochemical bases of personality and its disorders. *Psychological Science, 6*, 325–332.

Zuckerman, M. (1996). The psychobiological model for Impulsive Unsocialized Sensation Seeking: A comparative approach. *Neuropsychobiology, 34*, 125–129.

Zuckerman, M. (1999). *Vulnerability to psychopathology: A biosocial model*. Washington, DC: American Psychological Association.

Zuckerman, M. (2002a). Zuckerman-Kuhlman Personality Questionnaire (ZKPQ): An alternative five-factorial model. In B. De Raad & M. Perugini (Eds.), *Big five assessment* (pp. 377–396). Seattle, WA: Hogrefe & Huber.

Zuckerman, M. (2002b). Personality and psychopathy: Shared behavioral, and biological traits. In J. Glicksohn (Ed.) *The neurobiology of criminal behavior* (pp. 27–49). Boston, MA: Kluwer.

Zuckerman, M. (2003). Biological bases of personality. In T. Millon & M. J. Lerner (Eds.) *Handbook of psychology, Vol. 5, personality and social psychology* (pp. 85–116). Hoboken, NJ: Wiley.

Zuckerman, M., Buchsbaum, M. S., & Murphy, D. L. (1980). Sensation seeking and its biological correlates. *Psychological Bulletin, 88*, 187–214.

Zuckerman, M., & Cloninger, C. R. (1996). Relationships between Cloninger's, Zuckerman's, and Eysenck's dimensions of personality. *Personality and Individual Differences, 21*, 283–285.

Zuckerman, M., Eysenck, S., & Eysenck, H. J. (1978). Sensation seeking in England and America: Cross cultural, age, and sex comparisons.

Zuckerman, M., Joireman, J., Kraft, M., & Kuhlman, D. M. (1999). Where do motivational and emotional traits fit within three factor models of personality. *Personality and Individual Differences, 26*, 487–504.

Zuckerman, M., Kolin, E. A., Price, L., & Zoob, I. (1964). Development of a sensation seeking scale. *Journal of Consulting Psychology, 28*, 477–482.

Zuckerman, M., & Kuhlman, D. M. (2000). Personality and risk-taking: Common biosocial factors. *Journal of Personality, 68*, 999–1029.

Zuckerman, M., Kuhlman, D. M., & Camac, C. (1988). What lies beyond E and N? Factor analyses of scales believed to measure basic dimensions of personality. *Journal of Personality and Social Psychology, 54,* 96–107.

Zuckerman, M., Kuhlman, D. M., Joireman, J., Teta, P., & Kraft, M. (1993). A comparison of three structural models for personality: The big three, the big five, and the alternative five. *Journal of Personality and Social Psychology, 65,* 757–768.

Zuckerman, M., Kuhlman, D., Thornquist, M., & Kiers, H. (1991). Five (or three) robust questionnaire scale factors of personality without culture. *Personality and Individual Differences, 12,* 929–941.

Zuckerman, M., & Litle, P. (1986). Personality and curiosity about morbid and sexual events. *Personality and Individual Differences, 7,* 49–56.

Zuckerman, M., & Lubin, B. (1985). *Manual for the Multiple Affect Adjective Check-List, Revised (MAACL-R).* San Diego, CA: Educational and Industrial Testing Service.

Zuckerman, M., Murtaugh, T. T., & Siegel, J. (1974). Sensation seeking and cortical augmenting-reducing. *Psychophysiology, 11,* 535–542.

Zuckerman, M., Simons, R. F., & Como, P. G. (1988). Sensation seeking and stimulus intensity as modulators of cortical, cardiovascular, and electrodermal response: A cross-modality study. *Personality and Individual Differences, 9,* 361–372.

Zureik, J. L., & Meltzer, H. Y. (1988). Platelet MAO activity in hallucinating and paranoid schizophrenics: A review and meta-analysis. *Biological Psychiatry, 24,* 63–78.

Author Index

Subject Index

RAY COUNTY LIBRARY
215 E. Lexington
Richmond, MO 64085